AF825348

Compendium of Psychiatry

(Questions with Explanatory Answers)

Dr. Vinit Gupta

MBBS, M.D. (Psychiatry)

Peepee Publishers and Distributors Private Limited®

Compendium of Psychiatry

Published by:

Pawaninder P. Vij and Anupam Vij

Peepee Publishers and Distributors Private Limited

Head Office: 160, Shakti Vihar, Pitam Pura, Delhi-110 034

Correspondence Address:

7/31, First Floor, Ansari Road, Daryaganj

New Delhi-110002 (India)

Ph: 41512412, 23246245, 9811156083

e-mail: peepee160@yahoo.co.in

e-mail: peepee160@gmail.com

www.peepeepub.com

© 2024 Peepee Publishers and Distributors Private Limited®

All rights reserved

No part of this publication may be reproduced or transmitted in any form or by any means, electronic, mechanical, photocopy, recording, translated, or any information storage and retrieval system, without permission in writing from the publisher.

This book has been published in good faith that the material provided by authors/contributors is original. Every effort is made to ensure accuracy of material, but publisher, printer and author/editor will not be held responsible for any inadvertent errors. In case of any dispute, all legal matters to be settled under Delhi jurisdiction only.

First Edition: 2024

ISBN: 978-81-9651-874-5

Preface

Psychiatry stands at the crossroads of a fascinating journey that intertwines the mysteries of the mind with the intricate mechanisms of the brain. This book is an endeavor to guide students and practitioners through this complex yet captivating landscape, where the fields of psychiatry and neurology converge.

As the authors of this text, we have aimed to provide a comprehensive, yet accessible resource for MBBS and MD students specializing in psychiatry and neurology. We recognize that the journey through medical education is rigorous and demanding. Thus, we have meticulously designed this book to be both a reliable companion for in-depth learning and a quick reference for the busy practitioner.

We begin with an introduction to psychiatry – a field that, in its essence, seeks to understand, empathize, and heal the human mind. Recognizing the foundational importance of the central nervous system in understanding psychiatric conditions, we then delve into a concise exploration of neuroanatomy and neurophysiology, focusing on aspects most relevant to psychiatric practice.

The core of this book is dedicated to an extensive examination of various psychiatric disorders. Here, we discuss both adult and child psychiatry, acknowledging the unique challenges and approaches required in managing mental health across different life stages. Our approach is one of clarity and depth, addressing each condition with the dual lens of scientific rigor and clinical empathy.

We have also included specialized topics that are often at the forefront of psychiatric challenges in modern society – addiction, sexual disorders, the interplay of violence and mental health, and the critical understanding of seizures and their differential diagnoses, including Psychogenic Non-Epileptic Seizures (PNES). Furthermore, we have dedicated sections to diagnostic tools such as EEG, emphasizing their relevance and application in clinical practice.

In recognition of the ever-evolving nature of psychiatry, a section on recent advancements in the field has been included. This segment is not just about new discoveries or treatments, but also about evolving perspectives, emerging challenges, and the future direction of psychiatric care.

Lastly, we have endeavored to make this book a pleasant and engaging read. We understand the pressures of medical training and practice and hope to provide content that is as engaging as it is informative.

We extend our gratitude to our peers and mentors in the fields of psychiatry, whose insights and experiences have been invaluable in the creation of this book. Our hope is that this book will not only educate but also inspire a deep and compassionate understanding of psychiatry.

Happy reading and best wishes on your journey through the remarkable world of psychiatry.

Dr. Vinit Gupta

Acknowledgements

I am profoundly grateful to all my teachers and seniors whose invaluable guidance has imparted enduring wisdom, serving as a beacon of inspiration for both present and future generations.

I extend heartfelt appreciation to my parents for their unwavering support, which has been an essential cornerstone of my journey.

My sincere gratitude extends to the publishers, Peepee Publishers and Distributors Private Limited, whose dedication and efficiency facilitated the timely publication of this book, setting a commendable standard.

Dr. Vinit Gupta

Index

COMPENDIUM OF PSYCHIATRY

What is psychiatry?

Psychiatry is a medical specialty dedicated to the diagnosis, prevention, study, and treatment of mental disorders. These include various maladaptation's related to mood, behavior, cognition, and perceptions.

1. **Medical Discipline**: Psychiatrists are medical doctors (MDs or DOs) who specialize in mental health. This means they can prescribe medication, perform medical procedures, and understand the complex relationship between emotional illness and other medical illnesses.

2. **Scope of Practice**: The range of conditions treated by psychiatrists includes, but is not limited to, depression, anxiety disorders, bipolar disorder, schizophrenia, and developmental disorders such as autism. They also deal with acute conditions like psychosis and long-term conditions like dementia.

3. **Treatment Approaches**: Treatment by a psychiatrist may involve various modalities, including medications, psychotherapy, and other treatments like electroconvulsive therapy (ECT). The choice of treatment depends on the nature and severity of the mental illness.

4. **Psychotherapy:** Many psychiatrists are trained in providing psychotherapy, which involves talking with patients about their problems. Psychotherapy can be in various forms, such as cognitive-behavioral therapy (CBT), psychoanalytic therapy, or supportive therapy.

5. **Diagnostic Evaluation**: Psychiatrists often use diagnostic tests like psychological assessments or lab tests to understand a patient's mental health condition comprehensively.

6. **Interdisciplinary Collaboration**: Psychiatrists often work in collaboration with other healthcare professionals, including psychologists, social workers, occupational therapists, and primary care physicians, to provide holistic care to patients.

7. **Research and Academia**: Many psychiatrists are involved in research and teaching about the brain and behavior, contributing to advancements in the field.

8. **Ethical and Legal Aspects**: Psychiatrists must adhere to strict ethical and legal standards, especially regarding confidentiality and the rights of patients.

9. **Global Perspective**: The field of psychiatry varies in practice across different cultures and countries, reflecting diverse approaches to mental health.

What is anti-psychiatry?

Anti-psychiatry is a movement that emerged primarily in the 1960s as a response to perceived problems in the way mental illness was being diagnosed and treated, particularly in psychiatric institutions. It encompasses a diverse array of critiques and perspectives, but there are several common themes:

1. **Criticism of Psychiatric Diagnoses**: Anti-psychiatry proponents argue that psychiatric diagnoses are often subjective and not based on objective scientific criteria. They believe these diagnoses can stigmatize individuals and may not adequately reflect the complexity of their experiences.

2. **Opposition to Coercive Treatment**: A central concern is the use of involuntary commitment and coercive treatments in psychiatry, such as electroconvulsive therapy (ECT), lobotomies, and enforced medication. The movement views these practices as violations of human rights and personal autonomy.

3. **Challenging the Medical Model**: Anti-psychiatry often questions the medical model of mental illness, which treats mental disorders primarily as biological or neurological diseases. Critics argue that this approach neglects the social, cultural, and psychological dimensions of mental distress.

4. **Influence of Pharmaceutical Industry**: There is concern about the over-reliance on medication for treating mental disorders, often attributed to the influence of the pharmaceutical industry in psychiatry. This is seen as leading to an over-medication of patients and an underemphasis on psychotherapy and social support.

5. **Institutional Critique**: The movement has historically critiqued the conditions and practices in psychiatric institutions, arguing that they can be dehumanizing and counterproductive to the healing process.
6. **Emphasis on Patient Rights and Empowerment**: Advocates for anti-psychiatry often emphasize the importance of patient rights, informed consent, and the empowerment of individuals to make choices about their own treatment.
7. **Diverse Perspectives**: The movement includes a range of perspectives, from radical calls for the abolition of psychiatry to more moderate criticisms seeking reform and improvement of psychiatric practices.

It is important to note that the anti-psychiatry movement is not a unified or homogeneous group, and its influence has varied over time and across different regions. While some of its criticisms have led to significant reforms in psychiaric care and a greater emphasis on patient rights and holistic approaches, the movement has also been critiqued for sometimes oversimplifying complex medical and psychological issues.

What is history of psychiatry?

The history of psychiatry, the branch of medicine focused on the diagnosis, treatment, and prevention of mental illness, is long and complex, marked by evolving understanding and various treatment methods. Here is an overview:

Ancient Times

- **Early Beliefs**: In ancient times, mental illnesses were often viewed as supernatural or divine punishments. Treatments varied from religious rituals to more physical methods.
- **Hippocrates (460-377 BC)**: The Greek physician proposed that mental disorders had natural causes and should be treated like any other disease, focusing on diet and environment.

Middle Ages

- **Supernatural Views**: During this period, mental illness was often seen as witchcraft or possession. Treatments could be harsh, including exorcism or persecution.
- **Islamic Medicine**: Islamic scholars like Avicenna emphasized the psychological aspects of illness and advocated for more humane treatments.

17th and 18th Centuries

- **Asylums**: The establishment of asylums began, initially as places to confine the mentally ill, often in deplorable conditions.
- **Humanitarian Reform**: Pioneers like Philippe Pinel in France and William Tuke in England advocated for more humane treatment of asylum patients, focusing on compassion and moral therapy.

19th Century

- **Psychiatry as a Medical Discipline**: Psychiatry began to emerge as a distinct medical field. Asylums proliferated, some with a focus on moral treatment and rehabilitation.
- **Biological Theories**: Researchers started to seek physiological causes for mental illnesses, leading to various biological theories and treatments.

20th Century

- **Psychoanalysis**: Sigmund Freud developed psychoanalysis, focusing on the unconscious mind, which influenced psychiatry significantly.
- **Psychopharmacology Revolution**: The discovery of medications like chlorpromazine in the 1950s revolutionized treatment, allowing many patients to leave asylums and live in the community.
- **Deinstitutionalization**: This movement, particularly active in the 1960s and 1970s, aimed to close large asylums and treat people with mental illness in community settings.
- **DSM Development**: The Diagnostic and Statistical Manual of Mental Disorders, first published by the American Psychiatric Association in 1952, has been regularly updated, reflecting changes in understanding and classification of mental disorders.

21st Century

- **Biopsychosocial Model**: This model integrates biological, psychological, and social factors in understanding and treating mental illnesses.
- **Personalized Medicine**: Advances in genetics and neuroscience are leading towards more personalized treatment approaches.
- **Digital Psychiatry**: The use of digital tools and telepsychiatry has become more prevalent, especially highlighted during the COVID-19 pandemic.

Throughout its history, psychiatry has been influenced by broader social, cultural, and scientific trends, leading to ongoing debates and evolution in how mental health is understood and treated.

What are the general issues concerning neuro-psychiatry?

Neuro-psychiatry, which combines elements of neurology and psychiatry to treat disorders at the intersection of brain and behavior, faces several general issues:

1. **Complex Diagnostic Challenges**: Many neuro-psychiatric disorders present with overlapping symptoms, making accurate diagnosis challenging. Conditions like depression, bipolar disorder, schizophrenia, and neurological disorders such as Alzheimer's disease or Parkinson's disease can have similar symptoms.
2. **Treatment Difficulties**: Effective treatment is often complicated due to the complexity of the brain and the variability in how individuals respond to medications or therapies. Medications that are effective for some patients might not work for others, and side effects can vary greatly.
3. **Understanding Brain-Behavior Relationships**: The relationship between neurological function and psychiatric symptoms is not fully understood. This gap in knowledge makes it difficult to develop targeted treatments.
4. **Stigma and Misunderstanding**: Mental health and neurological disorders often carry a stigma, which can lead to patients being marginalized or misunderstood. This can impact their willingness to seek treatment or adhere to therapy.
5. **Ethical and Legal Concerns**: Neuropsychiatric conditions can raise complex ethical and legal issues, such as questions of consent, capacity, and involuntary treatment.
6. **Research Limitations**: While there have been advances in neuroimaging and genetics, there is still much to learn about the brain. Research in neuro-psychiatry is often expensive and time-consuming.
7. **Integration of Care**: Coordinating care between neurology and psychiatry services can be challenging. Integrated, multidisciplinary approaches are essential but not always available.
8. **Global Health Disparities**: Access to neuro-psychiatric care varies greatly around the world, with many regions lacking adequate resources, trained professionals, or awareness.

What is the future in psychiatry?

The future of psychiatry is likely to be shaped by advancements in various fields, including neuroscience, technology, and personalized medicine. While predicting the future with precision is challenging, several emerging trends and potential developments could significantly influence the practice of psychiatry:

1. **Integration of Technology:**
   - **Digital Psychiatry:** Use of mobile apps, wearables, and online platforms for monitoring mental health, delivering therapy (e.g., cognitive-behavioral therapy apps), and enhancing patient engagement.
   - **Telepsychiatry:** Wider adoption of telepsychiatry for remote consultations, which can increase access to care, particularly in underserved areas.
   - **Virtual Reality (VR):** Use of VR for exposure therapy in conditions like PTSD, anxiety disorders, and phobias.
2. **Advancements in Neuroscience:**
   - Better understanding of the brain's neurobiology could lead to more targeted treatments for psychiatric disorders.
   - Research in neuroplasticity might offer new therapeutic approaches to rewire the brain and alleviate symptoms.
3. **Personalized Medicine:**
   - Use of genetic testing to predict individual responses to psychiatric medications, minimizing trial-and-error in finding effective treatments.
   - Development of personalized treatment plans based on a patient's genetic profile, lifestyle, and environmental factors.
4. **AI and Machine Learning:**
   - AI could assist in diagnosing mental health conditions, predicting treatment outcomes, and identifying individuals at risk for mental illnesses.
   - Machine learning algorithms might analyze data from various sources, including electronic health records and wearable devices, to inform treatment decisions.
5. **Neuromodulation Techniques:**
   - Expansion of techniques like Transcranial Magnetic Stimulation (TMS) and Deep Brain Stimulation (DBS) for treating conditions resistant to medication and psychotherapy.

- Development of new, less invasive neuromodulation therapies.

6. **Collaborative and Integrative Care:**
   - Increased emphasis on integrative care models, combining psychiatry with other medical disciplines for a more holistic approach to mental health.
   - Collaboration with primary care providers to identify and manage mental health issues early.
7. **Focus on Prevention and Early Intervention:**
   - Greater emphasis on identifying and addressing mental health issues early, especially in children and adolescents, to prevent more severe problems later.
   - Community-based initiatives and public health approaches to promote mental well-being and resilience.
8. **Ethical and Legal Considerations:**
   - Ongoing discussions regarding the ethical implications of emerging technologies and treatments.
   - Addressing issues related to data privacy and the digital divide in access to technological tools.
9. **Evolving Therapies:**
   - Continued development and validation of new psychotherapeutic techniques.
   - Potential use of psychedelic-assisted therapy for conditions like depression, PTSD, and addiction, pending research outcomes and regulatory approval.
10. **Public Awareness and Stigma Reduction:**
    - Increased public education and awareness efforts to reduce the stigma associated with mental illness.

The future of psychiatry promises significant advancements and potential for improved patient care, though it also presents challenges that need to be carefully navigated, particularly in terms of ethics, equitable access, and maintaining the human aspect of mental health care.

What is psychoanalysis?

Psychoanalysis is a set of theories and therapeutic techniques related to the study of the unconscious mind, which together form a method of treatment for mental disorders. Developed by Sigmund Freud in the late 19th and early 20th centuries, it has since evolved and influenced many aspects of psychology and psychiatry.

1. **The Unconscious Mind**: Freud believed that many mental disorders result from thoughts, memories, and desires that are unconsciously repressed but continue to influence behavior and emotions. Psychoanalysis aims to bring these unconscious elements to conscious awareness.
2. **Free Association**: In therapy, patients are encouraged to speak freely about whatever thoughts come to mind, a process known as free association. This technique is intended to uncover hidden memories and desires.
3. **Dream Analysis**: Freud saw dreams as a window into the unconscious, filled with symbolism. Analyzing dreams is a crucial part of psychoanalytic therapy, aiming to understand the unconscious messages in them.
4. **Psychosexual Development**: Freud proposed that psychological development in childhood occurs in stages (oral, anal, phallic, latency, and genital stages). Each stage is characterized by the erogenous zone that is the source of the child's psychosexual energy.
5. **Defense Mechanisms**: Freud identified several defense mechanisms, such as repression, denial, and projection, which the ego uses to protect itself from anxiety-provoking thoughts and feelings.
6. **Transference**: This refers to the phenomenon where patients project feelings about important people in their lives onto the therapist. Understanding and analyzing this transference is considered important in psychoanalytic therapy.
7. **Long-term Therapy**: Psychoanalytic therapy is typically a long-term process, often involving several sessions per week over many years. It delves deeply into personal history and emotional development.
8. **Influence on Culture and Other Disciplines**: Psychoanalysis has had a profound impact not only on psychology and psychiatry but also on literature, art, film, and critical theory.
9. **Criticism and Evolution**: Psychoanalysis has been criticized for its lack of scientific rigor, overemphasis on sexuality, and the untestability of its theories. Despite this, it has evolved and influenced other therapeutic approaches, such as psychodynamic therapy, which retains key psychoanalytic principles but with modifications like a shorter duration and a focus on specific issues or symptoms.

10. **Contemporary Applications**: While traditional psychoanalysis is less common today, its concepts still influence many therapeutic practices, and it remains a significant part of the history of psychology and the study of the human mind.

What is Freudian psychoanalysis?

Freudian psychoanalysis is the original form of psychoanalysis as developed by Sigmund Freud in the late 19th and early 20th centuries. It is both a theory of the human psyche and a therapeutic practice.

1. **The Unconscious Mind**: Freud proposed that the unconscious mind plays a crucial role in human behavior. According to him, unconscious thoughts, feelings, and memories, especially those associated with trauma or conflict, influence our conscious experience and can lead to psychological distress.
2. **Psychosexual Development**: Freud believed that personality develops through a series of childhood stages in which the pleasure-seeking energies of the id become focused on certain erogenous zones. These stages are oral, anal, phallic, latency, and genital. Fixation at any stage can lead to specific character traits in adulthood.
3. **Structure of the Mind**: Freud's model of the mind comprises three main parts:
    - The **id** is the primal, unconscious part of the mind that seeks pleasure and avoids pain.
    - The **ego** functions as the rational part, mediating between the desires of the id and the constraints of reality.
    - The **superego** represents the moral conscience and societal norms.
4. **Defense Mechanisms**: The ego employs various defense mechanisms, such as repression, denial, and projection, to cope with stress and anxiety arising from internal conflicts.
5. **Dream Analysis**: Freud considered dreams to be the "royal road to the unconscious," expressing repressed desires and conflicts. He used dream interpretation as a key tool in his psychoanalytic practice.
6. **Free Association**: A fundamental technique in Freudian psychoanalysis, free association involves patients speaking freely about whatever comes to mind, allowing the therapist to explore the unconscious content of their thoughts.
7. **Transference and Countertransference**: Transference occurs when patients project feelings about significant people in their past onto the therapist. Countertransference is the therapist's emotional reaction to the patient. Both are considered important in the therapeutic process for understanding and resolving unconscious conflicts.
8. **Lengthy and Intensive Therapy**: Freudian psychoanalysis typically involves frequent sessions over an extended period, allowing for the in-depth exploration of the patient's psyche.
9. **Influence and Criticism**: Freud's theories have been immensely influential in psychology, psychiatry, and broader culture, but they have also attracted significant criticism for their lack of empirical support, perceived overemphasis on sexuality, and generalizability.
10. **Legacy**: Despite these criticisms, Freudian psychoanalysis laid the groundwork for modern psychotherapeutic and psychological theories, particularly in understanding the importance of early childhood experiences, the role of the unconscious, and the complexity of human behavior.

What is history of psychoanalysis?

The history of psychoanalysis is deeply intertwined with the life and work of its founder, Sigmund Freud, and it has evolved significantly over the years.

Late 19th Century

- **Sigmund Freud**: A neurologist in Vienna, Freud began developing the foundations of psychoanalysis based on his clinical observations and theories about the role of the unconscious mind in mental disorders.
- **Studies on Hysteria (1895)**: Freud, with his colleague Josef Breuer, published this work, introducing the concept of "talking cure" and "free association."

Early 20th Century

- **The Interpretation of Dreams (1900)**: Freud proposed that dreams are a form of wish fulfilment and a way to access the unconscious mind.
- **Development of Key Concepts**: Freud introduced the Oedipus complex, the psychosexual stages of development, and the structural model of the psyche (id, ego, superego).

1910s to 1930s

- **International Psychoanalytical Association (IPA)**: Founded in 1910 to advance psychoanalytic theory and practice.
- **Growing Influence and Expansion**: Psychoanalysis spread across Europe and to the United States, attracting followers and practitioners.
- **Divergences**: Figures like Carl Jung and Alfred Adler, initially part of Freud's circle, broke away due to theoretical disagreements, forming their own schools of thought.

Mid-20th Century

- **Incorporation into Psychiatry**: Psychoanalysis became a dominant force in American psychiatry and influenced clinical practice significantly.
- **Development of Neo-Freudian Theories**: Psychoanalysts like Anna Freud, Melanie Klein, and Donald Winnicott expanded and modified Freud's theories, focusing more on interpersonal relations and ego psychology.

Late 20th Century

- **Criticisms and Decline**: The rise of biological psychiatry, the advent of psychopharmacology, and increasing criticism of the scientific validity of Freudian theory led to a decline in the influence of traditional psychoanalysis.
- **Cultural Impact**: Despite the decline in clinical practice, psychoanalytic concepts remained influential in literature, film, and critical theory.

21st Century

- **Modern Adaptations**: Contemporary psychoanalysis has diversified and often integrates with other psychological theories and therapies.
- **Revival in Some Areas**: There is a renewed interest in psychoanalytic and psychodynamic therapies, focusing on their value in treating certain mental health issues and understanding human behavior.

Throughout its history, psychoanalysis has sparked intense debate and controversy. While criticized for its lack of empirical support and scientific rigor, its contributions to the understanding of the unconscious mind, dream interpretation, and the significance of early childhood experiences continue to be influential in various fields.

What is hypnotherapy, or hypnotism?

Hypnotherapy, or hypnotism, refers to the use of hypnosis as a therapeutic tool. Hypnosis is a trance-like state of heightened focus and concentration often accompanied by deep relaxation. This state is similar to being absorbed in a book, movie, music, or even one's own thoughts or meditations. In therapeutic settings, hypnosis can be used to help individuals explore painful thoughts, feelings, and memories they might have hidden from their conscious minds.

1. **Inducing Hypnosis**: Hypnosis typically involves the person experiencing a sense of deep relaxation with their attention narrowed down, and they focus on appropriate suggestions made by the therapist.
2. **Applications**: Hypnotherapy is used to help manage a variety of health conditions, such as pain, stress, anxiety, and mood disorders. It can also be used to overcome habits like smoking, improve sleep, and alleviate symptoms of certain gastrointestinal disorders.
3. **Mechanism of Action**: During hypnosis, a person is said to have heightened focus and concentration. The hypnotic state allows a person to be more open to discussion and suggestion. It can improve the success of other treatments for many conditions, including:
    - Phobias, fears, and anxiety
    - Sleep disorders
    - Depression
    - Stress
    - Post-trauma anxiety
    - Grief and loss
4. **Misconceptions**: Hypnosis is often misunderstood as a form of mind control or brainwashing. However, people under hypnosis are in full control of themselves and would generally not do anything in hypnosis that they would not do under normal circumstances.
5. **Self-Hypnosis**: Some individuals learn self-hypnosis, which they can use to reinforce and continue the benefits of formal sessions with a therapist.
6. **Qualified Practitioners**: It is important that hypnotherapy is conducted by a qualified and professionally trained therapist. In some countries, hypnotherapy is a regulated profession.
7. **Effectiveness**: The effectiveness of hypnotherapy can vary greatly from person to person. Some individuals are more 'hypnotizable' than others, and the approach has varying degrees of effectiveness for different conditions.

8. **Scientific Standing**: While hypnotherapy is widely used, it remains a topic of debate within some medical circles regarding its efficacy. However, numerous studies have shown its effectiveness in various conditions, particularly in pain management and anxiety disorders.

9. **Integration with Other Therapies**: Hypnotherapy is often used in conjunction with other forms of therapy, including cognitive-behavioral therapy (CBT), to enhance therapeutic outcomes.

Overall, hypnotherapy is a respected and valuable tool in the therapeutic arsenal, especially when used by skilled and qualified practitioners within an appropriate clinical framework.

What is the difference between psychiatry and neuropsychiatry?

Psychiatry and neuropsychiatry are closely related fields, but they focus on different aspects of mental health and neurological conditions.

Psychiatry

1. **Scope**: Psychiatry is a medical specialty focusing on the diagnosis, treatment, and prevention of mental, emotional, and behavioral disorders.

2. **Approach**: Psychiatrists use a variety of treatments, including psychotherapy, medications, and other interventions to treat mental health disorders like depression, anxiety, schizophrenia, bipolar disorder, and others.

3. **Training**: Psychiatrists are medical doctors (MDs or DOs) who have completed medical school, a residency in psychiatry, and possibly additional fellowship training in a psychiatric specialty.

4. **Broad Perspective**: While psychiatrists are knowledgeable about how neurological conditions affect behavior and mental functioning, their training emphasizes a broader range of mental health issues, including psychosocial, environmental, and biological factors.

Neuropsychiatry

1. **Scope**: Neuropsychiatry specializes in the interface between psychiatry and neurology, focusing on psychiatric disorders with a clear neurological component.

2. **Approach**: Neuropsychiatrists deal with mental illnesses that are understood to have a neurological basis, such as dementia, epilepsy-related psychiatric conditions, brain injuries, and neurodevelopmental disorders.

3. **Training**: Neuropsychiatrists are typically trained in both psychiatry and neurology, allowing them to understand and treat conditions that encompass both brain and mind.

4. **Neurological Emphasis**: The field emphasizes the understanding of brain-behavior relationships, and treatment approaches may be more biologically focused, often integrating neurology into psychiatric treatment.

Overlapping and Differences

- **Overlap**: Both psychiatrists and neuropsychiatrists are concerned with how mental processes and behaviors are related to brain function. They can prescribe medication, and both may use psychotherapy in treatment.

- **Differences**: The primary difference lies in their focus and training. Neuropsychiatry often deals with more complex clinical problems involving the nervous system and mental health, while psychiatry has a broader scope encompassing a wide range of mental health conditions, including those without a clear neurological basis.

In summary, while psychiatry broadly addresses mental health, neuropsychiatry is a subspecialty focusing on the overlap of psychiatric symptoms with neurological conditions.

What is the difference between neuropsychiatry and neuropsychology?

Neuropsychiatry and neuropsychology are both disciplines that explore the relationship between the brain and behavior, but they differ in their focus, methods, and the type of professionals who practice in each field.

Neuropsychiatry

1. **Focus**: Neuropsychiatry is a medical field primarily concerned with the interface between psychiatry and neurology. It deals with mental illnesses that have a clear neurological basis, such as brain injuries, dementia, seizure disorders, and neurodevelopmental disorders.

2. **Practitioners**: Neuropsychiatrists are medical doctors (MDs or DOs) who have completed training in psychiatry and often have additional training in neurology. They can prescribe medication and manage medical and neurological aspects of mental health conditions.

3. **Approach**: Neuropsychiatry often involves diagnosing and treating neurological conditions that manifest psychiatric symptoms. It integrates knowledge from both neurology and psychiatry to understand and treat these conditions.

Neuropsychology

1. **Focus**: Neuropsychology is a field within clinical psychology focused on understanding how the structure and function of the brain relate to specific psychological processes and behaviors. It often deals with the assessment and treatment of cognitive and behavioral changes resulting from brain disorders.
2. **Practitioners**: Neuropsychologists are psychologists (typically with a doctoral degree in psychology) who have specialized training in neuropsychology. They cannot prescribe medication but focus on assessing, diagnosing, and treating cognitive and behavioral aspects of neurological conditions.
3. **Approach**: Neuropsychologists use standardized tests and assessments to evaluate cognitive functions such as memory, attention, language, problem-solving, and personality. They often work with individuals who have experienced brain injury, stroke, neurological diseases, or developmental disorders.

Key Differences

- **Training and Qualifications**: Neuropsychiatrists are medical doctors with training in psychiatry (and often additional training in neurology), while neuropsychologists are psychologists with specialized training in brain-behavior relationships.
- **Prescription Rights**: Neuropsychiatrists can prescribe medication; neuropsychologists cannot.
- **Primary Functions**: Neuropsychiatrists diagnose and treat neurological and psychiatric disorders, often focusing on the medical management of these conditions. Neuropsychologists focus on assessing cognitive and behavioral functions and providing non-pharmacological interventions and rehabilitation strategies.
- **Tools and Methods**: Neuropsychologists extensively use cognitive and psychological assessments for diagnosis, while neuropsychiatrists may use these in addition to medical diagnostics like brain imaging and neurological evaluations.

In summary, while both neuropsychiatry and neuropsycho logy deal with the interplay between the brain and behavior, they differ in their professional training, methods, and approaches to treatment and assessment.

What is the difference between a psychiatrist and a neurologist?

Psychiatrists and neurologists are both medical doctors who specialize in studying and treating disorders related to the brain, but their areas of focus and approaches to treatment are distinct.

Psychiatrist

1. **Primary Focus**: Psychiatrists specialize in the diagnosis, treatment, and prevention of mental health disorders. This includes conditions like depression, anxiety, schizophrenia, bipolar disorder, and personality disorders.
2. **Medical Training**: Psychiatrists attend medical school and then complete a residency in psychiatry. They may also undergo additional training in a psychiatric subspecialty.
3. **Treatment Methods**: Psychiatrists use a variety of treatment methods, including medications (like antidepressants, antipsychotics, and mood stabilizers), psychotherapy (such as cognitive-behavioral therapy), and other treatments (like electroconvulsive therapy).
4. **Approach**: Psychiatrists focus on how mental health disorders affect thinking, emotion, and behavior. They often consider a combination of biological, psychological, and social factors in treatment.

Neurologist

1. **Primary Focus**: Neurologists specialize in disorders of the nervous system, which includes the brain, spinal cord, nerves, and muscles. This includes conditions like epilepsy, multiple sclerosis, Parkinson's disease, and stroke.
2. **Medical Training**: Neurologists also attend medical school followed by a residency in neurology. They may further specialize in areas like stroke care, neurodegenerative diseases, or epilepsy.
3. **Treatment Methods**: Neurologists primarily focus on diagnosing and treating neurological diseases. They use medications, physical therapy, and other medical interventions. They do not typically provide psychotherapy.
4. **Approach**: Neurologists focus on the physical and biological aspects of the nervous system, addressing conditions that affect motor skills, sensation, cognitive abilities, and other functions of the nervous system.

Key Differences

- **Scope of Practice**: Psychiatrists treat mental

health disorders, often with an emphasis on mood, behavior, and cognition. Neurologists treat conditions that affect the nervous system, focusing more on physical and neurological functions.

- **Treatment Approaches**: While both can prescribe medications, psychiatrists are more likely to provide psychotherapy, and their treatment often includes a focus on emotional and behavioral issues. Neurologists focus on physical and medical treatments for neurological disorders.
- **Overlap**: There is some overlap in the conditions they treat. For example, both may deal with dementia, head injuries, or conditions with both neurological and psychiatric components. In such cases, collaboration between a psychiatrist and a neurologist can be beneficial for the patient.

In summary, while both psychiatrists and neurologists deal with conditions related to the brain, their training, methods of diagnosis, and treatment approaches differ based on their respective focuses on mental health and neurological disorders.

When should a person go to a psychiatrist or a neurologist?

Deciding whether to see a psychiatrist or a neurologist can depend on the nature of your symptoms and concerns. Here is a general guideline to help determine which specialist might be more appropriate:

When to See a Psychiatrist

You might consider seeing a psychiatrist if you are experiencing:

1. **Mental Health Symptoms**: Such as prolonged sadness, excessive worries, mood swings, or feelings of hopelessness.
2. **Behavioral Changes**: Like withdrawal from social interactions, significant changes in sleep or appetite, or self-harming behaviors.
3. **Emotional Distress**: If emotional issues are significantly impacting your daily life, relationships, or work.
4. **Thought Disorders**: Symptoms such as hallucinations, delusions, or disorganized thinking.
5. **Psychiatric Disorders**: If you suspect or have been previously diagnosed with a psychiatric disorder like depression, anxiety disorders, bipolar disorder, schizophrenia, or personality disorders.
6. **Substance Abuse Issues**: Struggling with alcohol or drug use that affects your mental health.
7. **Management of Psychotropic Medications**: If you need medication for a mental health condition, psychiatrists are trained in prescribing and managing these drugs.
8. **Psychotherapy Needs**: If you are seeking therapy for mental health issues, trauma, life stresses, or relationship problems.

When to See a Neurologist

A visit to a neurologist might be more appropriate if you have:

1. **Neurological Symptoms**: Such as persistent headaches, migraines, seizures, or episodes of loss of consciousness.
2. **Movement Disorders**: Symptoms like tremors, difficulty with coordination, muscle weakness, or unexplained changes in movement.
3. **Cognitive or Memory Issues**: Significant memory loss, confusion, cognitive decline, or dementia symptoms.
4. **Neurological Conditions**: If you have a known or suspected neurological condition like epilepsy, multiple sclerosis, Parkinson's disease, stroke, or neuropathy.
5. **Sensory Impairments**: Unexplained changes in vision, hearing, smell, taste, or touch.
6. **Chronic Pain**: Especially if it is suspected to have a neurological origin, such as neuropathic pain.
7. **Sleep Disorders**: If you have sleep disturbances that might have a neurological basis, like narcolepsy or restless leg syndrome.

Overlapping Areas

There are some conditions where both specialties overlap, and in such cases, your primary care physician might guide you based on the predominant symptoms or refer you to both for a comprehensive evaluation. For example, conditions like dementia, traumatic brain injury, and certain types of headaches might involve both psychiatric and neurological aspects.

General Rule

As a general rule, if your concerns are primarily about your mood, emotions, thoughts, or behaviors, a psychiatrist is likely the appropriate specialist. If your symptoms are primarily physical or related to the functioning of the nervous system, a neurologist may be more suitable. However, your primary care physician can be a valuable resource in guiding you to the right specialist based on your specific symptoms and medical history.

What is the difference between psychology and psychiatry?

Psychology and psychiatry are related fields that both deal with mental health, but there are significant differences in their approach, training, and practice.

Psychology

1. **Education and Training**: Psychologists typically hold a doctoral degree in psychology (Ph.D., PsyD, or EdD). Their training emphasizes psychological theory, research, and the administration of psychological tests.

2. **Scope of Practice**: Psychologists focus on assessing, diagnosing, and treating mental and emotional disorders, primarily through psychotherapy and behavioral interventions. They often specialize in areas like clinical, counseling, educational, or developmental psychology.

3. **Non-Medical Approach**: Psychologists are not medical doctors and, in most jurisdictions, do not prescribe medication (with some exceptions in a few U.S. states where they can obtain additional training and certification for prescription privileges).

4. **Use of Psychological Testing**: Psychologists are trained in administering and interpreting psychological tests, which can assess cognitive ability, personality, interests, and other aspects of mental functioning.

Psychiatry

1. **Education and Training**: Psychiatrists are medical doctors (MDs or DOs) who specialize in mental health. They complete medical school and a residency in psychiatry, and may also have subspecialty training.

2. **Scope of Practice**: Psychiatrists diagnose and treat mental illnesses, and they can provide a range of treatments including medication, psychotherapy, and other biological treatments like electroconvulsive therapy (ECT).

3. **Medical Approach**: As medical doctors, psychiatrists understand the complex relationship between mental health and physical health, and they can evaluate and treat physical symptoms that may have a psychiatric origin.

4. **Prescription Authority**: Psychiatrists are licensed to prescribe medication, which is a major part of treatment for many mental illnesses, particularly those that are biological in nature, like major depression, bipolar disorder, and schizophrenia.

Key Differences

- **Training and Credentials**: Psychiatrists are medical doctors with a focus on mental health, while psychologists hold doctoral degrees in psychology and have extensive training in psychological research and psychotherapy.

- **Treatment Methods**: Psychiatrists can prescribe medication and provide a full range of medical treatments, while psychologists focus on providing psychotherapy and behavioral interventions and can conduct detailed psychological testing.

- **Approach to Mental Health**: While both can provide psychotherapy, psychiatrists often treat more severe mental health conditions that require medication, whereas psychologists deal more with emotional and behavioral issues, and conditions that can be treated effectively with psychotherapy and behavioral interventions.

Collaborative Care

In many cases, psychologists and psychiatrists work together to provide comprehensive mental health care. A patient might see a psychiatrist for medication management and a psychologist for psychotherapy. Both professions play a crucial role in the field of mental health, and their distinct but complementary skills and approaches enable a broad range of treatments for mental health issues.

What is hysteria?

"Hysteria" is a historical term used to describe a psychological disorder that was believed to manifest as a wide range of physical and psychological symptoms. The concept of hysteria dates back to ancient times and has evolved significantly over the centuries. The understanding and interpretation of hysteria have changed dramatically, especially in the last century, leading to its eventual discontinuation as a medical diagnosis.

Historical Perspective

1. **Ancient Views**: The term "hysteria" comes from the Greek word for uterus, "hystera." The Greeks believed hysteria was caused by disturbances in the uterus and was thus exclusive to women.

2. **Symptoms**: Historically, hysteria was said to present with a wide array of symptoms, including fainting, nervousness, insomnia, fluid retention, heaviness in the abdomen, muscle spasms, shortness of breath, irritability, loss of appetite for food or sex, and "a tendency to cause trouble."

Freudian Influence

1. **Psychoanalytic Theory**: Sigmund Freud, the

founder of psychoanalysis, played a significant role in shaping the understanding of hysteria in the late 19th and early 20th centuries. He linked hysteria to unconscious psychological conflicts and repressed emotions.

2. **Conversion Disorder**: Freud and his colleague Josef Breuer proposed that hysteria involved the conversion of psychological distress into physical symptoms.

Modern Understanding

1. **Disuse of the Term**: The term "hysteria" is no longer used in medical or psychological practice. It was officially removed from the Diagnostic and Statistical Manual of Mental Disorders (DSM) in 1980 with the publication of DSM-III.
2. **Replacement Diagnoses**: What was historically categorized as hysteria may now be diagnosed as specific conditions, such as conversion disorder (functional neurological symptom disorder), somatic symptom disorder, or other psychiatric conditions.
3. **Gender Bias**: The historical diagnosis of hysteria is now seen as having been heavily influenced by social and cultural biases, particularly against women.

Current Relevance

While the term "hysteria" is outdated and no longer used clinically, its history reflects the evolving understanding of mental health and the influence of sociocultural factors on psychiatric diagnoses. Today, conditions that might have been labeled as hysteria in the past are understood in more nuanced ways, with a focus on specific symptoms and underlying psychological mechanisms.

What is intelligence?

Intelligence is a complex and multifaceted concept that has been defined and studied in various ways in psychology and related fields. Generally, it refers to the ability to learn from experience, adapt to new situations, understand and handle abstract concepts, and use knowledge to manipulate one's environment.

Key Aspects of Intelligence

1. **Cognitive Abilities**: This includes memory, reasoning, problem-solving skills, and the ability to comprehend complex ideas.
2. **Adaptability**: The capacity to adjust to new challenges and environments.
3. **Knowledge Application**: The ability to apply learned knowledge effectively in different situations.
4. **Learning and Understanding**: The capability to absorb new information, understand it, and put it into practice.
5. **Abstract Thinking**: Involving the ability to understand and manipulate abstract concepts, not just concrete physical objects.

Theories of Intelligence

1. **Spearman's g Factor**: Charles Spearman proposed that intelligence is a single general ability (g factor) that influences performance on various cognitive tasks.
2. **Multiple Intelligences**: Howard Gardner's theory of multiple intelligences suggests there are several distinct types of intelligence, such as linguistic, logical-mathematical, musical, spatial, bodily-kinesthetic, interpersonal, intrapersonal, and naturalistic.
3. **Triarchic Theory of Intelligence**: Robert Sternberg's model divides intelligence into three types: analytical (problem-solving abilities), creative (ability to deal with new situations using past experiences and current skills), and practical (ability to adapt to a changing environment).

Measurement of Intelligence

- **IQ (Intelligence Quotient)**: Traditionally, intelligence has been measured with IQ tests, designed to assess a range of cognitive abilities. An average IQ score is set at 100.
- **Standardized Testing**: Tests like the Wechsler Adult Intelligence Scale (WAIS) and the Stanford-Binet Intelligence Scales are commonly used.

Critiques and Debates

- **Cultural Bias**: Some argue that IQ tests may be culturally biased, favoring certain linguistic and cultural groups.
- **Nature vs. Nurture**: There is ongoing debate about the extent to which intelligence is a product of genetics (nature) versus environmental factors (nurture).
- **Dynamic Nature**: Intelligence is increasingly seen as dynamic and malleable, not fixed at birth.

Applications

Understanding intelligence has important implications in education, psychology, and cognitive science.

It informs how we design educational programs; understand individual differences, and even how we approach artificial intelligence.

In summary, intelligence is a broad and complex concept that encompasses various cognitive abilities and adaptive skills. It is subject to ongoing research, debate, and reinterpretation in the light of new findings and societal changes.

What is emotional intelligence and their main components?

Emotional Intelligence (EI or EQ) refers to the ability to recognize, understand, and manage one's own emotions as well as the emotions of others. This concept involves several key skills:

1. **Self-Awareness:** This is the ability to recognize and understand your own emotions and how they affect your thoughts and behavior. It involves being aware of your strengths and weaknesses, and having self-confidence.
2. **Self-Regulation:** This refers to the ability to control and adapt your emotions, impulses, and behaviors. It involves being able to manage your emotional reactions in different situations, and includes skills such as impulse control, stress management, and adaptability.
3. **Motivation:** In the context of emotional intelligence, motivation is often driven by internal factors, rather than external rewards or pressures. It includes the drive to improve and achieve for the sake of personal satisfaction and effectiveness, rather than for external rewards.
4. **Empathy:** This is the ability to understand and share the feelings of others. It is crucial for building and managing relationships, effective communication, and understanding the needs and concerns of others.
5. **Social Skills:** This component involves the ability to manage relationships, influence others, and navigate social environments effectively. Key skills include effective communication, leadership, conflict resolution, collaboration, and the ability to build and maintain relationships.

Emotional intelligence is considered an essential factor in both personal and professional success. Unlike traditional measures of intelligence (IQ), which focus on logic and reasoning, EQ focuses on one's ability to navigate social complexities and make positive contributions to one's environment. It is a skill set that can be developed and enhanced over time with practice and self-reflection.

How can you develop EQ?

Developing Emotional Intelligence (EQ) involves intentional efforts to improve in the key areas of self-awareness, self-regulation, motivation, empathy, and social skills. Here are some strategies for each component:

1. **Improving Self-Awareness:**
   - **Reflect on Your Emotions:** Take time to recognize and understand what you are feeling and why. This might involve keeping a journal or simply taking a few moments each day to reflect on your emotional state.
   - **Ask for Feedback:** Sometimes, others can see aspects of our behavior that we can't. Ask trusted friends, family, or colleagues for honest feedback about your emotional responses and behavior.
2. **Enhancing Self-Regulation:**
   - **Practice Mindfulness:** Mindfulness techniques, such as meditation or focused breathing, can help you become more aware of your emotional state and give you the space to choose how to respond.
   - **Learn to Pause:** Before reacting, take a moment to pause. This can prevent impulsive responses and help you respond more thoughtfully.
3. **Boosting Motivation:**
   - **Set Personal Goals:** Setting and working towards personal goals that are important and meaningful to you can boost your intrinsic motivation.
   - **Stay Positive:** Try to maintain a positive attitude, especially during challenging times. This often involves reframing negative thoughts into more positive ones.
4. **Developing Empathy:**
   - **Active Listening:** Practice really listening to what others are saying, without immediately preparing your response. This helps in truly understanding the other person's perspective.
   - **Put Yourself in Others' Shoes:** Try to imagine how others feel in different situations. This can be done through reading, watching diverse stories, or simply imagining yourself in someone else's place.
5. **Improving Social Skills:**
   - **Practice Effective Communication:** Work on clearly expressing your thoughts and feelings in a respectful way and be open to hearing the perspectives of others.

- **Work on Conflict Resolution:** Learn strategies for resolving conflicts constructively, without causing further harm to your relationships.

In addition to these strategies, attending workshops or trainings on emotional intelligence, reading relevant books, or even seeking the guidance of a professional coach or therapist can be beneficial. Remember, developing EQ is a continuous process and involves ongoing learning and practice.

What is normal behavior?

"Normal behavior" is a concept that can vary widely based on cultural, social, and individual contexts. Generally, it refers to conduct or actions that are considered acceptable or typical within a particular society or group.

1. **Cultural Norms:** What is considered normal in one culture may be unusual in another. Cultural norms dictate many aspects of behavior, including how people communicate, dress, eat, and interact socially.
2. **Social Norms:** Within any given culture, there are also social norms that can vary among different groups. For instance, behavior that is normal in a professional workplace might be out of place at a casual family gathering.
3. **Age-Appropriate Behavior:** Normal behavior often depends on a person's age and developmental stage. For example, certain behaviors expected from an adult might not be expected from a child.
4. **Situational Norms:** The context or situation also plays a significant role in determining what behavior is considered normal. For example, shouting might be normal at a sports event but not in a library.
5. **Personal Norms:** On an individual level, what's normal can vary greatly. Personal norms are influenced by an individual's personality, experiences, and personal values.

It is important to note that the concept of "normal" is often subjective and can change over time as societal values and norms evolve. Also, the idea of normalcy can sometimes be used inappropriately to stigmatize or exclude those who do not conform to certain standards or norms. Therefore, it is crucial to approach the concept of normal behavior with an understanding of its relative and dynamic nature.

What is abnormal behavior?

Abnormal behavior refers to patterns of behavior, thought, or emotion that are considered atypical or significantly deviate from societal norms or expectations. It is important to note that determining what constitutes "abnormal" can be complex and subjective, as it often depends on cultural, contextual, and individual factors. However, in the field of psychology, certain criteria are generally used to help define abnormal behavior:

1. **Statistical Rarity:** If a behavior is rare or uncommon within a particular culture or society, it might be considered abnormal. However, rarity alone does not necessarily mean a behavior is abnormal in a clinical sense.
2. **Deviation from Social Norms:** Behaviors that significantly deviate from the accepted standards or rules of a society may be considered abnormal. These norms can vary greatly between different cultures and social groups.
3. **Personal Distress:** If a behavior causes significant distress to the individual—such as anxiety, depression, or other emotional pain—it may be considered abnormal.
4. **Maladaptiveness:** Behaviors that are maladaptive interfere with an individual's ability to function effectively in daily life. This could include difficulty in performing routine tasks, maintaining relationships, holding a job, etc.
5. **Unpredictability and Irrationality:** Behavior that is unpredictable, uncontrollable, or irrational (e.g., sudden, unprovoked outbursts) might be classified as abnormal.
6. **Violation of Moral and Ideal Standards:** In some cases, behavior may be considered abnormal if it violates moral or ideal standards of the society, though this criterion is highly subjective and culturally dependent.

It is essential to approach the concept of abnormal behavior with sensitivity and an awareness of its complexity. In mental health, professionals use specific criteria, such as those outlined in the Diagnostic and Statistical Manual of Mental Disorders (DSM), to assess and diagnose mental health conditions. This assessment is typically comprehensive, taking into account the individual's cultural, social, and personal background. Additionally, it is crucial to avoid stigmatizing people with labels and to understand that abnormal behavior can often be effectively managed or treated with the appropriate care.

What is brain?

The brain is a complex and vital organ in the human body, serving as the center of the nervous system. It is responsible for processing sensory information, regulating bodily functions, and forming the foundation of our thoughts, emotions, and behaviors.

1. **Structure and Composition:**

   - The human brain is made up of billions of nerve cells (neurons) and glial cells. Neurons are responsible for transmitting and processing information, while glial cells provide support and nutrition to neurons.
   - It is divided into several major parts, including the cerebrum, cerebellum, and brainstem.
   - The cerebrum, the largest part, is divided into two hemispheres (left and right) and is responsible for higher functions like thinking, decision-making, emotions, and language. It is further divided into lobes that specialize in different functions.
   - The cerebellum, located under the cerebrum, plays a key role in motor control and coordination.
   - The brainstem, connecting the brain and spinal cord, controls many vital life functions, such as breathing, heart rate, and blood pressure.

2. **Functionality:**

   - The brain processes sensory information it receives from the outside world (like sight, sound, and touch) and from within the body (like hunger, pain, and temperature).
   - It is responsible for cognitive functions such as thinking, memory, learning, and problem-solving.
   - Emotional responses and regulation are also governed by the brain.
   - It orchestrates voluntary movements, like walking and talking, and manages involuntary responses, like reflexes.

3. **Neuroplasticity:**

   - The brain has the remarkable ability to change and adapt. This plasticity allows for learning and memory formation and enables recovery from injuries to a certain extent.

4. **Communication:**

   - Neurons communicate with each other through electrical impulses and chemical signals (neurotransmitters).
   - This network of communication is fundamental to everything from basic reflexes to complex thoughts.

5. **Protection:**

   - The brain is protected by the skull, meninges (three layers of protective tissue), and cerebrospinal fluid, which cushions and provides nutrients.

Understanding the brain and its function is a vast and ongoing field of study in neuroscience. Advances in technology, such as neuroimaging and electrophysiological recording, continue to deepen our understanding of this complex organ. The brain's intricate workings are crucial to what makes us human, underpinning our thoughts, actions, and experiences.

How is brain structure organised?

The human brain is a highly complex and intricately organized organ. Its structure is organized into several distinct parts, each with specific functions. Here is a brief overview of the major components and their organization:

1. **Cerebrum:**

   - The cerebrum is the largest part of the brain and is divided into the left and right hemispheres.
   - Each hemisphere is further divided into four lobes: frontal, parietal, temporal, and occipital.
   - **Frontal Lobe:** Involved in cognitive functions like thinking, planning, problem-solving, and emotions.
   - **Parietal Lobe:** Processes sensory information such as touch, temperature, and pain.
   - **Temporal Lobe:** Important for processing auditory information and is also involved in memory and emotion.
   - **Occipital Lobe:** Primarily responsible for visual processing.
   - The cerebral cortex, the outer layer of the cerebrum, is involved in higher brain functions such as thought, language, and consciousness.

2. **Cerebellum:**

   - Located under the cerebrum, its primary function is to coordinate voluntary movements, posture, balance, coordination, and speech, resulting in smooth and balanced muscular activity.

3. **Brainstem:**

   - The brainstem connects the brain with the spinal cord and consists of the midbrain, pons, and medulla oblongata.
   - It regulates vital life functions, including breathing, heart rate, and blood pressure.

4. **Limbic System:**
   - This system includes structures such as the hippocampus, amygdala, and hypothalamus.
   - It is involved in emotional response, memory, and the regulation of the autonomic nervous system.
5. **Basal Ganglia:**
   - A group of structures linked to the thalamus in the base of the brain and involved in coordination of movement.
6. **Thalamus and Hypothalamus:**
   - The thalamus acts as a relay station for information coming to the brain.
   - The hypothalamus is involved in various functions of the autonomic nervous system, and it plays a significant role in hormone production and regulation.
7. **White Matter and Grey Matter:**
   - **Grey Matter:** Composed of neuronal cell bodies and is involved in processing and cognition.
   - **White Matter:** Consists of axons connecting different parts of grey matter to each other.
8. **Ventricular System:**
   - Filled with cerebrospinal fluid, the ventricles are a series of connected cavities within the brain.

Each part of the brain works in concert with others to regulate everything from basic bodily functions to complex cognitive processes. The brain's structure is both intricate and adaptable, capable of remarkable changes (neuroplasticity) in response to learning, experience, and injury.

What are the primary functions of the brain?

The brain, being the control center of the body, performs a multitude of critical functions. These functions can be broadly categorized into several primary areas:

1. **Processing of Sensory Information:**
   - The brain receives and interprets sensory information from the environment (like sight, sound, smell, taste, and touch) and from within the body (like pain, temperature, and hunger).
2. **Motor Function Control:**
   - It sends signals to muscles, coordinating voluntary movements such as walking, talking, writing, and involuntary movements like reflexes.
3. **Cognitive Functions:**
   - Higher cognitive processes including thinking, learning, memory, decision-making, problem-solving, and planning are centralized in the brain.
   - It is also involved in processing and understanding language.
4. **Emotional Regulation:**
   - The brain helps in regulating emotions and responses to stimuli. Structures within the limbic system, like the amygdala and hippocampus, play a key role in emotional response and memory.
5. **Regulation of Bodily Functions:**
   - The brain regulates numerous bodily functions, often without conscious awareness. This includes the autonomic nervous system, which controls things like heart rate, breathing, digestion, and blood pressure.
6. **Hormonal Regulation:**
   - Through the hypothalamus and its connection to the pituitary gland, the brain controls the release of hormones that regulate various bodily functions, including growth, metabolism, and the reproductive system.
7. **Sleep and Wakefulness:**
   - The brain regulates the sleep-wake cycle, controlling when we feel alert and when we feel sleepy.
8. **Homeostasis:**
   - It maintains homeostasis, the body's internal balance, by regulating temperature, pH levels, and other vital parameters.
9. **Social and Behavioral Responses:**
   - The brain plays a key role in social interaction and behavior, affecting how we communicate, form relationships, and respond to others.
10. **Creativity and Imagination:**
    - It is also responsible for creative thought, imagination, and dreaming.

These functions underscore the complexity and versatility of the brain, highlighting its role not just in basic survival, but also in aspects that are foundational to our identity and daily experience.

How does 'brain released hormones' cause psychiatric disorders?

The relationship between brain-released hormones and psychiatric disorders is complex and multifaceted. Hormones are chemical messengers released into the bloodstream by glands, including those in the brain, and they play a significant role in regulating mood, cognition, and behavior. Imbalances or dysregulation of these hormones can contribute to the development or exacerbation of psychiatric disorders.

1. **Stress Hormones (e.g., Cortisol):**
   - The hypothalamic-pituitary-adrenal (HPA) axis is a major neuroendocrine system that controls reactions to stress and regulates many body processes. Overactivity or dysregulation of the HPA axis, leading to abnormal cortisol levels, has been linked to disorders like depression, anxiety, and PTSD.
2. **Serotonin:**
   - Often referred to as a "feel-good hormone," serotonin influences mood, anxiety, and happiness. Imbalances in serotonin levels are associated with conditions like depression, anxiety disorders, and OCD.
3. **Dopamine:**
   - Dopamine plays a key role in reward, motivation, and pleasure. Dysregulation in dopamine levels and its pathways is implicated in various psychiatric disorders, including schizophrenia, bipolar disorder, and addiction.
4. **Norepinephrine (Noradrenaline):**
   - This hormone and neurotransmitter is involved in the body's stress response and is also thought to play a role in attention and emotion. Dysregulation can be associated with mood disorders like depression and anxiety.
5. **Thyroid Hormones:**
   - Thyroid hormone imbalances can have profound effects on mood and brain function. Both hypothyroidism and hyperthyroidism can manifest with symptoms resembling depression, anxiety, or other mood disorders.
6. **Sex Hormones (e.g., Estrogen and Testosterone):**
   - Fluctuations in sex hormones can affect mood and are linked to conditions such as premenstrual dysphoric disorder (PMDD), postpartum depression, and mood swings during menopause. They may also influence the course of other psychiatric disorders.
7. **Melatonin:**
   - Involved in regulating the sleep-wake cycle, imbalances in melatonin can affect sleep patterns, which is a critical factor in the development and maintenance of many psychiatric disorders.

It is important to note that the relationship between hormones and psychiatric disorders is not purely one-directional or causal. Psychiatric disorders are complex and result from a combination of genetic, environmental, psychological, and biological factors. Hormonal imbalances may contribute to the onset or severity of a disorder, but they are typically just one part of a larger picture. Additionally, the perception of stress, psychological factors, and individual differences in hormone sensitivity also play crucial roles in how hormonal changes affect mental health.

Understanding these interactions is a key area of research in psychiatry and neuroscience, aiming to develop more effective treatments and interventions for mental health disorders.

What is the stress hormone called?

The hormone commonly referred to as the "stress hormone" is cortisol. Cortisol is a glucocorticoid hormone produced by the adrenal glands, which are located on top of each kidney. It plays a crucial role in the body's stress response and is part of the broader hypothalamic-pituitary-adrenal (HPA) axis.

Cortisol serves several important functions in the body, especially in situations of stress:

1. **Mobilizes Energy:** It increases glucose in the bloodstream by stimulating gluconeogenesis in the liver and breaking down muscle protein and fat tissue, providing the body with immediate energy.
2. **Suppresses Non-Essential Functions:** During stress, cortisol helps to temporarily suppress functions that are non-essential in a fight-or-flight situation, such as the immune, digestive, and reproductive systems.
3. **Helps in Stress Response:** It enhances the brain's use of glucose and increases the availability of substances that repair tissues.
4. **Modulates Inflammation:** Cortisol has anti-inflammatory effects, modulating the body's immune response.

While cortisol is vital in managing stress and maintaining homeostasis in the body, chronic elevation of cortisol levels can lead to a range of health problems. These can include anxiety, depression, memory and concentration problems, trouble sleeping, weight gain, and increased risk for a variety of chronic conditions like hypertension and heart disease. Therefore, maintaining a balanced cortisol level is important for overall health and well-being.

What makes up the limbic system and what are their parts?

The limbic system is a complex set of structures located on both sides of the thalamus, right under the cerebrum. It is primarily responsible for our emotional life and has a significant role in the formation of memories. The key components of the limbic system include:

1. **Amygdala:** Plays a pivotal role in processing emotions, especially fear, anger, and pleasure. It is also involved in determining what memories are stored and where they are stored in the brain.
2. **Hippocampus:** Essential for the formation of new memories and is also involved in learning. The hippocampus helps connect emotions and senses, such as smell and sound, to memories.
3. **Thalamus:** Acts as a relay station, directing sensory signals to the appropriate areas of the cortex and other parts of the limbic system. It is involved in processing sensory information and consciousness.
4. **Hypothalamus:** Located below the thalamus, it regulates a variety of bodily functions including hunger, thirst, sleep, and sexual response. It also controls the body's endocrine system via the pituitary gland, influencing stress levels, metabolism, and emotional responses.
5. **Cingulate Gyrus:** Functions in processing emotions and behavior regulation. It also helps regulate autonomic motor function.
6. **Fornix:** A bundle of nerve fibers that acts as a major output tract of the hippocampus, involved in memory processing.
7. **Mammillary Bodies:** Involved in recollective memory. Damage to this area can lead to disorders of memory.
8. **Olfactory Bulbs:** Involved in the sense of smell. Olfactory information is sent to the limbic system, which explains why smell is often linked to emotional memories.

The limbic system is a functionally diverse and complex system that contributes to many aspects of our emotional and memory processes. Its structures are interconnected with various other parts of the brain, making it a central network for processing a wide range of neurological functions.

What does the limbic system control?

The limbic system, a complex set of brain structures located beneath the cerebrum, plays a pivotal role in controlling various aspects of human behavior and physiological responses. Its main functions include:

1. **Emotional Responses:** The limbic system is central to the processing and regulation of emotions, including fear, pleasure, anger, and affection. The amygdala, in particular, is critical for emotional learning and the formation of emotional memories.
2. **Memory Formation:** The hippocampus, a key component of the limbic system, is essential for the formation of new memories, especially those related to personal experiences (episodic memories) and spatial navigation (spatial memories).
3. **Olfactory Processing:** The limbic system has a primary role in processing olfactory (smell) signals. The olfactory bulbs are directly connected to the limbic system, explaining why smells are often strongly linked to memories and emotions.
4. **Regulation of Autonomic and Endocrine Functions:** The hypothalamus, part of the limbic system, regulates the autonomic nervous system (which controls involuntary bodily functions like heart rate, digestion, and respiratory rate) and the endocrine system (which releases hormones). This regulation is crucial for maintaining homeostasis and responding to stress.
5. **Behavioral Responses:** The limbic system influences a range of behaviors, from basic survival instincts like feeding and reproduction to complex social and motivational behaviors.
6. **Drive and Motivation:** It is involved in the regulation of hunger, thirst, sexual desire, and other primal drives. It also plays a role in reward-seeking behavior and pleasure.
7. **Decision Making and Problem Solving:** Although not the primary site for these cognitive functions, the limbic system contributes to decision making by integrating emotional information. This helps in making choices that are not just rational but also emotionally sound.
8. **Mood Regulation:** The limbic system's interaction with neurotransmitters and hormones can significantly impact mood and is implicated in mood disorders such as depression and bipolar disorder.

The limbic system's functions demonstrate its importance in linking cognitive functions with emotional and physiological responses, playing a significant role in both survival mechanisms and more complex behaviors that characterize human experience.

What is the main function of the limbic system?

The main function of the limbic system is to regulate emotions and to form and process memories. It plays a crucial role in emotional responses, mood regulation, and the formation of both long-term and short-term memories. The limbic system, through its interconnected structures, integrates emotional states with cognitive processes, ensuring that decision-making and behavioral responses are influenced by emotional cues and past experiences.

In addition to these primary functions, the limbic system is also involved in controlling various autonomic and physiological responses to emotional stimuli, such as changes in heart rate or hormonal adjustments in response to stress. This makes it a central player in linking the body's physiological states with psychological states, essential for survival and adaptation.

What is the limbic system of the brain responsible for?

The limbic system of the brain is responsible for several key functions, mainly related to emotions, memory, and basic drives. Here is a breakdown of its primary responsibilities:

1. **Emotion Regulation:** The limbic system is crucial in processing and regulating emotions. It is involved in the formation of emotional responses and determining the emotional content of memories. Structures like the amygdala play a vital role in fear responses and other emotional reactions.
2. **Memory Formation and Retrieval:** The hippocampus, a part of the limbic system, is essential for the formation of new memories and the retrieval of existing ones, particularly those related to personal experiences and spatial navigation.
3. **Drive and Motivation:** The limbic system is involved in regulating basic drives such as hunger, thirst, and sex drive. It also plays a role in motivation and reward-seeking behaviors, influencing how we perceive and pursue rewards.
4. **Olfactory Processing:** The limbic system has a significant role in processing olfactory (smell) information, which is why certain smells can trigger strong memories or emotions.
5. **Autonomic and Endocrine Control:** The hypothalamus, part of the limbic system, regulates the autonomic nervous system and the endocrine system. It helps maintain body homeostasis, controlling functions like body temperature, circadian rhythms, and the stress response.
6. **Social Behavior:** The limbic system influences social interaction and bonding. It affects our ability to form and maintain social relationships and plays a role in empathy and emotional intelligence.

Overall, the limbic system is integral to how we experience and interpret the world emotionally, how we form memories, and how we respond to various survival needs and social cues.

How does the limbic system work?

The limbic system, a complex set of structures in the brain, works through intricate interactions between its various components and with other parts of the brain to perform its functions.

1. **Emotion Processing and Regulation:**
   - The amygdala, often considered the emotional center of the brain, plays a key role in the detection and response to emotional stimuli, particularly those related to fear and pleasure. It helps process emotions and forms emotional memories.
   - These emotional responses can be influenced by past experiences, memories, and contextual information processed in other parts of the brain, like the cerebral cortex.
2. **Memory Formation and Retrieval:**
   - The hippocampus is crucial for the formation of new memories, especially those involving personal experiences (episodic memory) and spatial information.
   - It helps in consolidating short-term memories into long-term memories and plays a role in retrieving these memories based on cues or context.
3. **Drive and Motivation:**
   - The hypothalamus, which is part of the limbic system, regulates basic drives and needs like hunger, thirst, and the sleep-wake cycle. It also plays a role in sexual behavior and motivation.
   - The limbic system interacts with the brain's reward system, involving structures like the nucleus accumbens, influencing behaviors related to pleasure and reward.
4. **Olfactory Processing:**
   - The olfactory bulbs, which are directly connected

to areas of the limbic system, process information about smells. This is why certain smells can trigger emotional memories.

5. **Autonomic and Endocrine Control:**
   - The hypothalamus controls the autonomic nervous system, affecting physiological responses like heart rate, blood pressure, and stress response.
   - It also regulates the endocrine system through its connection to the pituitary gland, influencing hormonal responses.
6. **Interactions with Other Brain Regions:**
   - The limbic system is not isolated; it continuously interacts with other parts of the brain. For instance, the prefrontal cortex (involved in decision-making and cognitive control) works in tandem with the limbic system to regulate emotional responses in a context-appropriate manner.

By orchestrating these functions, the limbic system plays a critical role in our emotional life, memory processing, and the way we respond to various internal and external stimuli. It is a key contributor to the formation of our behaviors, motivations, and overall psychological experience.

What is thalamus?

The thalamus is a small but critically important structure in the brain. It serves as a central relay station for sensory and motor signals to the cerebral cortex, playing a significant role in regulating consciousness, sleep, and alertness. Here are some key aspects of the thalamus:

1. **Location and Structure:**
   - The thalamus is located in the center of the brain, just above the brainstem. It consists of two lobes connected by a bridge of nerve fibers.
   - It is part of the diencephalon, which also includes the hypothalamus, epithalamiums, and subthalamus.
2. **Function as a Relay Station:**
   - Most sensory information (like visual, auditory, and touch inputs) received by the body is relayed through the thalamus before being sent to the appropriate areas of the cerebral cortex for processing.
   - It plays a crucial role in processing and interpreting this sensory data.
3. **Role in Motor Control:**
   - The thalamus is involved in the coordination and control of motor activities. It receives information from the cerebellum and the basal ganglia and then relays this information to motor areas in the cerebral cortex.
4. **Regulation of Consciousness and Alertness:**
   - The thalamus has a significant role in regulating states of sleep and wakefulness. It is part of the system that controls the transitions between wakefulness, sleep, and different stages of sleep.
5. **Cognitive Functions:**
   - While primarily known for sensory and motor signal relay, the thalamus also has connections to the prefrontal cortex, playing a role in cognitive functions such as memory and attention.
6. **Pain Perception:**
   - The thalamus is involved in the perception of pain, processing pain signals before they are sent to the cerebral cortex.

Given its central location and the variety of inputs it processes, damage to the thalamus can have widespread effects, impacting sensory perception, motor skills, consciousness, and cognitive abilities. The thalamus's role as a relay and processing center makes it a fundamental component in the overall function of the brain.

Is the hypothalamus part of the limbic system?

Yes, the hypothalamus is considered a part of the limbic system. The limbic system is a group of interconnected structures in the brain that are crucial for emotional responses, memory processing, and autonomic regulation. The hypothalamus, although small, plays a significant role within this system.

1. **Emotion and Behavior Regulation:** The hypothalamus is involved in regulating various emotional responses and behaviors. It interacts with other parts of the limbic system, like the amygdala and hippocampus, to influence emotional states.
2. **Autonomic Control:** The hypothalamus plays a central role in controlling the autonomic nervous system, which manages involuntary bodily functions like heart rate, blood pressure, digestion, and body temperature.
3. **Endocrine Function:** The hypothalamus links the nervous system to the endocrine system via the pituitary gland. It synthesizes and secretes hormones that can influence mood, sleep, temperature regulation, appetite, and sex drive.
4. **Homeostasis:** The hypothalamus is key in maintaining homeostasis in the body. It constantly

monitors the body's internal conditions and initiates responses to maintain a balanced and stable internal environment.

5. **Appetite and Thirst Regulation:** The hypothalamus is involved in regulating hunger and thirst. It receives signals related to energy intake and body's hydration status and responds accordingly.

In summary, while the hypothalamus is often discussed in the context of its roles in autonomic and endocrine functions, its contributions to emotional processing and behavior as part of the limbic system are also critically important.

Is the amygdala in the limbic system?

Yes, the amygdala is a key component of the limbic system. Located deep within the temporal lobes of the brain, the amygdala plays a crucial role in processing and regulating emotions, particularly those related to survival, such as fear and aggression. It is also involved in the formation of emotional memories and helps in attaching emotional significance to memories.

In the context of the limbic system, the amygdala interacts with other structures such as the hippocampus, hypothalamus, and various regions of the cerebral cortex. This interaction is vital for coordinating a wide range of emotional responses and for integrating emotional information with cognition and memory. The amygdala's involvement in emotional learning and memory is particularly significant in understanding how we develop responses to various stimuli based on past experiences.

How to calm down the amygdala?

Calming down the amygdala, which is the brain's center for processing emotions like fear and anxiety, can be crucial for managing stress and anxiety. Here are several effective strategies:

1. **Deep Breathing Exercises:** Deep, controlled breathing can help activate the body's relaxation response. Techniques like diaphragmatic breathing or the 4-7-8 breathing method can be particularly effective.

2. **Mindfulness and Meditation:** Regular practice of mindfulness meditation has been shown to reduce the activity of the amygdala and increase connections to the prefrontal cortex, which helps regulate emotional responses.

3. **Progressive Muscle Relaxation:** This technique involves tensing and then relaxing different muscle groups in the body, which can help reduce the physical symptoms of stress and anxiety.

4. **Regular Exercise:** Physical activity can help reduce stress and anxiety. It releases endorphins, which are natural mood lifters, and can also help take your mind off worries.

5. **Adequate Sleep:** Quality sleep is crucial for emotional regulation and brain health. Poor sleep can exacerbate stress and anxiety, while good sleep can help soothe and reset the nervous system.

6. **Healthy Diet:** Eating a balanced diet can support overall brain health. Some foods, like those rich in omega-3 fatty acids, can be particularly beneficial for brain function.

7. **Cognitive Behavioral Therapy (CBT):** CBT and other forms of therapy can be effective in changing the thought patterns that trigger stress and anxiety, thus reducing amygdala activation.

8. **Exposure Therapy:** Gradually and repeatedly being exposed to the source of your fear, in a controlled way, can help reduce the amygdala's response over time. This is often used in treating phobias and anxiety disorders.

9. **Social Support:** Engaging in positive social interactions can stimulate the release of oxytocin, a hormone that decreases amygdala activity and promotes feelings of calm and safety.

10. **Mindfulness-Based Stress Reduction (MBSR):** This structured program combines mindfulness, meditation, and yoga to help reduce stress and anxiety.

It is important to note that what works for one person might not work for another, so it may take some experimentation to find what best helps you calm your amygdala.

Where is the seat of origin of normal or abnormal behavior in humans?

The origin of normal and abnormal behavior in humans is a complex and multifaceted topic, involving various structures and functions of the brain. There is not a single "seat" of origin, but rather a network of brain regions and neurobiological processes that collectively contribute to behavior. Key areas and aspects include:

1. **Frontal Lobes and Prefrontal Cortex:**
    - These areas are crucial for decision-making, problem-solving, impulse control, and social behavior. Abnormalities or damage here can lead to changes in personality, impulsivity, and difficulty in understanding social norms.

2. **Amygdala:**
   - Involved in processing emotions, especially fear and aggression. Abnormalities in the amygdala are linked to anxiety disorders, depression, and other mood disorders.
3. **Hippocampus:**
   - Important for memory formation. Disorders of the hippocampus can affect memory and are associated with conditions like Alzheimer's disease and PTSD.
4. **Basal Ganglia:**
   - Involved in motor control and reward. Dysfunctions here are associated with disorders like Parkinson's disease, Huntington's disease, and Tourette syndrome.
5. **Hypothalamus:**
   - Regulates basic drives such as hunger, thirst, and sexual behavior, as well as the stress response. Imbalances can affect these fundamental drives and emotional states.
6. **Neurotransmitter Systems:**
   - Chemical messengers like serotonin, dopamine, and norepinephrine are crucial for brain function. Imbalances in these systems can lead to a range of disorders, including depression, schizophrenia, and bipolar disorder.
7. **Cerebral Cortex:**
   - Involved in complex mental functions, sensory processing, and consciousness. Abnormalities in different cortical areas can lead to various cognitive, sensory, and perceptual disorders.
8. **Limbic System:**
   - This system, including the amygdala, hippocampus, and thalamus, is key for emotional regulation and memory. Dysfunctions in this system are often implicated in mood and anxiety disorders.
9. **Genetic Factors:**
   - Genetics play a significant role in predisposing individuals to certain mental health conditions, influencing how brain structure and chemistry develop.
10. **Environmental Factors:**
    - Experiences, especially in early life, can shape brain development and behavior. Trauma, stress, and social environments are crucial in this regard.

In summary, both normal and abnormal behaviors are the result of complex interactions between multiple brain regions, neurotransmitter systems, genetic predispositions, and environmental influences. Understanding these behaviors often requires a holistic view of the brain's structure and function, as well as the individual's experiences and context.

What is a receptor and types?

A receptor is a protein molecule that receives and responds to chemical signals in the body. Receptors are critical components in various physiological processes and are found in various types of cells. Their primary function is to bind to specific molecules, such as hormones, neurotransmitters, or drugs, and to initiate a response within the cell. Here are some key aspects of receptors:

1. **Types of Receptors:**
   - **Cell Surface Receptors:** Located on the cell membrane, these receptors interact with substances that cannot enter the cell directly. They are involved in processes like neurotransmission, immune responses, and hormone signaling.
   - **Intracellular Receptors:** Found within the cell, in the cytoplasm or nucleus, these receptors bind to substances that can cross the cell membrane, such as steroid hormones. They typically regulate gene expression.
2. **Binding and Activation:**
   - Receptors have specific sites where signaling molecules (ligands) bind. This binding usually causes a change in the receptor's shape, activating it and triggering a series of events inside the cell.
3. **Signal Transduction:**
   - Once activated, receptors initiate a process called signal transduction, converting the external signal into a cellular response. This can involve a cascade of biochemical reactions inside the cell.
4. **Roles in the Body:**
   - Receptors play a vital role in various systems, including the nervous system (neurotransmitter receptors), endocrine system (hormone receptors), and immune system (antigen receptors).
5. **Importance in Pharmacology:**
   - Many drugs work by interacting with receptors, either mimicking a natural ligand to activate the receptor or blocking the receptor to prevent it from being activated.

6. **Receptor Sensitivity:**
   - The sensitivity of receptors can change in response to various factors, such as prolonged exposure to a ligand, which can lead to receptor upregulation or downregulation.

In summary, receptors are essential for communication between cells and for the regulation of bodily functions. They are integral in the body's response to internal and external stimuli and are key targets in the development of many medications.

What do receptors do?

Receptors play a crucial role in cellular communication and function in the body. Their primary actions include:

1. **Signal Reception:**
   - Receptors are designed to recognize and bind to specific molecules called ligands, which can be hormones, neurotransmitters, or other signaling molecules. Each receptor has a unique binding site that is complementary to its specific ligand.
2. **Signal Transduction:**
   - Upon binding with their ligand, receptors undergo a conformational change that triggers a series of biochemical reactions inside the cell. This process, known as signal transduction, converts the external signal into a specific cellular response.
3. **Modulation of Cellular Activity:**
   - The activation of receptors leads to various cellular responses, such as changes in gene expression, alteration of ion channel activity, activation or inhibition of enzymes, and changes in cellular metabolism. These responses depend on the type of receptor and the cell in which it is located.
4. **Regulation of Physiological Processes:**
   - Receptors are key regulators of numerous physiological processes, including neurotransmission, immune responses, hormone regulation, growth and development, and sensory perception (such as vision and taste).
5. **Mediating the Effects of Drugs:**
   - Many drugs exert their effects by interacting with receptors, either mimicking (agonists) or blocking (antagonists) the action of natural ligands. Understanding how drugs interact with receptors is fundamental in pharmacology and medicine.
6. **Adaptation and Sensitization:**
   - Receptors can adapt to the presence of ligands through processes like desensitization (reduced response to a continuously present ligand) or sensitization (increased response).

In essence, receptors are essential for cells to communicate with each other and to respond appropriately to their internal and external environments. They are integral components in maintaining the body's homeostasis and overall function.

What are the two types of neuron receptors?

Neuron receptors, also known as neural receptors, can be broadly categorized into two main types based on their mode of action and structure: ionotropic receptors and metabotropic receptors.

1. **Ionotropic Receptors:**
   - Also known as ligand-gated ion channels.
   - These receptors are direct-acting; when a neurotransmitter (ligand) binds to the receptor, it causes the receptor to change shape and form an ion channel. This channel opens or closes, allowing specific ions (like Na^+, K^+, $Ca2^+$ or Cl^-) to pass through the cell membrane.
   - The movement of ions changes the electrical charge across the neuron's membrane, leading to either excitation or inhibition of the neuron.
   - Ionotropic receptors are known for their fast response but short duration of action.
   - Examples include NMDA, AMPA, and GABA_A receptors.
2. **Metabotropic Receptors:**
   - Also known as G-protein-coupled receptors (GPCRs).
   - These receptors are indirect-acting. When a neurotransmitter binds to a metabotropic receptor, it activates a G-protein located inside the cell membrane.
   - The activated G-protein then interacts with other intracellular molecules (like enzymes or ion channels), initiating a signaling cascade that results in changes within the cell. These changes can alter neuron excitability, modify the effectiveness of synaptic transmission, or influence various cellular processes.
   - Metabotropic receptors typically produce slower but longer-lasting effects compared to ionotropic receptors.
   - Examples include muscarinic acetylcholine receptors, metabotropic glutamate receptors, and various neuropeptide receptors.

Both ionotropic and metabotropic receptors are essential for neural communication, processing various types of signals received by neurons. They play crucial roles in numerous neurological functions and are important targets in pharmacology for treating various neurological and psychiatric disorders.

What are cellular receptors and types?

Cellular receptors are specialized protein molecules found on the surface of cells or within cells that bind to specific substances, like hormones, neurotransmitters, drugs, or other signaling molecules. These receptors are crucial in cellular communication and play a vital role in numerous physiological processes. Here are key aspects of cellular receptors:

1. **Location and Types:**
   - **Cell Surface Receptors:** These are embedded in the cell membrane and bind to external signaling molecules that cannot cross the lipid bilayer of the cell membrane. Examples include G-protein-coupled receptors (GPCRs), ion channel-linked receptors, and enzyme-linked receptors.
   - **Intracellular Receptors:** Found within the cell, usually in the cytoplasm or nucleus, these receptors bind to signaling molecules that can cross the cell membrane, like steroid hormones or thyroid hormones.
2. **Binding and Activation:**
   - Cellular receptors have specific binding sites that are complementary to their ligands. The binding of a ligand to its receptor typically triggers a change in the receptor's conformation (shape), activating it.
3. **Signal Transduction:**
   - Activation of receptors initiates a process called signal transduction, converting the external signal into a specific response inside the cell. This process can involve a cascade of biochemical reactions, ultimately leading to changes in cell function, such as altered gene expression, enzyme activity, or ion channel permeability.
4. **Roles in the Body:**
   - Receptors play key roles in various physiological functions, including growth and development, immune responses, neurotransmission, hormone regulation, and metabolic processes.
5. **Pharmacological Importance:**
   - Many drugs exert their effects by interacting with specific receptors. Understanding how drugs interact with these receptors is fundamental in pharmacology for developing new therapeutic agents and understanding drug actions and side effects.
6. **Adaptation Mechanisms:**
   - Cellular receptors can undergo changes in sensitivity and density in response to prolonged exposure to ligands, known as upregulation or downregulation, which can affect cellular responsiveness.

In summary, cellular receptors are essential for the communication between cells and their environment, enabling the body to respond appropriately to internal and external stimuli. They are critical targets in the treatment of various diseases and are a focus of extensive research in medicine and biology.

What are intracellular receptors?

Intracellular receptors are a type of cellular receptor located within the cell, typically in the cytoplasm or nucleus. Unlike cell surface receptors, intracellular receptors can directly interact with small, lipophilic (fat-soluble) signaling molecules that can easily pass through the cell membrane.

1. **Ligand Binding:**
   - Intracellular receptors bind to ligands that are able to diffuse across the cell membrane. These ligands are often hormones, such as steroid hormones (like cortisol, estrogen, and testosterone), thyroid hormones, and certain vitamins like vitamin D.
2. **Activation and Mechanism of Action:**
   - When a ligand binds to an intracellular receptor, it causes a conformational change in the receptor, activating it.
   - The activated receptor-ligand complex then often migrates to the cell nucleus where it can directly interact with the cell's DNA.
3. **Gene Regulation:**
   - In the nucleus, the receptor-ligand complex binds to specific DNA sequences, known as hormone response elements, and acts as a transcription factor.
   - This binding regulates the transcription of certain genes, either increasing or decreasing the synthesis of specific proteins.
4. **Roles and Impact:**
   - Intracellular receptors play significant roles in

regulating development, metabolism, and homeostasis.

- Because they directly influence gene expression, their effects are typically slower to manifest compared to those of cell surface receptors, but they are usually longer-lasting.

5. **Examples of Intracellular Receptors:**
   - The glucocorticoid receptor, which binds to glucocorticoids like cortisol.
   - The estrogen receptor, which binds to estrogen.
   - The thyroid hormone receptor, which binds to thyroid hormones.

Intracellular receptors are essential for the fine-tuned regulation of physiological processes and are also important targets in pharmacology and medicine, particularly in the treatment of hormone-related conditions and certain cancers. Understanding their function is key to developing targeted therapies for various diseases.

What are the receptors on the cell membrane?

Receptors on the cell membrane, also known as cell surface receptors, are protein molecules embedded in the plasma membrane of cells. They are crucial for transmitting signals from the outside environment to the inside of the cell. These receptors interact with specific external molecules (ligands), such as hormones, neurotransmitters, antigens, or drugs, leading to a variety of cellular responses. There are several major types of cell surface receptors:

1. **G-Protein-Coupled Receptors (GPCRs):**
   - These receptors are involved in a wide range of physiological processes and are the largest and most diverse group of membrane receptors in eukaryotic cells.
   - When a ligand binds to a GPCR, it causes a conformational change in the receptor, which then activates an associated G-protein. This activation leads to the initiation of intracellular signaling pathways or the production of secondary messengers like cAMP.
2. **Ion Channel-Linked Receptors (Ionotropic Receptors):**
   - These receptors act as gateways for specific ions, such as sodium, potassium, calcium, or chloride.
   - When the appropriate ligand binds to these receptors, the channel part of the receptor opens, allowing ions to flow across the membrane. This flow changes the electrical charge across the membrane, which can lead to cellular responses such as muscle contraction or neuronal signaling.
3. **Enzyme-Linked Receptors:**
   - These receptors have an extracellular domain that binds the ligand and an intracellular domain with enzyme activity, often a protein kinase that can phosphorylate specific target proteins.
   - The binding of the ligand activates the enzyme, triggering a cascade of intracellular reactions. A common example is the receptor tyrosine kinase (RTK) family.

Each type of cell surface receptor has a specific mechanism of action but generally functions to convert an extracellular signal into an intracellular signal, allowing the cell to respond to its external environment. This signaling is fundamental to many physiological processes, including immune responses, growth factor signaling, sensory perception, and neural communication. Due to their accessibility on the cell surface and their crucial role in numerous biological pathways, these receptors are often targeted by pharmaceutical drugs to treat a variety of diseases.

What are receptor proteins responsible for?

Receptor proteins are responsible for facilitating communication between the cell and its external environment, playing a crucial role in numerous physiological processes. Their primary functions include:

1. **Signal Transduction:**
   - Receptor proteins are key players in signal transduction, the process by which a cell responds to external stimuli. When a signaling molecule, like a hormone or neurotransmitter, binds to a receptor, it triggers a chain of biochemical reactions inside the cell.
2. **Regulating Cellular Activity:**
   - Activation of receptor proteins can regulate a wide range of cellular activities, including gene expression, metabolic pathways, cell growth, and apoptosis (programmed cell death).
3. **Mediating Interactions Between Cells:**
   - Certain receptor proteins facilitate cell-to-cell communication, which is essential in processes like immune responses, synaptic transmission in neurons, and inflammatory reactions.
4. **Sensing the Environment:**
   - Receptors are involved in sensing environmental changes, such as variations in light, temperature, and chemical signals. This is crucial in maintaining

homeostasis and responding appropriately to environmental changes.

5. **Controlling the Entry and Exit of Substances:**

   - Some receptor proteins function as ion channels or transporters, controlling the movement of ions or molecules across the cell membrane. This is vital for processes like nerve signal transmission and muscle contraction.

6. **Endocytosis and Cell Adhesion:**

   - Receptor-mediated endocytosis allows cells to internalize substances from their surroundings. Additionally, some receptors play a role in cell adhesion, helping cells to attach to each other or to the extracellular matrix.

7. **Target for Pharmaceuticals:**

   - Many drugs work by interacting with receptor proteins, either to mimic or inhibit the action of natural ligands. This makes receptor proteins important targets in the development of treatments for various diseases.

In summary, receptor proteins are essential for the proper functioning of cells and organisms, enabling cells to perceive and react to their internal and external environments. They are integral in processes ranging from basic cellular metabolism to complex behaviors in multicellular organisms.

What are receptor molecules?

Receptor molecules are specialized proteins typically located on the surface of cells or within cells that bind to specific molecules, known as ligands. These ligands can include hormones, neurotransmitters, drugs, or other signaling molecules. Receptor molecules play a critical role in communication between cells and in regulating a wide array of biological processes.

1. **Types of Receptor Molecules:**

   - **Cell Surface Receptors:** Embedded in the cell membrane, these receptors bind to substances that cannot readily cross the lipid bilayer of the cell membrane, such as peptide hormones and neurotransmitters.

   - **Intracellular Receptors:** Located within the cell, in the cytoplasm or nucleus, these receptors bind to small or lipid-soluble substances that can diffuse through the cell membrane, such as steroid hormones and thyroid hormones.

2. **Binding and Activation:**

   - Receptor molecules have specific binding sites that are complementary to their respective ligands. When a ligand binds to a receptor, it typically causes a change in the receptor's shape or structure, activating the receptor.

3. **Signal Transduction:**

   - The activation of receptors initiates a process called signal transduction, converting an external signal into a specific cellular response. This can involve a cascade of biochemical reactions, changes in gene expression, or alterations in cellular activity.

4. **Roles in the Body:**

   - Receptor molecules are involved in a vast array of physiological functions, including growth and development, immune responses, neurotransmission, and hormone regulation.

5. **Target for Pharmacological Interventions:**

   - Many drugs are designed to interact with specific receptor molecules, either to mimic a natural ligand (agonists) or to block the receptor and prevent it from being activated (antagonists). Understanding these interactions is crucial for the development of therapeutic agents.

6. **Adaptation and Sensitivity:**

   - The sensitivity of receptor molecules can change in response to various factors. For instance, prolonged exposure to a ligand can lead to a decrease in the number of receptors on the cell surface (downregulation), reducing the cell's responsiveness to that ligand.

In summary, receptor molecules are essential components of cellular communication and regulation, enabling cells to respond to their internal and external environments in a coordinated and efficient manner. They are fundamental to the functioning of biological systems and are key targets in the treatment of a wide range of diseases.

What are types of receptors in brief?

Receptors, vital for cellular communication and response mechanisms, come in various types. Here is a brief overview of the major types:

1. **Ion Channel-Linked Receptors (Ionotropic Receptors):**

   - These receptors act as gateways for specific ions (like Na^+, K^+, $Ca2^+$, Cl^-).

   - Binding of a ligand (like a neurotransmitter) to these receptors opens or closes the channel, altering the cell's electrical charge and triggering a rapid response.

2. **G-Protein-Coupled Receptors (GPCRs):**
   - Largest family of cell surface receptors.
   - When a ligand binds, it activates a G-protein inside the cell, leading to a cascade of intracellular signals.
   - Involved in many physiological processes and widely targeted by pharmaceuticals.
3. **Enzyme-Linked Receptors:**
   - These receptors have an extracellular ligand-binding domain and an intracellular domain that usually has enzymatic activity.
   - Commonly, the intracellular domain is a protein kinase that becomes active upon ligand binding and phosphorylates specific target proteins.
4. **Intracellular Receptors:**
   - Located inside the cell, these receptors bind to small, hydrophobic ligands that can diffuse across the cell membrane (like steroid hormones).
   - The receptor-ligand complex often acts as a transcription factor, directly affecting gene expression.
5. **Nuclear Receptors:**
   - A type of intracellular receptor found in the cell nucleus.
   - They also bind to small, lipophilic ligands and typically regulate gene transcription.

Each type of receptor plays a unique role in cellular function, responding to different kinds of stimuli and triggering specific cellular responses. Their diversity and specificity are key to the functioning of biological systems, making them crucial targets for therapeutic intervention in a wide range of diseases.

What are different types of opiate receptors?

Opiate receptors are a group of G-protein-coupled receptors that are targeted by opiates like morphine, heroin, and other opioid drugs. These receptors are primarily involved in pain modulation and reward, and they are found in the brain, spinal cord, and gastrointestinal tract. There are several types of opiate receptors, each with its own specific role and function:

1. **Mu (μ) Receptors**: These are the most well-known opiate receptors. They are responsible for the analgesic (pain-relieving) effects of opioids. Stimulation of mu receptors can also lead to euphoria, which is why opioids have a high potential for abuse. These receptors are also involved in respiratory depression, which is a common cause of death in opioid overdoses.
2. **Delta (δ) Receptors**: Delta receptors are less well understood than mu receptors. They also contribute to analgesia and are thought to play a role in mood regulation and emotional response. Some research suggests that delta receptors might modulate the effects of mu receptors and may have a role in developing opioid tolerance.
3. **Kappa (κ) Receptors**: Activation of kappa receptors generally produces analgesia, but without the euphoria associated with mu receptors. Instead, kappa receptor activation can lead to dysphoria (a state of unease or dissatisfaction) and hallucinations. These receptors are also thought to be involved in the regulation of stress and anxiety.
4. **Nociceptin/Orphanin FQ (NOP) Receptors**: Previously known as the opioid receptor-like (ORL1) receptor, NOP receptors are activated by the peptide nociceptin. They have complex effects, including roles in pain modulation, anxiety, and depression, but they do not respond to traditional opioid drugs like morphine.

Each of these receptor types has its own set of ligands (activating molecules), and they are distributed differently throughout the body. Research into these receptors has helped in the development of opioid drugs that target specific receptors to maximize pain relief while minimizing side effects like addiction and respiratory depression.

What is anatomy of neurotransmitter receptors?

The anatomy of neurotransmitter receptors, whether ionotropic or metabotropic, involves complex structures that enable them to bind neurotransmitters and initiate cellular responses.

1. **Ionotropic Receptors:**
   - **Subunit Structure**: Ionotropic receptors are typically composed of multiple subunits that come together to form an ion channel pore. These subunits are arranged symmetrically around the pore.
   - **Transmembrane Domains**: Each subunit usually has multiple transmembrane domains (regions of the protein that span the cell membrane).
   - **Ligand-Binding Site**: The part of the receptor where the neurotransmitter binds is usually located on the extracellular side of the neuron's membrane.

- **Ion Channel Pore**: When a neurotransmitter binds to the receptor, it causes a conformational change that opens the ion channel pore, allowing specific ions to pass through the cell membrane.
- **Regulatory Sites**: Many ionotropic receptors also have sites where other molecules, such as drugs or ions, can bind to modulate the receptor's activity.

2. **Metabotropic Receptors:**

- **Single Protein Structure**: Unlike ionotropic receptors, metabotropic receptors are typically composed of a single protein subunit.
- **Seven Transmembrane Domains**: These receptors characteristically have seven transmembrane domains, a structure typical of G protein-coupled receptors (GPCRs).
- **Extracellular Ligand-Binding Domain**: The neurotransmitter binding site is usually on the extracellular side of the receptor.
- **Intracellular G-Protein Binding Site**: The intracellular side of the receptor interacts with G proteins. When a neurotransmitter binds, it activates the G protein, triggering a signaling cascade within the cell.
- **Intracellular Signaling Pathways**: The activated G protein can influence various intracellular processes, such as the activation of enzymes, the opening or closing of ion channels, or changes in gene expression.

Both types of receptors are integral membrane proteins, meaning they are embedded within the cell membrane. Their specific structures enable them to perform their crucial roles in neurotransmission, translating the binding of neurotransmitters outside the cell into a functional response inside the cell. The intricate design of these receptors also makes them key targets for pharmacological intervention in numerous neurological and psychiatric conditions.

What are neurotransmitter receptors and their categories?

Neurotransmitter receptors are specialized proteins found on the surface of cells, particularly neurons in the brain and nervous system. Their main function is to receive and respond to chemical signals, specifically neurotransmitters, which are substances that transmit nerve impulses across synapses.

1. **Ionotropic Receptors:**

- **Structure**: These receptors are also known as ligand-gated ion channels. They are composed of several subunits that form a pore through the cell membrane.
- **Function**: When a neurotransmitter binds to these receptors, it causes a conformational change in the receptor, leading to the opening or closing of the ion channel. This allows specific ions (such as Na^+, K^+, Ca2+, or Cl^-) to flow across the membrane.
- **Response Time**: Ionotropic receptors typically produce a fast, direct, and short-lived response.
- **Examples**: Some well-known ionotropic receptors include the NMDA, AMPA, and kainate receptors for glutamate, the GABA_A receptor for GABA, and the nicotinic acetylcholine receptor.

2. **Metabotropic Receptors:**

- **Structure**: These receptors are part of the G protein-coupled receptor (GPCR) family. They do not form an ion channel themselves but are linked to one or more intracellular signaling pathways through G proteins.
- **Function**: When a neurotransmitter binds to a metabotropic receptor, it activates the associated G protein, which in turn can activate or inhibit various enzymes, ion channels, or other cellular components. This leads to a cascade of intracellular events.
- **Response Time**: Metabotropic receptors mediate slower, more prolonged responses compared to ionotropic receptors.
- **Examples**: Some examples include the muscarinic acetylcholine receptors, GABA_B receptors, and many of the receptors for serotonin and dopamine.

Both types of receptors are essential for neural communication and play distinct roles in the nervous system. Ionotropic receptors are typically involved in fast synaptic transmission, whereas metabotropic receptors modulate neuronal excitability and synaptic plasticity over longer periods. Their functions are not mutually exclusive, and they often work together to fine-tune neural responses and plasticity.

What are types of neurotransmitter receptors?

Neurotransmitter receptors are classified into various types based on different criteria such as the neurotransmitter they bind to, their mechanism of action, or their location. Here are some of the major types:

1. **Based on Neurotransmitter Type:**

- **Glutamate Receptors**: Including NMDA, AMPA, and Kainate receptors.

- **GABA Receptors**: Such as GABA_A and GABA_B receptors.
- **Acetylcholine Receptors**: Including Nicotinic and Muscarinic receptors.
- **Dopamine Receptors**: D1, D2, D3, D4, and D5 receptors.
- **Serotonin Receptors**: A large family including 5-HT1, 5-HT2, 5-HT3, etc.
- **Norepinephrine Receptors**: Including alpha and beta adrenergic receptors.

2. **Based on Mechanism of Action:**
   - **Ionotropic Receptors**: These are ligand-gated ion channels, which open to allow ions to pass through the membrane in response to the binding of a neurotransmitter.
   - **Metabotropic Receptors**: These are G protein-coupled receptors (GPCRs) that activate intracellular signaling cascades when a neurotransmitter binds.
3. **Based on Location:**
   - **Presynaptic Receptors**: Located on the presynaptic terminal of a neuron, these receptors can modulate the release of neurotransmitters.
   - **Postsynaptic Receptors**: Found on the postsynaptic membrane, they receive the neurotransmitter signal from the presynaptic neuron.
4. **Based on Ion Selectivity (specifically for ionotropic receptors):**
   - **Cationic Receptors**: Preferentially allow cations (like Na^+, K^+, $Ca2^+$) to pass through. Examples include nicotinic acetylcholine receptors and AMPA receptors.
   - **Anionic Receptors**: Allow anions (like Cl") to pass through. The GABA_A receptor is a key example.
5. **Based on Function:**
   - **Excitatory Receptors**: These receptors generally cause depolarization of the neuron, making it more likely to fire an action potential. Glutamate receptors are typically excitatory.
   - **Inhibitory Receptors**: These receptors often cause hyperpolarization of the neuron, making it less likely to fire. GABA and glycine receptors are typically inhibitory.

Each type of neurotransmitter receptor has a unique role in the nervous system, contributing to the complex process of neural communication and modulation. Their diversity is key to the wide range of physiological processes and behaviors mediated by the nervous system.

What is catecholamine?

Catecholamines are a group of neurotransmitters and hormones that play a vital role in the body's stress response and help regulate various physiological functions. The primary catecholamines are dopamine, norepinephrine (noradrenaline), and epinephrine (adrenaline). They share a common chemical structure that includes a catechol group (a benzene ring with two hydroxyl groups) and an amine group (nitrogen-containing group).

1. **Dopamine:**
   - **Function in the Brain**: Dopamine plays a crucial role in the brain's reward and pleasure systems, motor control, and regulation of mood. It is also involved in cognitive functions like attention and learning.
   - **Dopamine Pathways**: There are several major dopamine pathways in the brain, including the mesolimbic pathway (associated with reward and pleasure) and the nigrostriatal pathway (involved in movement control).
2. **Norepinephrine (Noradrenaline):**
   - **Role in the Nervous System**: Norepinephrine acts as a neurotransmitter in the brain and is involved in arousal, alertness, and attention. It is a part of the fight-or-flight response.
   - **Function as a Hormone**: Outside the brain, it acts as a hormone, increasing heart rate, releasing glucose from energy stores, and increasing blood flow to skeletal muscle.
3. **Epinephrine (Adrenaline):**
   - **Hormonal Role**: Primarily acts as a hormone released by the adrenal glands. It plays a significant role in the fight-or-flight response by increasing heart rate, dilating airways, and boosting energy availability.
   - **Neurotransmitter Function**: While its role as a neurotransmitter is less prominent, it does have some neurotransmitter activity, particularly in the brain.

Catecholamines are synthesized from the amino acid tyrosine and their levels can be influenced by both physiological factors and psychological states, especially stress. Imbalances in catecholamines have been associated with various medical conditions, including heart diseases, mood disorders, and Parkinson's disease. The understanding of catecholamines is crucial in both neuroscience and medicine, as they have profound effects on both the brain and the body.

What is an agonist?

An agonist is a chemical substance that binds to a specific receptor and activates the receptor to produce a biological response. In the context of neurotransmission and pharmacology, agonists are crucial because they can mimic or enhance the actions of naturally occurring substances in the body, such as hormones or neurotransmitters. Here is a more detailed explanation:

1. **Binding to Receptors**: Agonists bind to receptors on the surface of cells. These receptors are typically proteins and are specific to certain molecules.
2. **Activation of Receptors**: Upon binding to the receptor, the agonist induces a conformational change in the receptor, which activates it. This activation triggers a series of events inside the cell, leading to a physiological response.
3. **Types of Agonists**:
   - **Full Agonists**: These substances bind to and fully activate the receptor, resulting in a maximal biological response.
   - **Partial Agonists**: They bind to the same receptors as full agonists but produce a weaker biological response, even at full binding capacity.
   - **Inverse Agonists**: These substances bind to the same receptor as agonists but produce the opposite effect, reducing the activity of the receptor below its baseline level.
4. **Therapeutic Use**: Many drugs are agonists and are used therapeutically to mimic or enhance the action of endogenous substances. For example, morphine is an agonist at opioid receptors and is used for pain relief.
5. **Selective and Non-selective Agonists**: Some agonists are selective, bind only to specific types of receptors, while others are non-selective, and can bind to multiple types of receptors, potentially leading to a broader range of effects.
6. **Contrast with Antagonists**: Agonists are often contrasted with antagonists, which also bind to receptors but do not activate them. Instead, antagonists block or dampen the action of agonists or the endogenous substance that normally activates the receptor.

Agonists play a crucial role in both the functioning of the body's natural processes and in pharmacology, where they are used to treat a variety of conditions by mimicking or enhancing the actions of naturally occurring substances.

What is an antagonist for a receptor?

An antagonist is a type of chemical substance that binds to a receptor but does not activate it. Instead, it blocks or dampens the normal biological response that would be triggered by an agonist at that receptor. Antagonists are important in both understanding physiological processes and in the development of various drugs.

1. **Binding to Receptors**: Antagonists bind to the same receptors as agonists but have a different effect. While agonists activate receptors to produce a biological response, antagonists prevent this activation.
2. **Blocking Agonist Binding**: By binding to the receptor, antagonists can prevent agonists (such as neurotransmitters or hormones) from binding to that receptor. This can be done either by occupying the binding site (competitive antagonism) or by binding to a different part of the receptor and altering its shape (non-competitive antagonism).
3. **No Intrinsic Activity**: Unlike agonists, antagonists do not have intrinsic activity to stimulate a receptor. Their primary role is to prevent or diminish the receptor's activation by agonists.
4. **Therapeutic Uses**: Antagonists are widely used in medicine to inhibit the action of endogenous substances or other drugs. For example, antihistamines are antagonists of histamine receptors and are used to treat allergies, and beta-blockers are antagonists of beta-adrenergic receptors and are used to manage heart conditions.
5. **Selective and Non-selective Antagonists**: Some antagonists are highly selective, affecting only one type of receptor, while others are non-selective and can block multiple receptor types. Selectivity is an important factor in determining the therapeutic usefulness and side effect profile of a drug.
6. **Reversible and Irreversible Antagonists**: Some antagonists bind reversibly to receptors, meaning their effects are temporary and diminish when the drug is metabolized or excreted. Others bind irreversibly, leading to longer-lasting effects.

In summary, antagonists are crucial in modulating the activity of various physiological systems and are extensively used in pharmacotherapy to control or alter biological responses by blocking specific receptors. Their ability to inhibit the actions of agonists makes them valuable tools in both research and medicine.

What are examples of agonist and antagonist drugs?

Agonist and antagonist drugs are widely used in medicine for various therapeutic purposes.

Agonist Drugs

1. **Morphine**:
   - **Target**: Opioid receptors.
   - **Use**: Pain relief.
2. **Salbutamol (Albuterol in the US)**:
   - **Target**: Beta-2 adrenergic receptors.
   - **Use**: Treatment of asthma and COPD by relaxing bronchial muscles.
3. **Nicotine**:
   - **Target**: Nicotinic acetylcholine receptors.
   - **Use**: Smoking cessation aids (although nicotine is also the addictive component in tobacco).
4. **Ropinirole**:
   - **Target**: Dopamine receptors.
   - **Use**: Treatment of Parkinson's disease and restless legs syndrome.
5. **Clonidine**:
   - **Target**: Alpha-2 adrenergic receptors.
   - **Use**: Treatment of hypertension, ADHD, and certain pain conditions.

Antagonist Drugs

1. **Losartan**:
   - **Target**: Angiotensin II receptor.
   - **Use**: Treatment of high blood pressure and heart failure.
2. **Naloxone**:
   - **Target**: Opioid receptors.
   - **Use**: Counteracts opioid overdose by blocking the effects of opioids like morphine and heroin.
3. **Propranolol**:
   - **Target**: Beta adrenergic receptors.
   - **Use**: Treatment of hypertension, anxiety, and certain heart conditions.
4. **Omeprazole**:
   - **Target**: Proton pumps in stomach lining.
   - **Use**: Reduces stomach acid, treating conditions like GERD and peptic ulcers. It is technically a proton pump inhibitor, which is a type of antagonist.
5. **Diphenhydramine (Benadryl)**:
   - **Target**: Histamine H1 receptors.
   - **Use**: Treatment of allergic reactions.

These examples illustrate the wide range of applications for both agonist and antagonist drugs in managing various health conditions. Agonists are typically used to mimic or enhance the body's natural processes, while antagonists are employed to block or dampen these processes.

What is receptor agonist?

A receptor agonist is a type of chemical that binds to a specific receptor and activates it, triggering a biological response. In simpler terms, an agonist can be thought of as a "key" that fits into a "lock" (the receptor), and upon fitting, it turns the lock to initiate a specific action or series of actions within the cell.

1. **Activation of Receptors**: When an agonist binds to its receptor, it induces a conformational change in the receptor that activates it. This activation can initiate various cellular processes and physiological responses.
2. **Mimicking Natural Ligands**: Often, receptor agonists mimic the action of a naturally occurring substance in the body, such as a hormone or neurotransmitter. For example, morphine is an agonist of the opioid receptors in the nervous system, mimicking the effects of endogenous opioids like endorphins.
3. **Types of Agonists**:
   - **Full Agonists**: They bind to the receptor and produce a maximal response compared to the body's natural ligand.
   - **Partial Agonists**: These agonists bind to the receptor but produce a weaker, or partial, response compared to a full agonist.
   - **Inverse Agonists**: These bind to the same receptors as agonists but induce an opposite

effect, reducing the receptor's activity below the baseline level.

4. **Therapeutic Uses**: Agonists are widely used in medicine to treat various conditions. For instance, some asthma medications are agonists of the beta-2 adrenergic receptor, helping to relax and open the airways in the lungs.

5. **Selective and Non-selective Agonists**: Some agonists are highly selective, acting only on specific types of receptors, while others are non-selective and can affect multiple receptor types.

Receptor agonists play a critical role in pharmacology and medicine, as they can be used to modulate body functions in a controlled way, either by mimicking the natural activation of receptors or by enhancing their activity. Their understanding and development are key to creating effective treatments for a wide range of medical conditions.

Is amphetamine an agonist or antagonist?

Amphetamine is primarily an agonist, although its mode of action is somewhat different from typical receptor agonists. Instead of directly activating receptors by binding to them (as most agonists do), amphetamine works primarily by increasing the release of certain neurotransmitters in the brain, particularly dopamine and norepinephrine. How it works:

1. **Increasing Neurotransmitter Release**: Amphetamine enters neurons and triggers the release of dopamine and norepinephrine from their storage vesicles into the synaptic cleft (the space between neurons).

2. **Reuptake Inhibition**: It also blocks the reuptake of these neurotransmitters by inhibiting their transporters. This results in increased levels of dopamine and norepinephrine in the synaptic cleft.

3. **Reverse Transport**: Amphetamine can induce the transporters for dopamine and norepinephrine to work in reverse, further increasing the concentration of these neurotransmitters in the synaptic cleft.

4. **Indirect Agonist Action**: Due to these actions, amphetamine indirectly leads to the activation of dopamine and norepinephrine receptors by increasing the availability of their natural ligands (dopamine and norepinephrine). Thus, while it does not bind to and activate these receptors directly, it enhances their activation by increasing neurotransmitter levels.

Amphetamine's stimulant effects, including increased alertness, concentration, and energy, as well as its potential for abuse, are primarily due to its impact on dopamine levels. It is used therapeutically in certain medical conditions like attention deficit hyperactivity disorder (ADHD) and narcolepsy, where these stimulant effects can be beneficial when used under medical supervision.

What are the examples of serotonin antagonists?

Serotonin antagonists are drugs that block the action of serotonin, a key neurotransmitter, at various serotonin receptors. These antagonists have diverse therapeutic uses, ranging from the treatment of depression and anxiety to the management of migraine headaches.

1. **Cyproheptadine:**
   - **Target**: Primarily a 5-HT2 receptor antagonist.
   - **Uses**: Used for allergies, as an appetite stimulant, and sometimes in the treatment of serotonin syndrome.

2. **Ondansetron:**
   - **Target**: 5-HT3 receptor antagonist.
   - **Uses**: Commonly used to prevent nausea and vomiting, especially in chemotherapy and post-surgery patients.

3. **Methysergide:**
   - **Target**: 5-HT2 receptor antagonist.
   - **Uses**: Previously used for migraine prevention, though less common now due to potential side effects.

4. **Risperidone:**
   - **Target**: 5-HT2A receptor antagonist, among others.
   - **Uses**: Used as an antipsychotic for the treatment of schizophrenia, bipolar disorder, and irritability associated with autism.

5. **Ketanserin:**
   - **Target**: 5-HT2A receptor antagonist.
   - **Uses**: Mainly used in research; has been investigated for the treatment of hypertension and certain cardiovascular diseases.

6. **Trazodone:**
   - **Target**: 5-HT2A and 5-HT2C receptor antagonist.
   - **Uses**: Primarily used as an antidepressant and often prescribed for its sedating effects, helpful in treating insomnia.

7. **Mirtazapine:**
    - **Target**: 5-HT2 and 5-HT3 receptor antagonist.
    - **Uses**: An antidepressant that is also effective in treating anxiety and insomnia.

These serotonin antagonists work by blocking different subtypes of serotonin receptors, which can have varying effects on mood, gastrointestinal function, and other bodily processes. Their use in medicine is based on the specific action they have at these receptor sites, making them valuable in treating a range of conditions.

What is an example of an inverse agonist?

An inverse agonist is a type of drug that not only blocks a receptor but also causes the opposite action of a typical agonist. Unlike antagonists, which simply block a receptor's activity, inverse agonists decrease the receptor's activity below its baseline level.

Flumazenil:

- **Target**: GABA_A receptors.
- **Action**: Flumazenil is an inverse agonist at the benzodiazepine site of the GABA_A receptor. The GABA_A receptor is an ion channel that, when activated, typically causes inhibitory effects in the brain. Benzodiazepines are agonists at this site and enhance the inhibitory effects of GABA, leading to sedation and anxiolytic effects.
- **Uses**: Flumazenil is used to reverse the sedative effects of benzodiazepines, particularly in cases of overdose or when it is necessary to awaken a patient after surgery.

Flumazenil's inverse agonist properties make it effective in counteracting the actions of benzodiazepines, essentially reducing the activity of the GABA_A receptor below its normal level when benzodiazepines are present. This is a clear example of how inverse agonists can have significant clinical applications, particularly in situations where reversing the action of agonists is required.

What is the difference between alpha and beta-receptors?

Alpha and beta-receptors are types of adrenergic receptors, which are activated by the neurotransmitters norepinephrine (noradrenaline) and epinephrine (adrenaline). These receptors are part of the sympathetic nervous system and play key roles in the body's "fight or flight" response. The main differences between alpha and beta-receptors lie in their locations, functions, and the specific effects they mediate:

1. **Location:**
    - **Alpha Receptors**: Found primarily in the blood vessels, eyes, bladder, and smooth muscles. There are two main types, alpha-1 and alpha-2 receptors, each with different locations and functions.
    - **Beta-receptors**: Located in the heart, lungs, blood vessels, muscles, and fat cells. Beta-receptors are subdivided into beta-1, beta-2, and beta-3 receptors.
2. **Function and Effects:**
    - **Alpha-1 Receptors**: When activated, these receptors cause vasoconstriction (narrowing of blood vessels), increase blood pressure, and dilate the pupils.
    - **Alpha-2 Receptors**: They inhibit the release of norepinephrine and can lead to vasodilation and decreased blood pressure. They also play a role in platelet aggregation and smooth muscle contraction.
    - **Beta-1 Receptors**: Primarily found in the heart. Their activation increases heart rate and the force of heart contractions, and they are also involved in the release of renin in the kidneys, which regulates blood pressure.
    - **Beta-2 Receptors**: Located in the lungs, blood vessels, and muscles. Activation leads to bronchodilation (expansion of the bronchi), vasodilation, decreased uterine tone, and increased metabolism.
    - **Beta-3 Receptors**: Mainly found in fat cells and are involved in lipolysis (the breakdown of fats).
3. **Pharmacological Importance:**
    - **Alpha Blockers**: Drugs that block alpha-receptors are used to treat conditions like hypertension, benign prostatic hyperplasia, and Raynaud's disease.
    - **Beta Blockers**: These drugs are used to manage cardiac arrhythmias, angina, hypertension, and anxiety. They work by blocking beta-1 receptors in the heart.
4. **Response to Adrenaline and Noradrenaline:**
    - Both alpha and beta-receptors respond to adrenaline and noradrenaline, but their sensitivity to these neurotransmitters can vary. For example, noradrenaline is more effective at activating alpha-1 receptors, while adrenaline has a greater effect on beta-2 receptors.

Understanding the differences between alpha and beta-receptors is crucial in physiology and pharmacology, as they are targets for various drugs used to treat a range of cardiovascular, respiratory, and other conditions.

What is the biochemistry and pharmacology of receptors?

The biochemistry and pharmacology of receptors involve understanding how receptors, which are specialized protein molecules on the surface of cells, interact with various substances, including neurotransmitters, hormones, and drugs, to elicit specific physiological responses.

Biochemistry of Receptors

1. **Structure**: Receptors are typically made of protein or glycoprotein and are often embedded in the cell membrane. They have specific sites where ligands (molecules that bind to receptors) can attach.
2. **Types of Receptors**:
   - **Ionotropic Receptors**: These are ligand-gated ion channels that open or close in response to a ligand binding, allowing ions to pass through the membrane.
   - **Metabotropic Receptors**: These are usually G protein-coupled receptors (GPCRs) that, upon ligand binding, activate a G protein, which then initiates a series of intracellular signaling cascades.
   - **Intracellular Receptors**: Located inside the cell, these receptors typically bind to lipid-soluble ligands, such as steroid hormones, which can cross the cell membrane.
3. **Signal Transduction**: The process by which a receptor translates an extracellular signal (ligand binding) into an intracellular response, often involving secondary messengers.
4. **Regulation**: Receptor activity can be modulated through various mechanisms, such as desensitization, internalization, and down-regulation.

Pharmacology of Receptors

1. **Agonists and Antagonists:**
   - **Agonists** bind to receptors and mimic the action of the natural ligand, activating the receptor.
   - **Antagonists** bind to receptors but do not activate them; they block or dampen the action of agonists or the natural ligand.
2. **Drug-Receptor Interactions:** The study of how drugs interact with receptors, including binding affinity and efficacy.
3. **Therapeutic Application:** Receptors are targets for many drugs. Understanding receptor pharmacology is crucial for developing new therapeutic agents and predicting drug effects and side effects.
4. **Dose-Response Relationship:** The relationship between the concentration of a drug and the biological response it elicits, which is fundamental in determining the efficacy and potency of a drug.
5. **Selective and Non-selective Drug Actions:** Some drugs are selective and act only on specific types of receptors, while others are non-selective and can influence multiple receptor types.
6. **Receptor Polymorphisms:** Variations in receptor genes among individuals can affect responses to drugs, contributing to personalized medicine approaches.

The biochemistry and pharmacology of receptors are central to understanding how drugs work in the body and are fundamental in medical research, drug development, and clinical therapeutics. This knowledge helps in designing drugs that can effectively target specific receptors to treat various diseases while minimizing side effects.

What is dopamine system and their functions?

The dopamine system refers to the pathways in the brain in which the neurotransmitter dopamine plays a central role. Dopamine is a critical neurotransmitter involved in many functions, including motivation, reward, attention, mood, and movement. Understanding the dopamine system is essential in many areas of neuroscience and medicine, particularly in the context of psychiatric and neurological disorders.

Key Components of the Dopamine System

1. **Neurons Producing Dopamine:** Dopamine is synthesized by specific neurons located primarily in the midbrain. The synthesis of dopamine involves several steps, starting with the amino acid tyrosine.
2. **Major Dopamine Pathways:**
   - **Mesolimbic Pathway:** Originating in the ventral tegmental area (VTA) and projecting to the nucleus accumbens, this pathway is associated with reward, pleasure, and addiction. It plays a key role in the reinforcement of certain behaviors.

- **Mesocortical Pathway:** Also originating in the VTA but projecting to the prefrontal cortex, it is involved in cognition, decision-making, and motivation.
- **Nigrostriatal Pathway:** Running from the substantia nigra to the striatum, this pathway is primarily involved in motor control. Degeneration of neurons in this pathway is a hallmark of Parkinson's disease.
- **Tuber infundibular Pathway:** This pathway projects from the hypothalamus to the pituitary gland and is involved in the regulation of prolactin secretion.

Functions of Dopamine

1. **Motor Control:** Dopamine is essential for coordinating movement, and its deficiency in certain brain regions leads to motor symptoms as seen in Parkinson's disease.
2. **Reward and Pleasure:** Dopamine is often referred to as the "feel-good" neurotransmitter because it is crucial for the brain's reward system. It reinforces behaviors that are pleasurable and contributes to the feelings of enjoyment and reinforcement.
3. **Cognition and Executive Function:** Dopamine in the prefrontal cortex is important for cognitive functions like attention, problem-solving, and working memory.
4. **Mood Regulation:** Imbalances in dopamine levels have been associated with various psychiatric disorders, including schizophrenia, depression, and bipolar disorder.
5. **Hormonal Regulation:** The tuber infundibular pathway influences the release of hormones from the pituitary gland.

Clinical Relevance

1. **Parkinson's disease:** Caused by the loss of dopamine-producing neurons in the nigrostriatal pathway.
2. **Schizophrenia:** Linked to excessive dopamine activity in certain brain regions.
3. **Addiction:** Many addictive substances increase dopamine activity in the mesolimbic pathway, reinforcing addictive behaviors.
4. **Treatment of Disorders:** Various medications used in psychiatry and neurology target the dopamine system, either by mimicking dopamine, blocking its receptors, or influencing its production and degradation.

Understanding the dopamine system is crucial for comprehending not just normal brain function but also the pathophysiology of numerous neurological and psychiatric disorders, paving the way for effective treatments.

What is the mesolimbic dopaminergic pathway?

The mesolimbic dopaminergic pathway is one of the major dopamine pathways in the brain and is critically involved in the brain's reward system. It plays a central role in the sensation of pleasure, reward, and reinforcement, which are essential for motivation and desire. This pathway has been extensively studied for its role in addiction, as well as in certain psychiatric disorders.

Anatomy of the Mesolimbic Pathway

1. **Origin:** The pathway originates in the ventral tegmental area (VTA), located in the midbrain.
2. **Projection:** The neurons in the VTA send their axons to several areas in the brain, most notably to the nucleus accumbens, located in the ventral striatum.
3. **Neurotransmitter:** Dopamine is the primary neurotransmitter involved in this pathway. The dopaminergic neurons release dopamine at their synapses in the nucleus accumbens and other target areas.

Functions of the Mesolimbic Pathway

1. **Reward and Pleasure:** The pathway is activated by rewarding stimuli, including natural rewards like food and social interactions, as well as artificial rewards like drugs of abuse. Activation of this pathway is thought to produce the feelings of pleasure and reward.
2. **Reinforcement Learning:** It is crucial for reinforcement learning, where the brain learns to repeat actions that result in rewarding outcomes. This learning process is essential for motivation and goal-directed behavior.
3. **Addiction:** Because of its role in reward and reinforcement, the mesolimbic pathway is central to the process of addiction. Drugs of abuse such as opioids, cocaine, and amphetamines produce their addictive effects primarily by increasing dopamine levels in this pathway.

4. **Mood Regulation:** Dysfunction in the mesolimbic pathway has been implicated in mood disorders. For example, decreased activity in this pathway may contribute to anhedonia, the inability to feel pleasure, a symptom often seen in depression.

Clinical Relevance

1. **Addiction Treatment:** Understanding the mesolimbic pathway has been crucial in developing treatments for addiction. Therapies often focus on modifying dopamine activity to reduce the reinforcing effects of addictive substances.

2. **Psychiatric Disorders:** The pathway's role in mood and motivation makes it a target for studying psychiatric disorders like depression and schizophrenia. Antipsychotic drugs, for example, can act on dopamine receptors in this and other pathways.

3. **Reward Deficiency Syndrome:** This theoretical model suggests that dysfunctions in the mesolimbic pathway might underlie certain behavioral disorders characterized by impulsivity and poor decision-making.

In summary, the mesolimbic dopaminergic pathway is a fundamental component of the brain's reward system, influencing behavior by reinforcing rewarding experiences. Its study is vital for understanding and treating addiction and various psychiatric conditions.

How does dopamine affect mood?

Dopamine significantly influences mood and emotional well-being, acting as a key neurotransmitter in brain circuits that regulate these aspects of mental health. The relationship between dopamine and mood can be understood in the following contexts:

1. **Role in the Brain's Reward System:** Dopamine is centrally involved in the brain's reward circuit, particularly in the mesolimbic pathway, which includes areas like the ventral tegmental area (VTA) and the nucleus accumbens. This pathway is activated by rewarding and pleasurable experiences, and dopamine release in these areas is associated with feelings of enjoyment and reinforcement. The anticipation of pleasure, as well as the pleasure itself, often results in increased dopamine release, contributing to an elevated mood.

2. **Motivation and Drive:** Dopamine is also linked to motivation, drive, and goal-oriented behavior. Adequate dopamine levels are essential for feeling energized, enthusiastic, and motivated. Low dopamine levels can lead to a lack of motivation and interest, which are common symptoms in depressive disorders.

3. **Mood Disorders:** Imbalances in dopamine levels and function are implicated in various mood disorders. For example:

   - **Depression:** Patients with depression often exhibit altered dopamine function, particularly in areas of the brain involved in reward and motivation, which may contribute to the anhedonia (inability to feel pleasure) and lack of motivation commonly seen in depression.
   - **Bipolar Disorder:** In the manic phases of bipolar disorder, dopamine activity may be increased, contributing to heightened mood, energy, and a reduced need for sleep.

4. **Stress Response:** Dopamine plays a role in the body's response to stress. Chronic stress can affect dopamine signaling, which may lead to changes in mood and an increased risk of depression.

5. **Cognitive Effects and Mood:** Dopamine in the prefrontal cortex is crucial for cognitive processes like attention and executive function. Impairments in these functions can negatively affect mood and emotional regulation.

6. **Interaction with Other Neurotransmitters:** Dopamine's effect on mood is not isolated; it interacts with other neurotransmitter systems, such as serotonin and norepinephrine, which also play significant roles in mood regulation. The balance and interaction between these systems are crucial for emotional stability.

In summary, dopamine affects mood through its roles in the reward system, motivation, response to stress, and cognitive functions. Both excesses and deficiencies in dopamine can lead to mood disturbances, illustrating its complex and crucial role in mental health. Understanding these dynamics is important for the development of treatments for mood disorders and other mental health conditions.

What happens when dopamine is low in the brain?

Low dopamine levels in the brain can lead to a range of physical and psychological symptoms, as dopamine is a crucial neurotransmitter involved in many key functions. The effects of reduced dopamine can vary depending on which part of the brain is affected and to what extent. Here are some of the common consequences of low dopamine levels:

1. **Motor Control Difficulties:** Dopamine plays a vital role in coordinating movement. Low levels, particularly in the nigrostriatal pathway, are associated with motor symptoms like those seen in Parkinson's disease. This can include tremors, muscle stiffness, bradykinesia (slowness of movement), and balance problems.
2. **Reduced Motivation and Pleasure:** Dopamine is essential in the brain's reward system, particularly in the mesolimbic pathway. Low dopamine can lead to a decrease in motivation, enthusiasm, and the drive to pursue activities that are typically rewarding or enjoyable, a condition known as anhedonia.
3. **Cognitive Impairment:** Dopamine is important for cognitive processes like attention, learning, and memory. Reduced levels in certain areas of the brain, like the prefrontal cortex, can lead to difficulties with concentration, executive functioning, and decision-making.
4. **Mood Disorders:** Dopamine deficiencies are linked to certain mood disorders. Low levels can contribute to symptoms of depression, such as feelings of sadness, hopelessness, and a lack of interest in life.
5. **Fatigue and Lack of Energy:** People with low dopamine levels often experience chronic fatigue and a lack of energy. This is not just physical tiredness but can also manifest as mental fatigue.
6. **Sleep Problems:** Dopamine plays a role in regulating sleep-wake cycles. Low levels can lead to sleep disturbances or disorders.
7. **Increased Pain Sensitivity:** Dopamine has been implicated in pain processing. A deficiency may increase sensitivity to pain or exacerbate chronic pain conditions.
8. **Changes in Blood Flow and Heart Function:** Dopamine also affects blood vessels and heart function. Low levels can lead to changes in blood pressure and heart rate.

It is important to note that low dopamine levels can be due to various factors, including genetic predispositions, neurological diseases, lifestyle factors, and certain medications. Treatment and management of low dopamine levels depend on the underlying cause and can involve medication, lifestyle changes, and other therapeutic approaches. If symptoms suggestive of low dopamine are present, it is advisable to consult a healthcare professional for a proper diagnosis and treatment plan.

What happens when dopamine is high in the brain?

Elevated levels of dopamine in the brain can have various effects, many of which are linked to certain psychiatric conditions, behavioral changes, and physiological responses. It is important to note that the impact of high dopamine levels can vary depending on the specific brain regions involved and individual differences. Here are some common effects and associated conditions:

1. **Schizophrenia and Psychosis:** One of the leading theories in the pathophysiology of schizophrenia and other forms of psychosis suggests an over activity of dopamine, especially in the mesolimbic pathway. Symptoms such as hallucinations, delusions, and disordered thinking have been linked to excessive dopamine activity.
2. **Mania:** High levels of dopamine can contribute to symptoms of mania, as seen in bipolar disorder. These symptoms include increased energy, reduced need for sleep, grandiosity, increased risk-taking behaviors, and racing thoughts.
3. **Addiction and Reward-seeking Behavior:** Dopamine plays a key role in the reward system of the brain. Elevated levels, particularly in response to certain stimuli like drugs of abuse, can lead to addictive behaviors and a preoccupation with reward-seeking activities.
4. **Impulsivity and Compulsive Behaviors:** High dopamine levels can be associated with increased impulsivity, lack of inhibitory control, and compulsive behaviors. This is evident in conditions such as certain types of addiction and impulse control disorders.
5. **Increased Energy and Alertness:** Elevated dopamine can lead to heightened energy levels, alertness, and wakefulness, but in extreme cases, it might also contribute to agitation and restlessness.
6. **Improved Mood and Motivation:** In the right context and within certain limits, increased dopamine levels can enhance mood, motivation,

and focus. This is why dopamine-targeting medications are used in conditions like ADHD and certain forms of depression.

7. **Motor System Effects:** In the nigrostriatal pathway, unusually high levels of dopamine can lead to abnormal involuntary movements, as sometimes seen as a side effect of medication in Parkinson's disease (dopamine dysregulation syndrome).
8. **Physiological Effects:** Apart from neurological and psychiatric effects, elevated dopamine can influence bodily functions such as heart rate and blood pressure.

It is important to understand that the effects of high dopamine are not inherently positive or negative; they depend on the context, the specific brain pathways involved, and how much dopamine is increased. In clinical practice, managing dopamine levels is a delicate balance, particularly in the treatment of conditions like Parkinson's disease, schizophrenia, and various mood disorders. Excessively high levels of dopamine can be just as problematic as low levels, highlighting the importance of regulation in both pharmacological and non-pharmacological treatments.

What are symptoms of low Serotonin Levels?

Low serotonin levels in the brain can affect both mental and physical health, as serotonin is a key neurotransmitter involved in a wide range of physiological processes. The symptoms of low serotonin can vary and may affect mood, behavior, and several bodily functions. Common symptoms include:

1. **Mood Changes:** One of the most well-known effects of low serotonin is on mood. It can lead to feelings of depression, sadness, hopelessness, or irritability.
2. **Anxiety:** Low levels of serotonin are often associated with increased anxiety, including generalized anxiety disorder, panic attacks, and social anxiety.
3. **Sleep Problems:** Serotonin plays a role in regulating sleep cycles. Low serotonin can lead to insomnia, disrupted sleep, or unsatisfying sleep.
4. **Appetite Changes:** Serotonin impacts appetite control. Changes in serotonin levels can lead to altered eating patterns, often causing either increased appetite, particularly for carbohydrates, or a lack of appetite.
5. **Cognitive Impairments:** Individuals with low serotonin may experience difficulty concentrating, memory problems, and reduced cognitive function.
6. **Fatigue and Low Energy:** Even in the absence of sleep problems, low serotonin can lead to persistent fatigue, lethargy, and a lack of energy.
7. **Low Libido:** Serotonin is involved in sexual desire and function, and decreased levels can result in reduced libido.
8. **Physical Symptoms:** These can include headaches, nausea, and digestive issues, as serotonin also plays a role in regulating the gastrointestinal tract.
9. **Pain Sensitivity:** Increased sensitivity to pain or chronic pain conditions can be exacerbated by low serotonin levels.

It is important to note that these symptoms can be caused by a variety of factors, not just serotonin levels. Moreover, symptoms can vary greatly from person to person. If you suspect an imbalance in serotonin or are experiencing these symptoms, it is advisable to seek medical advice. A healthcare professional can provide a proper assessment and recommend appropriate treatment, which may include lifestyle changes, psychotherapy, and possibly medication like selective serotonin reuptake inhibitors (SSRIs).

What are symptoms of high serotonin levels in brain?

High levels of serotonin in the brain, a condition sometimes referred to as serotonin syndrome, can lead to a range of symptoms. Serotonin syndrome is typically caused by the use of certain medications or drug interactions that increase serotonin levels. It is important to recognize that while serotonin is generally beneficial and associated with positive mood and behavior, excessively high levels can be harmful. The symptoms of high serotonin levels can vary in severity and include:

1. **Mental Status Changes:** Agitation, restlessness, confusion, rapid mood swings, and hallucinations.
2. **Autonomic Dysfunction:** Symptoms include high blood pressure, rapid heart rate, fever, sweating, flushing, and dilated pupils.
3. **Neuromuscular Abnormalities:** This can include muscle rigidity, twitching, tremors, and coordination problems. In severe cases, there can be uncontrollable muscle spasms.
4. **Gastrointestinal Symptoms:** Nausea, vomiting, and diarrhea are common as serotonin has a significant role in regulating the digestive system.
5. **Headache:** A common symptom which can range from mild to severe.
6. **Shivering and Goosebumps:** Even in the absence of a cold environment.

7. **Insomnia:** Difficulty falling or staying asleep despite high levels of fatigue.

In severe cases, serotonin syndrome can be life-threatening and requires immediate medical attention. It is most commonly triggered by a combination of medications that increase serotonin levels, such as a mix of SSRIs (selective serotonin reuptake inhibitors) and MAOIs (monoamine oxidase inhibitors), or SSRIs and certain migraine medications like triptans.

If you suspect that you or someone else has serotonin syndrome, it is crucial to seek medical attention immediately. Treatment typically involves discontinuing the medications causing the syndrome, managing the symptoms, and in some cases, hospitalization for more severe reactions.

What is prostaglandin system and their types and roles?

The prostaglandin system refers to a group of physiologically active lipid compounds called prostaglandins, which are derived from fatty acids and have diverse hormone-like effects in animals. Prostaglandins are part of a larger family of substances known as eicosanoids. Here is an overview of the prostaglandin system:

Synthesis

- **Origin:** Prostaglandins are synthesized from arachidonic acid, a type of fatty acid.
- **Enzymes Involved:** The key enzymes in the synthesis of prostaglandins are cyclooxygenase (COX) enzymes, particularly COX-1 and COX-2. These enzymes convert arachidonic acid to prostaglandin H2, the precursor of other prostaglandins.

Types and Roles

- **Diverse Types:** There are various types of prostaglandins, each with distinct roles, including prostaglandin E2 (PGE2), prostaglandin D2 (PGD2), prostaglandin F2α (PGF2α), and others.
- **Regulation of Physiological Processes:** Prostaglandins are involved in regulating numerous physiological processes, including:
  - o **Inflammation and Pain:** They mediate inflammatory responses and are associated with the symptoms of pain and fever.
  - o **Gastric Mucosa Protection:** Prostaglandins help protect the lining of the stomach from damage by promoting mucus production and regulating acid secretion.
  - o **Blood Flow and Clotting:** Certain prostaglandins are involved in vasodilation or vasoconstriction and play roles in blood clotting processes.
  - o **Reproductive System Functions:** Prostaglandins are involved in processes like ovulation, uterine contraction, and regulation of menstrual cycle.

Clinical Significance

- **Therapeutic Targets:** Many anti-inflammatory drugs, like nonsteroidal anti-inflammatory drugs (NSAIDs), target the COX enzymes to reduce the production of prostaglandins, thereby alleviating pain and inflammation.
- **Role in Diseases:** Abnormal prostaglandin activity is implicated in various diseases, including cardiovascular diseases, certain types of cancer, and arthritis.
- **Reproductive Health:** Prostaglandins are used in certain medications for inducing labor and for the treatment of ulcers.

Regulation

- **Complex Regulation:** The production and action of prostaglandins are tightly regulated by the body, as they can have potent and sometimes opposing effects depending on their type and the context of their release.

Research and Therapeutics

- Ongoing research is focused on understanding the diverse roles of prostaglandins and their potential as therapeutic targets in various diseases, beyond just their role in pain and inflammation.

The prostaglandin system is a critical component of many biological processes and understanding it is essential for the development of various pharmacological treatments. Due to their wide-ranging effects, prostaglandins are a focus of considerable medical research.

What do endocannabinoid receptors do?

Endocannabinoid receptors are part of the endocannabinoid system, a complex and widespread network in the body that plays a key role in regulating various physiological processes. This system includes the endocannabinoids (cannabinoid-like substances produced by the body), their receptors, and the enzymes involved in their synthesis and degradation. The primary endocannabinoid receptors are the CB1 and CB2 receptors.

CB1 Receptors

- **Location:** Predominantly found in the brain and central nervous system, but also present in some peripheral tissues and organs.
- **Functions:**
    - o **Neurological Effects:** Regulate neurotransmitter release, influencing processes like pain sensation, memory, appetite, and mood.
    - o **Motor Control:** Involved in the regulation of movement, and their alteration is linked to various motor disorders.
    - o **Thermoregulation:** Play a role in regulating body temperature.

CB2 Receptors

- **Location:** Mainly found in the peripheral tissues, especially in immune cells.
- **Functions:**
    - o **Immune System Regulation:** Modulate immune cell function, playing a significant role in inflammation and autoimmune diseases.
    - o **Pain Management:** Involved in the reduction of pain and inflammation in peripheral tissues.

General Functions of Endocannabinoid Receptors

- **Homeostasis:** The endocannabinoid system helps maintain homeostasis by regulating several bodily functions, including pain, mood, appetite, memory, and sleep.
- **Stress Response:** It plays a role in modulating the body's response to stress and anxiety.
- **Digestive System:** Influences appetite control and gastrointestinal motility.

Clinical Implications

- **Therapeutic Targets:** The endocannabinoid system is a target for the treatment of various conditions, including chronic pain, inflammation, epilepsy, and certain psychiatric disorders.
- **Cannabis and Pharmaceuticals:** Compounds derived from cannabis, like THC and CBD, exert their effects primarily by interacting with endocannabinoid receptors. Synthetic cannabinoids and other drugs that target these receptors are being developed for medical use.

Understanding the functions of endocannabinoid receptors is crucial for exploring therapeutic strategies for a range of diseases and conditions. The system's wide-reaching effects on many aspects of human physiology make it an area of significant interest in medical research.

Does the human body produce cannabinoids?

Yes, the human body does produce cannabinoids. These naturally occurring compounds, known as endo-cannabinoids, are part of the body's endocannabinoid system (ECS). The ECS is a complex cell-signaling system identified in the early 1990s by researchers exploring THC, a well-known cannabinoid found in marijuana. Endocannabinoids are similar to the cannabinoids found in cannabis but are produced by the human body. Here is a brief overview:

Key Endocannabinoids

The two most studied endocannabinoids are:

1. **Anandamide (AEA):** Often referred to as the "bliss molecule," anandamide plays a role in regulating mood, memory, appetite, pain, and other functions.
2. **2-Arachidonoylglycerol (2-AG):** This endocannabinoid is involved in the regulation of appetite, immune system functions, and pain management.

Functions of Endocannabinoids

- **Maintaining Homeostasis:** Endocannabinoids help maintain biological balance in response to environmental changes. They are involved in a variety of physiological processes including pain sensation, mood regulation, memory, and appetite.
- **Neurotransmitter Regulation:** They modulate the release of neurotransmitters, affecting how messages are sent, received, and processed by the brain and body.
- **Immune System Regulation:** Endocannabinoids play a role in modulating the immune system, influencing inflammation and immune cell activity.

Endocannabinoid System Components

Apart from endocannabinoids, the ECS includes:

- **Cannabinoid Receptors:** Primarily CB1 and CB2 receptors, which are found throughout the body. Endocannabinoids bind to these receptors to signal the ECS to take action.
- **Enzymes:** Enzymes that synthesize and degrade endocannabinoids, like fatty acid amide hydrolase (FAAH) which breaks down anandamide, and MAGL (monoacylglycerol lipase) which breaks down 2-AG.

Clinical Implications

- **Therapeutic Potential:** The ECS is a target for the treatment of various conditions, such as chronic pain, inflammation, epilepsy, and mood disorders. Understanding how the ECS works and how compounds from cannabis (like THC and CBD) interact with this system is crucial for developing new therapies.

In summary, the human body produces its own cannabinoids (endocannabinoids), which play a vital role in regulating a wide range of physiological and cognitive processes. The study of the endocannabinoid system continues to reveal its significance in health and disease, opening up possibilities for novel therapeutic approaches.

How do opioids activate receptors?

Opioids activate receptors by binding to specific opioid receptors in the brain, spinal cord, and other parts of the body. These receptors are part of a larger family known as G protein-coupled receptors (GPCRs). The interaction of opioids with these receptors triggers a cascade of biochemical reactions that lead to the effects associated with opioid use, such as pain relief, sedation, and euphoria.

Types of Opioid Receptors

There are three main types of opioid receptors: mu (μ), delta (δ), and kappa (κ). Each has different functions:

- Mu Receptors: Primarily responsible for opioid-induced analgesia (pain relief) and euphoria. They are also involved in respiratory depression, physical dependence, and constipation.
- Delta Receptors: Their role is less understood, but they are thought to contribute to analgesic effects and also play a role in mood regulation.
- Kappa Receptors: Primarily associated with spinal analgesia and sedation. Activation of kappa receptors can also produce dysphoria and hallucinations.

Activation Mechanism

1. **Binding to Receptors:** When opioids enter the body, they bind to opioid receptors. Different opioids have varying affinities for these receptors. For example, morphine has a high affinity for mu receptors.
2. **Receptor Activation:** Upon binding, opioids induce a conformational change in the receptor. This activates the G protein that is coupled to the receptor.
3. **Signal Transduction:** The activated G protein inhibits adenylate cyclase activity, leading to a decrease in the production of cAMP (cyclic adenosine monophosphate), a critical secondary messenger in cells.
4. **Neuronal Effects:** This leads to the opening of potassium channels and the closing of calcium channels in neurons. As a result, there is hyperpolarization of the neuron (making it less likely to fire) and a reduction in the release of neurotransmitters.
5. **Inhibition of Pain Signals:** In the context of pain management, this process diminishes the transmission of pain signals through the spinal cord to the brain and alters the brain's perception of pain, providing relief.
6. **Other Effects:** Besides analgesia, the activation of opioid receptors can result in a range of effects, including euphoria, sedation, reduced gastrointestinal motility, and respiratory depression.

Therapeutic and Adverse Effects

- **Pain Management:** Opioids are effective analgesics and are used to treat moderate to severe pain.
- **Risks:** However, they also have significant risks, including the development of tolerance, physical dependence, addiction, and potentially life-threatening respiratory depression.

Understanding how opioids activate receptors has been crucial in developing pain management strategies and addressing the challenges of opioid misuse and dependence. It has also spurred research into creating safer pain-relief medications that target opioid receptors with fewer adverse effects.

What is the function of serotonin hormone?

Serotonin, commonly known as a neurotransmitter in the brain, also functions as a hormone in other parts of the body. It is a versatile molecule with a variety of roles:

In the Brain

1. **Mood Regulation:** Serotonin is best known for its role in regulating mood. Adequate levels are associated with feelings of happiness and well-being. It is a key target for many antidepressant drugs.
2. **Anxiety and Stress Response:** Serotonin helps to regulate anxiety and the body's response to stress.

3. **Sleep Regulation:** It plays a role in sleep cycles by influencing the body's internal clock and sleep-wake cycles, largely through its conversion to melatonin, a hormone that regulates sleep.

In the Body

1. **Gastrointestinal Function:** Serotonin is involved in controlling the movement of the digestive system. It helps regulate bowel function and movements.
2. **Blood Clotting:** Released by platelets in the blood, serotonin aids in the constriction of blood vessels and formation of blood clots after a vascular injury.
3. **Bone Density:** Serotonin has a role in bone metabolism. High levels of serotonin in the bones can lead to decreased bone density.
4. **Sexual Function:** It plays a complex role in sexual function, and changes in serotonin levels can affect libido and sexual performance.
5. **Heart and Lung Function:** Serotonin can affect cardiovascular and pulmonary systems, influencing blood pressure and respiratory function.

As a Hormone

As a hormone, serotonin acts as a signaling molecule, sending messages between different parts of the body. It is synthesized from the amino acid tryptophan and is found in various body tissues, including the brain, digestive system, and blood platelets.

Overall Function

Overall, serotonin's function is multifaceted, affecting mood, digestion, sleep, bone health, and cardiovascular and pulmonary systems. Due to its wide range of actions, imbalances in serotonin levels can contribute to numerous physical and mental health conditions, making it a significant focus in medical research and pharmacology.

What is the difference between adrenaline and noradrenaline?

Adrenaline (also known as epinephrine) and noradrenaline (norepinephrine) are closely related hormones and neurotransmitters that play significant roles in the body's stress response, but they have different functions and effects.

1. **Chemical Structure:** Although similar, adrenaline and noradrenaline have slightly different chemical structures. This difference in structure influences how they interact with different receptors in the body.
2. **Produced By:** Adrenaline is primarily produced in the adrenal glands, especially in the medulla (the inner part of the adrenal glands). Noradrenaline is produced both in the adrenal glands and in the nerve endings of the sympathetic nervous system.
3. **Roles in the Body:**
   - Adrenaline is more involved in the body's "fight-or-flight" response. It is released in response to stress and increases heart rate, expands air passages of the lungs, enlarges the pupil in the eye, redistributes blood to muscles, and alters the body's metabolism to maximize blood glucose levels (primarily for the brain).
   - Noradrenaline acts primarily as a neurotransmitter in the nervous system and also plays a role in the fight-or-flight response. It is more involved in the body's reaction to stress, increasing blood pressure by causing blood vessels to constrict. It also increases mental alertness and readiness for action.
4. **Receptors:** They interact with different receptors in the body. Adrenaline interacts with alpha and beta-receptors relatively equally, while noradrenaline has a greater affinity for alpha receptors. This difference in receptor interaction leads to different physiological effects.
5. **Overall Effect:** The overall effect of adrenaline is to prepare the body for immediate physical exertion, whereas noradrenaline has a more specific role in increasing blood pressure and heart rate, leading to increased alertness and preparedness.

Both hormones are critical in stress responses, adrenaline is more focused on preparing the body for immediate physical activity, and noradrenaline is more involved in maintaining alertness and increasing blood pressure.

What is norepinephrine responsible for?

Norepinephrine, also known as noradrenaline, is a hormone and neurotransmitter that plays a key role in the body's stress response and general functioning of the nervous system. Here are some of the primary functions and responsibilities of norepinephrine:

1. **Fight-or-Flight Response:** Norepinephrine is crucial in the body's fight-or-flight response, a physiological reaction to perceived harmful events,

attacks, or threats to survival. It prepares the body for action, increasing alertness and focus.

2. **Increases Blood Pressure and Heart Rate:** As a hormone, norepinephrine increases blood pressure by causing blood vessels to constrict. This action helps to redirect blood flow to areas where it is needed during stress, such as muscles and vital organs. It also increases heart rate and the force of heart contractions, which aids in the rapid delivery of blood throughout the body.

3. **Mental Focus and Alertness:** In the brain, as a neurotransmitter, norepinephrine is involved in regulating attention, focus, and alertness. It helps in maintaining a state of wakefulness and can enhance cognitive abilities like concentration and memory, particularly in stressful or demanding situations.

4. **Mood Regulation:** Norepinephrine has a role in regulating mood. Imbalances in norepinephrine levels have been linked to mood disorders such as depression and anxiety. Some antidepressant medications work by altering the levels of norepinephrine in the brain.

5. **Regulation of Blood Sugar Levels:** It helps regulate blood sugar levels by stimulating the breakdown of stored glucose (glycogen) in the liver, increasing blood glucose levels, and providing energy during stress responses.

6. **Response to Cold:** Norepinephrine is also involved in the body's response to cold. It triggers the constriction of blood vessels in the skin, reducing blood flow to the skin, and helps in generating heat.

7. **Pain Modulation:** In the spinal cord, norepinephrine can modulate pain signals, playing a role in the perception of pain and potentially reducing pain sensitivity under certain conditions.

Overall, norepinephrine is a critical neurotransmitter and hormone that helps the body respond to stress, maintain alertness and focus, regulate mood, and perform various other important physiological functions. Its balance and regulation are essential for both physical and mental well-being.

What is the difference between a Neuro-transmitters and a hormone?

Neurotransmitters and hormones are both chemical messengers used in the human body, but they differ in their mechanisms of action, the areas where they exert their effects, and how they are released and transported.

1. **Origin and Secretion:**
   - Neurotransmitters are produced by nerve cells (neurons) and are released at the nerve endings in response to an electrical impulse. They are secreted into the synaptic cleft (a very small gap between neurons) and act locally.
   - Hormones are secreted by glands (such as the pituitary, thyroid, or adrenal glands) and released directly into the bloodstream. They are not restricted to local action but can exert effects on distant organs and tissues that have the appropriate receptors.

2. **Mode of Transport:**
   - Neurotransmitters travel very short distances across the synapse to act on adjacent neurons, muscle cells, or gland cells.
   - Hormones are carried by the circulatory system throughout the entire body, reaching various distant targets.

3. **Speed of Action:**
   - Neurotransmitters usually act quickly, within milliseconds, because they do not have far to travel and the response is often immediate (e.g., muscle contraction or change in neuron firing).
   - Hormones generally have slower effects, ranging from a few seconds to several hours or even days, as they need time to be transported through the bloodstream and often initiate longer-term processes (like growth or metabolism regulation).

4. **Types of Effects:**
   - Neurotransmitters typically have localized and specific effects, such as muscle contraction, heart rate modulation, or mood regulation in a particular part of the brain.
   - Hormones can have widespread and diverse effects on many different bodily functions, including growth, metabolism, sexual function, reproduction, and mood.

5. **Feedback Mechanisms:**
   - Neurotransmitter levels and activity are primarily regulated by reuptake mechanisms (where the neurotransmitter is reabsorbed by the

neuron that released it) and enzymatic degradation.

- Hormone levels are often regulated by complex feedback systems, usually involving the brain and other endocrine glands (e.g., the hypothalamic-pituitary axis).

6. **Examples:**

- Neurotransmitters include substances like dopamine, serotonin, norepinephrine, and glutamate.
- Hormones include insulin, cortisol, thyroid hormones, and estrogen.

Both neurotransmitters and hormones are essential for communication within the body, they differ significantly in how they are produced, transmitted, the speed of their action, and the range of effects they exert.

What is pathology of receptors?

The term "pathology of receptors" refers to the study of abnormalities or dysfunctions in cell receptors that can lead to diseases or contribute to their progression. Receptors are proteins located on the surface of cells or within cells, and they play a crucial role in cell signaling by binding to specific molecules like hormones, neurotransmitters, or drugs, and triggering a response in the cell. When these receptors malfunction due to various reasons, it can lead to a wide range of pathologies.

Several aspects fall under the umbrella of receptor pathology:

1. **Genetic Mutations:** Mutations in the genes encoding receptors can alter their structure and function. This can lead to a variety of genetic disorders. For example, mutations in hormone receptors can lead to endocrine disorders.

2. **Autoimmune Disorders:** Some autoimmune diseases are characterized by the production of antibodies that mistakenly target the body's own receptors. For instance, in Graves' disease, antibodies bind to and stimulate the thyroid-stimulating hormone receptor, leading to overproduction of thyroid hormones.

3. **Downregulation and Upregulation:** Chronic exposure to high levels of a ligand (like a hormone or neurotransmitter) can lead to receptor downregulation, where the number of receptors on the cell surface decreases. This can diminish the cell's response to the ligand. Conversely, decreased ligand availability can lead to upregulation, increasing receptor numbers and potentially making cells overly sensitive.

4. **Desensitization:** Receptors can become less responsive or desensitized after prolonged exposure to a ligand. This is commonly seen with drugs, such as the decreased effectiveness of narcotics with prolonged use due to opioid receptor desensitization.

5. **Altered Receptor Signaling Pathways:** Changes in the internal signaling pathways activated by receptors can lead to diseases. This may be due to mutations in the receptor itself or in the proteins involved in the signaling pathway.

6. **Receptor Blockage:** Drugs or endogenous molecules can block receptors, preventing them from binding to their natural ligands. This can be therapeutic (as with many drugs) or pathological (as with certain toxins).

7. **G-protein Coupled Receptor (GPCR) Disorders:** Many receptors are GPCRs, and abnormalities in these receptors or their associated G-proteins can lead to various diseases, including cancer, heart disease, and psychiatric disorders.

8. **Receptor Overexpression:** Overexpression of certain receptors can lead to enhanced cell activity and is often seen in cancers. For example, overexpression of the HER2 receptor is associated with certain types of breast cancer.

The pathology of receptors is a significant area of study in medical research, as it has implications for understanding disease mechanisms and developing targeted treatments, such as drugs that specifically modulate receptor activity.

What is a Neurotransmitter?

A neurotransmitter is a type of chemical messenger that plays a key role in transmitting signals across a chemical synapse, such as between a neuron and another neuron, a muscle cell, or a gland cell. These substances are essential for the proper functioning of the nervous system and influence a wide range of both physical and psychological functions.

1. **Production and Storage:** Neurotransmitters are synthesized in the neuron, often in the nerve terminal. They are stored in small vesicles (sac-like structures) at the end of neurons.

2. **Release Mechanism:** When an electrical signal (nerve impulse or action potential) reaches the

end of a neuron, it triggers the release of neurotransmitters into the synaptic cleft, which is the small gap between neurons.

3. **Receptor Binding:** Once released, neurotransmitters travel across the synaptic cleft and bind to specific receptors on the surface of the adjacent neuron (or muscle or gland cell). This binding can either stimulate or inhibit the function of the receiving cell.

4. **Types of Action:**

   - **Excitatory Neurotransmitters:** These neurotransmitters increase the likelihood that the neuron will fire an action potential. An example is glutamate, which is the most common excitatory neurotransmitter in the brain.
   - **Inhibitory Neurotransmitters:** These reduce the likelihood of the neuron firing an action potential. Gamma-aminobutyric acid (GABA) is a well-known inhibitory neurotransmitter in the brain.
   - **Modulatory Neurotransmitters:** Some neurotransmitters can modify the effects of other neurotransmitters. They often have a more widespread and less direct effect on neuronal activity.

5. **Removal from Synapse:** After their release and action, neurotransmitters are quickly removed from the synaptic cleft to stop their action. This can happen through reuptake into the neuron, enzymatic degradation, or diffusion away from the synapse.

6. **Examples and Functions:** Common neurotransmitters include:

   - **Dopamine:** Involved in reward, motivation, and motor control.
   - **Serotonin:** Plays a role in mood regulation, appetite, and sleep.
   - **Norepinephrine (Noradrenaline):** Involved in alertness, arousal, and the stress response.
   - **Acetylcholine:** Important for muscle contraction and also involved in learning and memory.

7. **Role in Diseases and Disorders:** Imbalances or dysfunctions in neurotransmitter systems can lead to various neurological and psychiatric disorders. For example, a deficiency in dopamine is associated with Parkinson's disease, while imbalances in serotonin and norepinephrine are linked to depression.

In summary, neurotransmitters are fundamental in the communication between neurons and between neurons and other types of cells. They are integral to the functioning of the nervous system, affecting everything from heart rate and digestion to mood and perception.

What are neuromodulators?

Neuromodulators are a type of chemical messenger in the nervous system that alter the way neurons communicate with each other. They differ from neurotransmitters in several key ways, particularly in their mode of action and the scope of their effects.

1. **Broad Impact on Neuronal Networks:** Unlike neurotransmitters, which typically have immediate and localized effects, neuromodulators can affect large numbers of neurons at once. They are often released into wider areas of the brain and can influence many neurons simultaneously.

2. **Modulation of Neural Activity:** Neuromodulators don't directly cause neurons to fire or inhibit their firing, as neurotransmitters do. Instead, they modify the strength or effectiveness of synaptic transmission. This means they can adjust or regulate the way neurons respond to neurotransmitters.

3. **Longer-lasting Effects:** The actions of neuromodulators are generally slower and more prolonged than those of neurotransmitters. While neurotransmitters are involved in rapid, millisecond-by-millisecond transmission of signals, neuromodulators can alter neural circuitry over longer periods, ranging from seconds to hours.

4. **Examples of Neuromodulators:**

   - **Dopamine:** Involved in reward, motivation, and motor control, dopamine can modulate the activity of large groups of neurons in the brain.
   - **Serotonin:** Affects mood, appetite, and sleep, and plays a role in regulating the overall excitability of brain regions.
   - **Norepinephrine (Noradrenaline):** Influences attention, arousal, and the stress response, modulating the sensitivity of neurons to input.
   - **Acetylcholine:** Apart from being a neurotransmitter, it also acts as a neuromodulator in the central nervous system, affecting processes like learning and memory.

5. **Mechanism of Action:** Neuromodulators typically act through G-protein coupled receptors (GPCRs), which can initiate a series of intracellular events leading to long-term changes in cell function.

6. **Role in Plasticity and Learning:** Neuromodulators are crucial for synaptic plasticity—the ability of synapses to strengthen or weaken over time, which is essential for learning and memory.

7. **Influence on Behavior and Emotion:** By modulating the activity of neural circuits, neuromodulators play a significant role in shaping behavior, emotional states, and cognitive processes.

8. **Clinical Importance:** Imbalances or disruptions in neuromodulatory systems are implicated in various psychiatric and neurological disorders, making them targets for therapeutic interventions.

Neuromodulators play a vital role in the nervous system by fine-tuning the activity of neural networks, influencing a wide range of physiological and psychological processes, and contributing to the brain's ability to adapt and learn.

What is the difference between a neurotransmitter and a neuromodulator?

Neurotransmitters and neuromodulators are both chemical messengers used in the nervous system, but they differ in their mechanisms of action, the scope of their effects, and how they influence neural activity.

1. **Mode of Action:**
   - Neurotransmitters are released from neurons and quickly bind to receptors on adjacent neurons (or muscle/gland cells), typically causing immediate, short-lived, and localized effects. They directly induce or inhibit action potentials in the target cells.
   - Neuromodulators, on the other hand, act more broadly and indirectly. They do not necessarily cause immediate changes in the target neuron's membrane potential but rather modify the neuron's response to neurotransmitters. This modulation can enhance or diminish the effectiveness of synaptic transmission.

2. **Area of Influence:**
   - Neurotransmitters generally act on very specific sites, namely the synapse between two neurons. Their effects are confined to the immediate area of release.
   - Neuromodulators often have a more widespread effect. They can be released into the neuronal environment and affect multiple neurons within an area, modulating the activity of entire neural circuits or brain regions.

3. **Duration of Effect:**
   - Neurotransmitters typically produce rapid, short-term responses, acting within milliseconds.
   - Neuromodulators usually induce slower, longer-lasting effects, often persisting for seconds to minutes or even longer. Their influence extends over a broader timescale.

4. **Examples:**
   - Neurotransmitters include substances like glutamate (excitatory), GABA (inhibitory), acetylcholine, dopamine, serotonin, and norepinephrine.
   - Some chemicals, like dopamine and serotonin, can act as both neurotransmitters and neuromodulators, depending on where and how they are released and the types of receptors they bind to.

5. **Role in Neural Processing:**
   - Neurotransmitters are primarily involved in transmitting signals and information across synapses, crucial for immediate responses and reflexes.
   - Neuromodulators play a role in altering the overall 'state' or 'tone' of neural circuits, thereby influencing processes like arousal, attention, learning, and mood over longer periods.

6. **Receptor Interaction:**
   - Neurotransmitters typically bind to ionotropic receptors (which directly control ion channels) or metabotropic receptors (which work through second messenger systems) for fast-acting effects.
   - Neuromodulators often bind to metabotropic receptors, which can initiate a cascade of intracellular events, leading to more gradual and prolonged changes in neural function.

In essence, while neurotransmitters are involved in the rapid and specific transmission of signals across synapses, neuromodulators regulate and modify the overall patterns of neural activity and synaptic strength, contributing to the fine-tuning of neural networks and brain functions.

What are some examples of neuromodulators?

Neuromodulators are chemicals in the nervous system that modify the way neurons communicate with each other. They play a crucial role in regulating a wide array of physiological functions and behaviors. Some well-known examples of neuromodulators include:

1. **Dopamine:** Perhaps one of the most famous neuromodulators, dopamine is involved in reward, motivation, and motor control. It plays a critical role in the brain's reward system and is associated with feelings of pleasure and reinforcement. Dopamine also has significant roles in motor control and is implicated in disorders such as Parkinson's disease.

2. **Serotonin:** This neuromodulator is involved in regulating mood, appetite, and sleep. Serotonin is also important for cognitive functions including memory and learning. Imbalances in serotonin levels are linked to depression, anxiety, and other mood disorders.

3. **Norepinephrine (Noradrenaline):** Norepinephrine acts as both a hormone and a neuromodulator. It is involved in the body's stress response, increasing alertness and arousal, and preparing the body for action. It also plays a role in attention and responding to new or challenging situations.

4. **Acetylcholine:** Acetylcholine is involved in muscle activation as a neurotransmitter, but it also acts as a neuromodulator in the central nervous system. It plays a key role in arousal, attention, memory, and motivation.

5. **Endorphins:** These are peptides that act as neuromodulators in the brain. Endorphins are involved in pain relief and are also associated with feelings of pleasure. They are often referred to as natural painkillers of the body.

6. **GABA (Gamma-Aminobutyric Acid):** GABA is the main inhibitory neurotransmitter in the brain, but it also acts as a neuromodulator. It helps regulate neuronal excitability throughout the nervous system and is important in reducing anxiety and promoting relaxation.

7. **Glutamate:** While primarily known as the main excitatory neurotransmitter in the brain, glutamate also functions as a neuromodulator. It plays a key role in synaptic plasticity, the ability of synapses to strengthen or weaken over time, which is crucial for learning and memory.

8. **Substance P:** This peptide is involved in the pain pathway as a neuromodulator. It is released in response to stress or injury and plays a role in transmitting pain signals to the brain.

Each of these neuromodulators influences various neural circuits and processes, thereby playing a significant role in shaping behavior, mood, cognitive functions, and physiological responses. Their balance and interaction are crucial for the normal functioning of the nervous system.

Why are receptors and neurotransmitters so important for psychiatry?

Receptors and neurotransmitters are fundamental to psychiatry because they are at the heart of how the brain functions, particularly in relation to mood, thought processes, and behavior—all of which are central to mental health and psychiatric disorders. Understanding their roles and interactions is crucial for several key reasons:

1. **Neural Communication:** Neurotransmitters are the chemicals that neurons use to communicate with each other. They are released by one neuron and bind to receptors on another neuron, influencing whether that neuron will become more or less active. This process of neural communication underlies all mental processes, from basic sensory perception to complex emotions and thoughts.

2. **Regulation of Mood and Thought:** Specific neurotransmitters are associated with different aspects of mood and cognitive function. For example, serotonin is closely linked to mood regulation and is implicated in the pathology of depression and anxiety disorders. Dopamine plays a key role in reward, motivation, and focus, and is involved in conditions such as schizophrenia and ADHD.

3. **Target for Medications:** Many psychiatric medications work by altering the levels of neurotransmitters in the brain or by modifying their interaction with receptors. Antidepressants, for instance, often target the serotonin system (e.g., SSRIs - Selective Serotonin Reuptake Inhibitors), while antipsychotics primarily affect dopamine pathways.

4. **Understanding Psychiatric Disorders:** Many mental health disorders are believed to involve imbalances or dysfunctions in neurotransmitter systems. For instance, depression has been linked with reduced levels of serotonin and

norepinephrine, while schizophrenia involves dysregulation in dopamine transmission.

5. **Personalized Medicine:** Knowledge about specific neurotransmitter and receptor dysfunctions in individuals can lead to more personalized and effective treatment plans. As psychiatric research advances, it is becoming possible to tailor treatments based on individual neurochemical profiles.
6. **Development of New Therapies:** Understanding how neurotransmitters and receptors work not only helps in refining existing treatments but also in developing new ones. Research in this area can lead to the discovery of novel therapeutic targets for conditions that are currently difficult to treat.
7. **Neuroplasticity and Recovery:** Neurotransmitters and receptors are involved in neuroplasticity—the brain's ability to change and adapt. This is fundamental for recovery from mental illness, as therapeutic interventions, including medications and psychotherapy, can lead to changes in neural pathways and synapses.
8. **Prevention Strategies:** Understanding the role of neurotransmitters and receptors can help in developing strategies for preventing certain psychiatric conditions, especially in individuals at high risk.

Receptors and neurotransmitters are central to the field of psychiatry because they provide the biochemical foundation for understanding how the brain regulates mood, thought, and behavior, and they offer pathways for effective treatments and potentially for the prevention of mental health disorders.

What are components of mental state examination of a patient?

The Mental State Examination (MSE) is a structured way of observing and describing a patient's current state of mind, primarily in terms of their cognitive, emotional, and behavioral functioning. It is an essential part of the assessment process in psychiatry and psychology. The MSE is used to gather important information about an individual's mental functioning at the time of the evaluation and includes the following components:

1. **Appearance:** Observations about the patient's physical appearance, including dress, grooming, and visible signs of health or illness.
2. **Behavior:** Noting the patient's actions, level of activity, and cooperation. This may include observations of any unusual movements, restlessness, agitation, or signs of lethargy.
3. **Speech:** Assessing the rate, volume, fluency, and tone of speech. This includes noting whether the speech is coherent, pressured, slow, or slurred.
4. **Mood and Affect:**
   - **Mood:** This is the patient's self-reported emotional state, often described in their own words.
   - **Affect:** The observable emotional state, including the range, intensity, and appropriateness of emotional expression.
5. **Thought Process:** Evaluating the form of thought, looking at how the patient thinks. This includes assessing the rate, continuity, coherence, and logical progression of thoughts.
6. **Thought Content:** This involves what the patient is actually thinking about, including beliefs, preoccupations, and the presence of delusions or suicidal/homicidal ideation.
7. **Perceptual Disturbances:** Checking for any hallucinations or illusions. This involves determining if the patient is experiencing distortions or misinterpretations of reality.
8. **Cognition:** Assessing cognitive functions such as memory, concentration, attention, and orientation (to time, place, person, and situation). This may involve asking the patient to perform certain tasks or answer questions.
9. **Insight:** The patient's awareness and understanding of their own condition and situation.
10. **Judgment:** The ability to understand the consequences of actions and to make reasoned decisions, which is often assessed through hypothetical questions.

The MSE is not a checklist but a nuanced exploration of the patient's current mental state. The information gathered can help in diagnosing mental health conditions, formulating a treatment plan, and assessing risk. It is important to note that the MSE is a snapshot of how the patient presents at a specific time and may change over time or in different contexts.

What are disorders of behavior?

Disorders of behavior refer to a range of psychiatric, psychological, or developmental conditions characterized by behavioral symptoms that are abnormal, maladaptive, or significantly impair functioning. These disorders can affect both children and adults, and they encompass a wide array of issues, often requiring clinical attention. Some of the key categories and examples include:

1. **Disruptive, Impulse-Control, and Conduct Disorders:**
   - **Attention-Deficit/Hyperactivity Disorder (ADHD):** Characterized by a persistent pattern of inattention and/or hyperactivity-impulsivity.
   - **Conduct Disorder:** Involving patterns of behavior in which the basic rights of others or major age-appropriate societal norms are violated.
   - **Oppositional Defiant Disorder (ODD):** A pattern of angry/irritable mood, argumentative/defiant behavior, or vindictiveness.
   - **Impulse-Control Disorders:** Including conditions like intermittent explosive disorder, where individuals fail to resist aggressive impulses.
2. **Neurodevelopmental Disorders:**
   - Autism Spectrum Disorders (ASD): Characterized by deficits in social interaction and communication, and the presence of restrictive and repetitive behaviors.
   - Intellectual Disabilities: Involving deficits in intellectual and adaptive functioning.
3. **Mood Disorders:** Although primarily affecting emotions, mood disorders can also significantly impact behavior.
   - **Major Depressive Disorder:** Can lead to behavioral symptoms like withdrawal from activities, reduced social interaction, or slowed movements.
   - **Bipolar Disorders:** Characterized by manic or hypomanic episodes that include behaviors such as increased activity, rapid speech, and impulsive actions.
4. **Anxiety Disorders:** While primarily impacting emotional states, anxiety disorders can manifest in behaviors such as avoidance, repetitive compulsions, or restlessness.
5. **Personality Disorders:** These involve enduring patterns of behavior, cognition, and inner experience that deviate markedly from the expectations of the individual's culture.
   - Examples include Borderline Personality Disorder, Antisocial Personality Disorder, and Narcissistic Personality Disorder.
6. **Psychotic Disorders:** Disorders like schizophrenia can lead to disorganized behavior, which may manifest as unpredictable or inappropriate actions, a lack of impulse control, or difficulties with routine activities.
7. **Substance-Related and Addictive Disorders:** These disorders involve behaviors centered around the excessive use of substances like alcohol, drugs, or addictive activities like gambling.
8. **Eating Disorders:** Such as anorexia nervosa, bulimia nervosa, and binge-eating disorder, involving maladaptive behaviors related to food intake and body image.
9. **Sleep-Wake Disorders:** Abnormal behaviors related to sleep, such as insomnia, narcolepsy, or sleepwalking.
10. **Obsessive-Compulsive and Related Disorders:** Including obsessive-compulsive disorder (OCD), where repetitive behaviors (compulsions) are performed in response to uncontrollable thoughts (obsessions).

It is important to note that many behavioral disorders are complex and may overlap with other mental health conditions. Diagnosis and treatment often require a comprehensive evaluation by mental health professionals. Additionally, the manifestation of these disorders can vary widely among individuals, and the nature of behavioral symptoms can change over time.

What is disorder of thought?

A disorder of thought refers to a disturbance in the way a person thinks, organizes, and expresses their thoughts. This can manifest in various ways and is a key feature in several psychiatric conditions. Thought disorders typically affect the form, flow, and content of thought. Some common manifestations:

1. **Form of Thought:**
   - **Disorganized Thinking:** This is evident when a person has difficulty organizing their thoughts, leading to incoherent or illogical speech. It is often seen in schizophrenia.
   - **Tangential Thinking:** The individual goes off on tangents and never returns to the original point or topic.

- **Circumstantial Thinking:** Excessive detail and digressions in speech before eventually getting to the point.
- **Flight of Ideas:** Rapidly shifting from one topic to another, often based on superficial connections. It is commonly observed in manic episodes of bipolar disorder.

2. **Flow of Thought:**
   - **Thought Blocking:** An abrupt stop in the middle of a train of thought, which the person may be unable to resume.
   - **Poverty of Thought:** Limited thought content; the individual says very little.
   - **Pressure of Speech:** Rapid, frenzied speech, often seen in manic episodes.
3. **Content of Thought:**
   - **Delusions:** False beliefs that are not based in reality and are not typical of the person's cultural background. Delusions can be paranoid, grandiose, somatic, or of other types.
   - **Obsessions:** Persistent, intrusive, and unwanted thoughts that cause distress or anxiety.
4. **Perception:**
   - **Hallucinations:** Perceiving things that are not present in reality, such as hearing voices or seeing things that others do not see. Although primarily a perceptual disturbance, hallucinations can significantly affect the content and organization of thought.

Thought disorders are a hallmark of several psychiatric conditions, including schizophrenia, bipolar disorder, and major depressive disorder with psychotic features. They can also occur in other medical and neurological conditions, such as brain injuries, infections, and substance abuse.

Diagnosing and treating thought disorders typically requires a comprehensive evaluation by mental health professionals, and the treatment may include medications, psychotherapy, or a combination of both. It is important to address these issues as they can significantly impact an individual's ability to function and their quality of life.

Which disorder shows disorder of thought?

Disorders of thought are primarily associated with several psychiatric conditions. Some of the key disorders where disturbances in thought processes are prominently featured:

1. **Schizophrenia:** This is perhaps the most well-known disorder associated with thought disorders. Individuals with schizophrenia may exhibit disorganized thinking, delusions (fixed, false beliefs), and hallucinations. Their speech might be incoherent or illogical, and they may have difficulty organizing their thoughts.
2. **Bipolar Disorder**: Especially during manic or mixed episodes, individuals may experience a flight of ideas, where their thoughts and speech rapidly jump from one topic to another. Delusions can also occur in severe cases.
3. **Major Depressive Disorder with Psychotic Features:** In severe cases of depression, individuals may have psychotic symptoms, including delusions and hallucinations, which represent a significant disturbance in thought content.
4. **Schizoaffective Disorder:** This disorder features symptoms of both schizophrenia (such as disorganized thinking and delusions) and mood disorder symptoms (like depression or mania).
5. **Delusional Disorder:** Characterized by the presence of one or more delusions for a duration of one month or longer. The delusions often involve real-life situations that could be true but aren't, like being followed, poisoned, or having a disease.
6. **Brief Psychotic Disorder:** This involves sudden, short-term displays of psychotic behavior, such as hallucinations or delusions, which can often be triggered by extreme stress.
7. **Borderline Personality Disorder:** While not primarily known as a thought disorder, individuals with this condition can experience transient, stress-related paranoid ideation or severe dissociative symptoms.
8. **Neurocognitive Disorders:** Disorders such as Alzheimer's disease and other forms of dementia can lead to disorganized thinking, especially in the later stages.
9. **Substance-Induced Psychotic Disorder**: Substance abuse (including alcohol, drugs, and certain medications) can lead to psychotic symptoms, including disordered thoughts.
10. **Organic Brain Syndromes:** Conditions like brain tumors, cerebrovascular disease, or encephalitis

can lead to cognitive disturbances, including impaired thought processes.

It is important to note that the manifestation of thought disorders can vary greatly among individuals and over time. Accurate diagnosis and effective treatment of these conditions typically require a comprehensive evaluation by mental health professionals. Treatment may involve a combination of medication, psychotherapy, and other supportive measures.

What is disorder of mood?

A mood disorder is a mental health condition characterized by disturbances in a person's emotional state or mood. These disorders can significantly impact an individual's daily functioning and quality of life. Mood disorders can range from feelings of intense sadness to extreme happiness and can be chronic or episodic in nature. The main types of mood disorders include:

1. **Major Depressive Disorder (MDD):** Characterized by persistent and intense feelings of sadness, hopelessness, and a lack of interest or pleasure in activities. It may also be accompanied by physical symptoms such as changes in sleep, appetite, energy level, concentration, daily behavior, or self-esteem.

2. **Bipolar Disorder:** This disorder involves episodes of mood swings ranging from depressive lows to manic highs. The depressive episodes are similar to those in MDD, while manic episodes are characterized by high energy, reduced need for sleep, and a loss of touch with reality.

3. **Cyclothymic Disorder:** A milder form of bipolar disorder, consisting of cyclical mood swings. However, the symptoms are less severe than full-blown manic or depressive episodes.

4. **Dysthymia (Persistent Depressive Disorder):** A chronic form of depression where a person's mood is regularly low. However, the symptoms are not as severe as major depression.

5. **Seasonal Affective Disorder (SAD):** A type of depression that is related to changes in seasons, SAD begins and ends at about the same times every year, often worsening in the winter months.

6. **Postpartum Depression:** A type of mood disorder that women can experience after childbirth, characterized by feelings of extreme sadness, anxiety, and exhaustion.

7. **Premenstrual Dysphoric Disorder (PMDD):** A severe form of premenstrual syndrome (PMS) characterized by significant mood swings, irritability, and depression in the lead-up to menstruation.

8. **Disruptive Mood Dysregulation Disorder (DMDD):** Seen in children and adolescents, DMDD is characterized by severe and recurrent temper outbursts that are out of proportion to the situation or provocation.

9. **Substance/Medication-Induced Mood Disorder:** Mood disturbances directly attributable to the physiological effects of a substance (such as a drug of abuse, a medication, or toxin exposure).

10. **Mood Disorder Due to Another Medical Condition:** Characterized by mood symptoms (depression or mania) that are the direct physiological result of another medical condition.

Mood disorders are complex conditions that involve a combination of genetic, biological, environmental, and psychological factors. Treatment often includes medication (like antidepressants or mood stabilizers), psychotherapy, and lifestyle changes. Early diagnosis and intervention can significantly improve outcomes for individuals with mood disorders.

Which disorder shows disorder of memory?

Disorders of memory involve significant impairment in the ability to encode, store, retain, and subsequently recall information. Various medical, neurological, and psychiatric conditions can lead to memory disorders. Some of the key disorders that prominently feature memory impairments include:

1. **Alzheimer's Disease:** This is the most common cause of dementia and is characterized by a progressive decline in memory, language, problem-solving, and other cognitive skills.

2. **Other Dementias:** Besides Alzheimer's, other forms of dementia such as vascular dementia, Lewy body dementia, and frontotemporal dementia also involve memory loss as a central symptom, along with other cognitive impairments.

3. **Amnestic Disorders:** These are characterized primarily by memory dysfunction. Amnestic disorder can be caused by brain injury, stroke, alcohol abuse (as seen in Wernicke-Korsakoff syndrome), or certain illnesses.

4. **Mild Cognitive Impairment (MCI):** MCI represents a slight but noticeable and measurable

decline in cognitive abilities, including memory and thinking skills. It is more severe than normal age-related decline but not severe enough to be classified as dementia.

5. **Traumatic Brain Injury (TBI):** Depending on the severity and location of the injury, TBI can lead to short-term or long-term memory problems.
6. **Stroke:** A stroke can damage brain tissue and impair memory, depending on the stroke's location and severity.
7. **Parkinson's Disease and Huntington's Disease:** While primarily known for their motor symptoms, these neurological diseases can also affect memory, especially in their later stages.
8. **Depressive Disorders:** Severe depression can sometimes lead to difficulties with memory and concentration, although these symptoms are typically reversible with treatment.
9. **Post-Traumatic Stress Disorder (PTSD):** This condition can affect the way the brain processes and recalls memories, particularly those associated with the traumatic event.
10. **Substance Abuse and Addiction:** Prolonged use of certain substances like alcohol and drugs can lead to deficits in memory function.
11. **Normal Pressure Hydrocephalus:** Caused by the build-up of cerebrospinal fluid in the brain, leading to symptoms including memory loss, along with difficulty walking and impaired bladder control.

It is important to note that memory issues can have many causes and may not always signify a serious condition like dementia. However, significant or rapidly progressing memory problems should be evaluated by a healthcare professional to determine the underlying cause and appropriate treatment.

What disorders result in poor or total loss of insight?

Loss of insight, or the inability to understand and acknowledge one's own condition and symptoms, is a notable feature in several psychiatric and neurological disorders. This lack of awareness can range from poor insight to complete anosognosia, where the person is entirely unaware of their condition. Some of the disorders commonly associated with a loss of insight include:

1. **Schizophrenia and Other Psychotic Disorders:** One of the most prominent examples is schizophrenia, where individuals may lack insight into their psychotic experiences, such as delusions or hallucinations. This is also common in other psychotic disorders.
2. **Bipolar Disorder:** During manic episodes, individuals may lack insight into their behavior and the consequences thereof. They may not recognize the severity or abnormality of their actions and decisions.
3. **Alzheimer's Disease and Other Dementias:** As these conditions progress, individuals often lose insight into their declining cognitive abilities, including memory loss and impaired judgment.
4. **Severe Major Depressive Disorder:** Particularly when accompanied by psychotic features, individuals may lack insight into their condition, believing their depressive thoughts to be accurate reflections of reality.
5. **Anosognosia in Stroke and Brain Injuries:** This is a specific condition where a person who has suffered a stroke or brain injury remains unaware of or denies the existence of their paralysis or disabilities.
6. **Frontotemporal Dementia (FTD):** Early in the disease, individuals may show a lack of insight into their changing behaviors and personalities.
7. **Obsessive-Compulsive Disorder (OCD):** Some individuals with OCD have poor insight regarding the irrational nature of their obsessions or compulsions.
8. **Substance Use Disorders:** Individuals may lack insight into the extent of their substance use and its impact on their life, health, and relationships.
9. **Anorexia Nervosa:** Often, individuals with anorexia nervosa do not recognize the severity of their weight loss and continue to perceive themselves as overweight.
10. **Body Dysmorphic Disorder:** Individuals may have little to no insight into the irrationality of their beliefs about perceived flaws in their physical appearance.
11. **Delusional Disorder:** People with delusional disorder firmly hold onto beliefs despite evidence to the contrary, often lacking insight into the implausibility of their delusions.

Loss of insight significantly affects treatment compliance and outcomes, as individuals may not believe they need help or may not adhere to prescribed treatment plans. This characteristic poses unique challenges in the management and care of such conditions, often requiring tailored therapeutic approaches and, in some cases, the involvement of caregivers or legal interventions for the safety and well-being of the individual.

Are disorders of behavior, thinking, mood, insight and judgment along with other symptoms exclusive to certain diseases?

Disorders of behavior, thinking, mood, insight, and judgment, along with other psychiatric symptoms, are not exclusive to any single disease. Instead, these symptoms can overlap across a wide range of psychiatric, neurological, and even medical conditions. This overlapping nature of symptoms makes diagnosis and treatment in mental health complex. Here is a broader view:

1. **Overlap Across Different Conditions:**
   - Many psychiatric conditions share similar symptoms. For example, disorders of mood can be seen in major depressive disorder, bipolar disorder, and some personality disorders.
   - Cognitive symptoms like impaired judgment or insight can occur in dementia, schizophrenia, and brain injuries.
   - Disorders of thinking, such as delusions or disorganized thought, can be present in schizophrenia, severe bipolar disorder, and some neurological conditions.
2. **Comorbidity:**
   - It is common for individuals to have more than one mental health disorder. For instance, someone with a primary diagnosis of bipolar disorder may also struggle with substance abuse or anxiety disorders.
   - Comorbid conditions can complicate the clinical picture and require comprehensive treatment approaches.
3. **Spectrum of Disorders:**
   - Mental health disorders often exist on a spectrum, with varying degrees of severity and symptom presentations. For instance, autism spectrum disorder encompasses a wide range of symptoms and levels of impairment.
4. **Influence of External Factors:**
   - Symptoms can be exacerbated or influenced by external factors such as stress, physical health, substance use, and environmental conditions.
5. **Neurological and Medical Conditions:**
   - Certain neurological conditions (like Parkinson's disease or multiple sclerosis) and medical issues (such as thyroid disorders or vitamin deficiencies) can manifest with psychiatric symptoms.
6. **Age-Related Factors:**
   - Symptoms may present differently across the lifespan. For example, disorders of behavior in children may be indicative of developmental disorders, while in older adults, they might signal the onset of dementia.
7. **Cultural and Individual Differences:**
   - The expression and interpretation of symptoms can vary significantly based on cultural background and individual differences.

Given this complexity, accurate diagnosis often requires a comprehensive assessment, including a detailed medical and psychiatric history, physical examination, and sometimes neuropsychological testing. Treatment is equally multifaceted, potentially involving medication, psychotherapy, lifestyle changes, and support from healthcare professionals and caregivers.

It is also crucial to approach mental health with a holistic perspective, understanding that symptoms can be interconnected and influenced by a wide array of factors.

What is abnormal behavior?

Abnormal behavior refers to patterns of behavior, thoughts, or emotions that are atypical, significantly deviate from societal norms, and can be disruptive to the individual's or others' functioning. Determining what constitutes "abnormal" can be complex, as it often depends on context, cultural norms, and subjective judgment. However, in the field of psychology and psychiatry, abnormal behavior is generally characterized by several key components:

1. **Statistical Rarity:** Behaviors that are uncommon or rare in the general population may be considered abnormal. However, rarity alone does not necessarily mean a behavior is abnormal; some rare behaviors can be positive or desirable.
2. **Deviation from Social Norms:** Behaviors, thoughts, or emotions that significantly deviate from the accepted standards or rules of a society or culture may be seen as abnormal. However, this criterion can vary greatly across different cultures and time periods.

3. **Personal Distress:** When behavior causes significant distress to the individual, it may be considered abnormal. This distress can manifest as depression, anxiety, or other emotional turmoil.

4. **Maladaptive Behavior:** Behaviors that are harmful or prevent an individual from functioning effectively in daily life are considered maladaptive. This can include an inability to perform routine tasks, maintain relationships, hold a job, or care for oneself.

5. **Irrationality or Unpredictability:** Behavior that is irrational (not logically understandable) or highly unpredictable without apparent reason can be seen as abnormal.

6. **Violation of Moral and Ethical Standards:** Sometimes, behaviors that significantly violate societal moral or ethical standards are considered abnormal.

7. **Danger to Self or Others:** Behaviors that pose a threat to the safety of the individual or others may also be classified as abnormal.

It is important to note that the concept of abnormal behavior is subjective and can be influenced by various factors, including cultural values, context, and individual perceptions. Mental health professionals typically use standardized diagnostic criteria, such as those outlined in the Diagnostic and Statistical Manual of Mental Disorders (DSM) or the International Classification of Diseases (ICD), to assess and diagnose abnormal behavior more objectively.

Furthermore, labeling a behavior as "abnormal" does not necessarily imply a mental disorder. A comprehensive assessment by qualified professionals is required to understand the context and causes of the behavior and to determine if it is part of a broader mental health condition.

What is the difference between a behavioral disorder and a mental disorder?

The terms "behavioral disorder" and "mental disorder" are often used interchangeably, but they can denote slightly different aspects of mental health. Understanding the distinction between them is important for accurate diagnosis and treatment.

1. **Behavioral Disorder:**

   - **Primarily Involves Behavior:** Behavioral disorders are characterized mainly by behaviors that are disruptive, inappropriate, or harmful, either to the individual or to others. These behaviors significantly deviate from socially accepted behaviors, especially considering the person's age and culture.

   - **Examples:** Common examples include Attention Deficit Hyperactivity Disorder (ADHD), Oppositional Defiant Disorder (ODD), and Conduct Disorder. These disorders are often diagnosed in childhood or adolescence and involve persistent patterns of disruptive, impulsive, or aggressive behavior.

   - **Focus on Observable Actions:** The diagnosis of behavioral disorders often relies on observable actions and behaviors rather than on internal psychological processes or emotional states.

2. **Mental Disorder:**

   - **Broader Spectrum:** Mental disorders encompass a wide range of conditions that can affect mood, thinking, behavior, and perception. They are characterized by alterations in thinking, mood, or behavior associated with distress and/or impaired functioning.

   - **Includes Internal Processes:** Mental disorders include not only external behaviors but also internal psychological and emotional processes. For instance, conditions like depression, anxiety disorders, schizophrenia, and bipolar disorder involve disturbances in emotions, thoughts, perceptions, and behaviors.

   - **Examples:** Mental disorders include a vast array of conditions like Major Depressive Disorder, Generalized Anxiety Disorder, Schizophrenia, Eating Disorders, and Personality Disorders.

3. **Overlap:**

   - Behavioral disorders are a subset of mental disorders. All behavioral disorders are mental disorders, but not all mental disorders are primarily behavioral disorders.

   - For instance, while ADHD is classified as a behavioral disorder due to its primary symptoms of hyperactivity and impulsivity, depression is classified as a mood disorder due to its primary symptoms of persistent sadness and loss of interest.

4. **Treatment and Management:**

   - Behavioral disorders often require specific interventions focused on modifying disruptive or harmful behaviors. This can include behavioral therapy, social skills training, and, in some cases, medication.

- Mental disorders have a broader range of treatments depending on the specific condition, including psychotherapy, medication, lifestyle changes, and support groups.

In summary, while behavioral disorders focus more specifically on problematic behaviors, mental disorders cover a broader spectrum that includes internal psychological states as well as external behaviors. Accurate diagnosis and tailored treatment plans are essential for both types of disorders, often requiring the expertise of mental health professionals.

What are the most common disruptive behaviors?

Disruptive behaviors refer to actions that are inappropriate for the setting or situation and interfere with the normal functioning of a group, such as a classroom, workplace, or social setting. These behaviors can be particularly common in children and adolescents but can occur in adults as well. Some of the most common disruptive behaviors include:

1. **Aggression:** This includes physical violence, threatening behavior, or verbal abuse towards others. Aggression can be reactive, proactive, or a combination of both.
2. **Non-compliance:** Refusing to follow rules or instructions, disobeying authority figures, and not adhering to social norms or expectations.
3. **Temper Tantrums:** Especially common in younger children, tantrums are outbursts of anger and frustration that can involve crying, screaming, and physical actions like kicking or hitting.
4. **Hyperactivity:** Excessive energy that might manifest as constant movement, fidgeting, inability to sit still, or impulsively moving about in inappropriate situations.
5. **Impulsivity:** Acting without thinking about the consequences, often resulting in risk-taking behavior or interrupting others.
6. **Inattention:** Difficulty focusing, not paying attention, or being easily distracted, which can disrupt learning and social interactions.
7. **Defiance:** Deliberately arguing, talking back, or refusing to cooperate with adults or authority figures.
8. **Bullying:** Intimidating or harassing others through physical, verbal, or psychological means.
9. **Social Withdrawal:** Although not disruptive in the traditional sense, extreme social withdrawal can be a concern in group settings, especially if it impacts group dynamics or the individual's social development.
10. **Destruction of Property:** Deliberately damaging or destroying objects or property.
11. **Lying or Cheating:** Deceptive behaviors that disrupt the trust and functioning of a social or educational environment.
12. **Inappropriate Language or Humor:** Using foul language, sexual comments, or offensive jokes in inappropriate settings.

These behaviors are considered disruptive because they can significantly impact the functioning of the individual exhibiting them, as well as those around them. In children and adolescents, such behaviors can interfere with learning and social development. It is important to address these behaviors appropriately, which may involve behavioral interventions, psychotherapy, family counseling, and, in some cases, medication. Understanding the underlying causes, such as emotional distress, environmental factors, or mental health disorders, is crucial for effective management and support.

What are most Common Mental Illnesses and Disorders?

Common mental illnesses and disorders encompass a wide range of psychological conditions that affect people's mood, thinking, and behavior. These disorders can vary in severity and impact on daily life.

1. **Anxiety Disorders:** This group of disorders involves excessive fear or anxiety. It includes generalized anxiety disorder (GAD), panic disorder, social anxiety disorder, specific phobias, and separation anxiety disorder.
2. **Mood Disorders:** These disorders primarily affect a person's mood, leading to periods of intense sadness or excessively elevated mood. Common examples are major depressive disorder (MDD), bipolar disorder, and dysthymia (persistent depressive disorder).
3. **Obsessive-Compulsive and Related Disorders:** Characterized by obsessive thoughts and compulsive behaviors. The most well-known

of these is obsessive-compulsive disorder (OCD), but the category also includes body dysmorphic disorder, trichotillomania (hair-pulling disorder), and hoarding disorder.

4. **Post-Traumatic Stress Disorder (PTSD):** This can develop following exposure to a traumatic event and is characterized by symptoms such as flashbacks, nightmares, severe anxiety, and uncontrollable thoughts about the event.
5. **Eating Disorders:** These disorders involve preoccupation with food, body weight, and shape, leading to dangerous eating behaviors. Common eating disorders include anorexia nervosa, bulimia nervosa, and binge-eating disorder.
6. **Schizophrenia and Other Psychotic Disorders:** These are characterized by distortions in thinking, perception, emotions, language, sense of self, and behavior. Schizophrenia is the most well-known of these disorders.
7. **Personality Disorders:** These are characterized by enduring patterns of behavior, cognition, and inner experience, exhibited across many contexts and deviating markedly from those accepted by the individual's culture. Examples include borderline personality disorder, antisocial personality disorder, and narcissistic personality disorder.
8. **Attention-Deficit/Hyperactivity Disorder (ADHD):** Marked by ongoing patterns of inattention and/or hyperactivity-impulsivity that interferes with functioning or development.
9. **Autism Spectrum Disorder (ASD):** A developmental disorder characterized by difficulties with social interaction and communication, and by restricted and repetitive behavior.
10. **Substance Use Disorders:** These disorders involve the excessive use of substances like alcohol, drugs, and tobacco, leading to significant impairment or distress.
11. **Neurocognitive Disorders:** This category includes cognitive decline associated with conditions like Alzheimer's disease, dementia, and traumatic brain injury.

It is important to note that mental health disorders can affect anyone, regardless of age, gender, socioeconomic status, or background. Effective treatments, including psychotherapy, medications, and lifestyle adjustments, are available for most mental health disorders, and early intervention can significantly improve outcomes. Mental health is an integral part of overall health, and seeking help for mental health issues is as important as addressing physical health concerns.

What is Mental Retardation?

"Mental retardation" is an outdated term previously used to describe a condition characterized by significantly below-average intellectual functioning and a lack of skills necessary for daily living. This term has largely been replaced by more respectful and accurate terms such as "intellectual disability" or "intellectual developmental disorder."

Intellectual disability is defined by the following key features:

1. **Significantly Impaired Intellectual Functioning:** This typically includes difficulties with reasoning, problem-solving, planning, abstract thinking, judgment, academic learning, and learning from experience. Intellectual functioning is often measured by standardized intelligence tests, where a score approximately two standard deviations below the mean (an IQ score of about 70 or below) is a common criterion.
2. **Deficits in Adaptive Functioning:** This refers to limitations in the ability to carry out everyday activities such as communication, social participation, and independent living. Adaptive functioning covers a range of skills, from self-care and domestic skills to social and interpersonal abilities.
3. **Onset During the Developmental Period:** These impairments in intellectual and adaptive functioning must be evident during the developmental period, typically considered to be before the age of 18.

The severity of intellectual disability can vary greatly among individuals and is usually classified based on the level of impairment in adaptive functioning, not just IQ scores. The four levels of severity recognized in the DSM-5 (Diagnostic and Statistical Manual of Mental Disorders, 5th Edition) are:

- Mild
- Moderate
- Severe
- Profound

It is important to note that people with intellectual disabilities can often learn new skills, but they may learn them more slowly. There is a strong emphasis on providing support and interventions that enable individuals to live as independently as possible.

The change in terminology from "mental retardation" to " intellectual disability" reflects a broader shift towards person-first language and respect for individuals with disabilities. This shift emphasizes the person, not the disability, and is part of a broader cultural and professional recognition of the dignity and capabilities of individuals with disabilities.

What are the levels of mental retardation?

The term "mental retardation" is no longer commonly used; it has been replaced with the term "intellectual disability" to more accurately and respectfully describe the condition. Intellectual disability is characterized by significant limitations in both intellectual functioning and adaptive behavior, which covers many everyday social and practical skills. This condition is identified during the developmental period, typically before 18 years of age.

Intellectual disability is classified into four levels based on the severity of the impairment in intellectual and adaptive functioning. These levels are:

1. **Mild Intellectual Disability:**
   - IQ range typically between 50-70.
   - Individuals can often acquire academic skills up to the sixth-grade level.
   - With appropriate support, they can usually live independently or in minimally supervised settings.
2. **Moderate Intellectual Disability:**
   - IQ range typically between 35-49.
   - Individuals may develop basic literacy and mathematical skills.
   - They often require moderate levels of support and may work in sheltered or supervised employment settings.
3. **Severe Intellectual Disability:**
   - IQ range typically between 20-34.
   - Marked developmental delays during childhood.
   - Individuals often require more intensive support and supervision and may learn basic self-care and communication skills.
4. **Profound Intellectual Disability:**
   - IQ below 20.
   - Significant developmental delays are evident in early childhood.
   - Individuals require close supervision and extensive support, often including assistance with basic physical needs.

It is important to note that IQ scores are only a part of the overall assessment for intellectual disability. The person's adaptive behaviors, which include a wide range of skills such as communication, self-care, home living, social skills, and community use, are equally important for the diagnosis and determination of the severity level.

Additionally, people with intellectual disabilities have a diverse range of abilities and potential. With appropriate support, education, and inclusive opportunities, many individuals with intellectual disabilities can lead fulfilling lives, contribute to their communities, and achieve significant personal goals.

What are the causes of mental retardation?

The causes of intellectual disability (formerly known as mental retardation) are diverse and can occur at any time during development, from before birth up to the age of 18 years. These causes can be broadly categorized into genetic conditions, problems during pregnancy and childbirth, and health problems and environmental factors.

1. **Genetic Conditions:** Certain genetic disorders can cause intellectual disability. These include:
   - **Down Syndrome:** Caused by an extra copy of chromosome 21.
   - **Fragile X Syndrome:** A genetic condition causing intellectual disability, especially in males.
   - **Phenylketonuria (PKU):** A metabolic disorder that, if untreated, leads to intellectual disability.
   - **Williams Syndrome:** A developmental disorder that affects many parts of the body.
2. **Problems During Pregnancy and Childbirth:** Factors that can affect brain development during pregnancy and childbirth include:
   - **Maternal Alcohol or Drug Abuse:** Exposure to alcohol (Fetal Alcohol Spectrum Disorders), certain drugs, or toxins in utero can impact brain development.
   - **Malnutrition:** Maternal malnutrition during pregnancy can affect fetal brain development.

- **Preeclampsia:** A condition in pregnancy characterized by high blood pressure, which can affect fetal growth and brain development.
- **Birth Complications:** Problems during labor and delivery, such as oxygen deprivation (birth asphyxia) or premature birth.

3. **Health Problems and Environmental Factors:** Certain health issues and environmental factors after birth can contribute to intellectual disability, such as:
    - **Infections:** Certain infections like meningitis or encephalitis can cause brain damage leading to intellectual disability.
    - **Lead poisoning:** Exposure to high levels of lead, which is toxic to the nervous system.
    - **Severe and chronic malnutrition:** Lack of essential nutrients can significantly impair brain development.
    - **Traumatic brain injury:** Injuries to the brain, especially at a young age, can affect cognitive development and function.
4. **Other Causes:**
    - Certain medical conditions present at birth that can interfere with normal brain development.
    - Chromosomal abnormalities other than Down syndrome can also cause intellectual disability.
    - In many cases, the cause remains unknown, especially in mild cases of intellectual disability.

It is important to recognize that intellectual disability is not a disease but a condition of reduced cognitive and adaptive abilities. Early intervention, educational strategies, and supportive environments can significantly improve functioning and quality of life for individuals with intellectual disabilities. Moreover, genetic counseling can provide valuable information to prospective parents, especially if there is a known genetic risk or a family history of intellectual disability.

What are the different types of mental retardation?

The term "mental retardation" is an outdated and no longer accepted term; it has been replaced by "intellectual disability" in medical, educational, and psychological communities. Intellectual disability describes a condition characterized by significant limitations in both intellectual functioning and adaptive behavior, which includes many everyday social and practical skills. The condition is diagnosed during the developmental period, generally before 18 years of age.

Intellectual disability is not a single, uniform condition but varies widely in its severity and the abilities of each individual. It is commonly categorized into four levels based on the severity of intellectual and adaptive functioning impairments:

1. **Mild Intellectual Disability:**
    - Represents about 85% of people with intellectual disabilities.
    - IQ level typically between 50-70.
    - Individuals may develop social and communication skills during the preschool years.
    - They usually acquire adequate academic skills up to 6th-grade level by late adolescence.
    - As adults, they can often live independently and maintain gainful employment.
2. **Moderate Intellectual Disability:**
    - Accounts for about 10% of individuals with intellectual disabilities.
    - IQ level typically between 35-49.
    - During the school years, individuals can learn basic academic skills but usually not beyond an elementary level.
    - They often benefit from vocational training and, with moderate support, can perform semi-skilled work.
3. **Severe Intellectual Disability:**
    - Comprises about 3-4% of people with intellectual disabilities.
    - IQ level typically between 20-34.
    - Individuals may learn some basic self-care and communication skills with support.
    - They may perform simple tasks in closely supervised settings.
4. **Profound Intellectual Disability:**
    - Makes up approximately 1-2% of individuals with intellectual disabilities.
    - IQ level below 20.
    - Significant developmental delays are evident in early childhood.

- Individuals require close supervision and help with self-care activities.
- They may have additional physical limitations and often require a high level of support.

It is important to note that the classification based on IQ levels is a general guideline and does not capture the full range of abilities and potential of an individual. People with intellectual disabilities have diverse skills and aptitudes. Moreover, a supportive environment, early intervention, and tailored educational and training programs can significantly help individuals with intellectual disabilities to develop essential life skills and contribute meaningfully to their communities.

What is the most common genetic cause of mental retardation?

The most common genetic cause of intellectual disability (formerly referred to as mental retardation) is Down syndrome. Down syndrome is caused by a trisomy of chromosome 21, meaning that individuals with this condition have three copies of chromosome 21 instead of the usual two. This extra genetic material affects the typical course of development and leads to the characteristics and health issues associated with the syndrome.

Key characteristics of Down syndrome include:

1. **Physical Features:** Distinctive facial features (such as a flat face, upward slanting eyes, a short neck), poor muscle tone, and a shorter stature.
2. **Cognitive Impairment:** Varying degrees of intellectual disability, typically in the mild to moderate range.
3. **Health Issues:** Increased risk of congenital heart defects, respiratory and hearing problems, Alzheimer's disease, leukemia, and thyroid conditions.
4. **Developmental Delays:** Delays in physical growth, and language and speech development.
5. **Learning and Social Engagement:** While learning may be slower and more challenging, individuals with Down syndrome can often participate in regular educational settings and many engage actively in social activities.

Down syndrome is not hereditary in the traditional sense, as it usually results from a random error in cell division during the formation of reproductive cells. However, the likelihood of having a child with Down syndrome increases with maternal age, particularly after the age of 35.

Despite the challenges associated with Down syndrome, many individuals with this condition lead fulfilling lives, participating in educational, social, and vocational activities. Early intervention programs, inclusive education, and supportive community environments can greatly enhance the quality of life and development for individuals with Down syndrome.

What are Down syndrome symptoms?

Down syndrome, a genetic condition caused by the presence of an extra copy of chromosome 21, is associated with a range of physical, developmental, and intellectual symptoms. While the severity of these symptoms can vary widely among individuals, common characteristics include:

1. **Physical Features:**
   - **Distinctive facial appearance:** This often includes a flat facial profile, an upward slant to the eyes, a short neck, and a small head.
   - **Hypotonia:** Decreased muscle tone at birth.
   - **Small stature:** Individuals with Down syndrome often have a shorter height.
   - **Short fingers and hands:** Often with a single crease across the palm (single transverse palmar crease).
   - Excess skin at the nape of the neck.
   - **Almond-shaped eyes:** Often with Brushfield spots (small white or grayish/brown spots on the periphery of the iris).
   - A small mouth, which may lead to the tongue sticking out.
   - Small ears.
2. **Developmental and Intellectual Delays:**
   - Delays in reaching developmental milestones such as sitting, standing, and speaking.
   - Mild to moderate intellectual disability, affecting cognitive development and learning.
   - Speech and language delays.
   - Short attention span.
3. **Health Issues:**
   - **Congenital heart defects:** Around half of individuals with Down syndrome are born with heart conditions.
   - **Vision problems:** Including cataracts, near- or farsightedness, and an increased risk of eye infections.
   - **Hearing loss:** Due to fluid build-up in the middle ear or structural problems of the ear.

- **Hypothyroidism:** A common occurrence in people with Down syndrome.
- Increased susceptibility to infections, particularly respiratory infections.
- **Gastrointestinal issues:** Such as gastroesophageal reflux or celiac disease.
- Increased risk of certain types of leukemia.

4. **Behavioral and Emotional Aspects:**
    - Generally sociable, affectionate, and happy demeanor.
    - Some individuals may exhibit stubbornness, impulsivity, or issues with attention.
5. **Later Life Health Concerns:**
    - Early aging: Individuals with Down syndrome may show signs of aging earlier than the general population.
    - Increased risk of developing Alzheimer's disease, often appearing in their 50s or 60s.

It is important to recognize that individuals with Down syndrome can lead fulfilling and productive lives. Early intervention, including physical, occupational, and speech therapy, along with inclusive educational opportunities, can greatly assist in development and skill acquisition. Regular health check-ups and appropriate medical care are also essential to manage the various health issues associated with the condition.

Is mental retardation considered a disability?

Yes, intellectual disability (formerly known as mental retardation) is considered a disability. It is characterized by significant limitations in both intellectual functioning (such as learning, problem solving, and judgment) and adaptive behavior (which includes practical, everyday social and life skills). This disability originates before the age of 18.

Intellectual disability is recognized as a disability under various laws and statutes in many countries, which entitles individuals with this disability to certain rights and protections. For example, in the United States, individuals with intellectual disabilities are protected under the Americans with Disabilities Act (ADA), ensuring they have access to accommodations in the workplace, in educational settings, and in other areas of public life.

Moreover, intellectual disability is a recognized condition in the Diagnostic and Statistical Manual of Mental Disorders (DSM) used by mental health professionals, and it is also included in the International Classification of Diseases (ICD) used by the World Health Organization.

As a disability, intellectual disability varies greatly in severity and in the impact it has on an individual's daily life. People with this disability can often lead fulfilling lives, especially when they receive appropriate support and accommodations. These may include special education programs, vocational training, life skills coaching, and community support services. The focus is often on maximizing the individual's independence and quality of life.

What are the different types of behavioral problems in children?

Children can exhibit a range of behavioral problems, which may be indicative of normal developmental stages, responses to stressors, or signs of underlying psychological or developmental issues. Common types of behavioral problems in children include:

1. **Aggression:** This includes hitting, biting, or kicking others, and can be a response to frustration, a way to express anger, or a learned behavior from the environment.
2. **Tantrums and Emotional Outbursts:** Common in toddlers and pre-schoolers, tantrums can include crying, screaming, and physical actions like throwing objects. They often occur when a child is trying to assert independence or express frustration.
3. **Defiance and Oppositional Behaviors:** This includes saying "no" to requests, deliberately disobeying rules, and talking back to adults. It is typical in the toddler years and also common in the adolescent stage.
4. **Hyperactivity:** Characterized by excessive energy and movement, difficulty sitting still, and impulsivity. Hyperactivity is a key feature of Attention-Deficit/Hyperactivity Disorder (ADHD), but can also occur in typical development.
5. **Inattention:** Difficulty focusing, not paying attention, or being easily distracted. This can be a sign of ADHD or could occur due to environmental factors or stress.
6. **Anxiety-Related Behaviors:** Such as excessive worry, nervousness, avoidance of certain activities or situations, and physical symptoms like stomach-aches or headaches.
7. **Social Withdrawal:** Avoiding or showing little interest in social interactions with peers or adults, which can be a sign of anxiety, depression, or other issues.

8. **Bullying or Mean Behavior to Peers:** Including physical or verbal abuse, exclusion of others, and spreading rumors.
9. **Lying or Stealing:** Dishonest behaviors that can be a normal part of development but may also indicate underlying issues.
10. **Learning Difficulties:** Struggling with academic tasks, which can lead to avoidance and behavior problems in the classroom.
11. **Eating Disorders:** Unusual eating habits or attitudes toward food, although these are more common in adolescents than young children.
12. **Regression:** Returning to earlier developmental stages, such as bedwetting or baby talk, often in response to stress or change.
13. **Obsessive-Compulsive Behaviors:** Repeatedly engaging in certain rituals or behaviors, or having intrusive thoughts that they cannot control.
14. **Self-Harm:** Behaviors like cutting or burning oneself, more common in older children and adolescents and often associated with emotional distress.

It is important to recognize that some behavioral issues are a normal part of childhood development and may not necessarily indicate a serious problem. However, if behaviors are persistent, cause significant distress, affect the child's ability to function in daily life, or disrupt family or school environments, it may be advisable to seek guidance from a pediatrician, psychologist, or other mental health professional. Early intervention can be crucial in addressing behavioral problems effectively.

What is oppositional defiant disorder (ODD)?

Oppositional Defiant Disorder (ODD) is a behavioral disorder primarily diagnosed in childhood and characterized by a persistent pattern of angry, irritable mood, argumentative, defiant behavior, and vindictiveness. This disorder goes beyond occasional rebellious or defiant behavior that is commonly seen in children and teenagers. Children with ODD show these behaviors more frequently and intensely than is typical for their age.

Key features and behaviors associated with ODD include:

1. **Angry and Irritable Mood:**
   - Frequent and persistent loss of temper.
   - Easily annoyed or irritated by others.
   - Often feeling angry or resentful.
2. **Argumentative and Defiant Behavior:**
   - Frequent arguments with authority figures or adults (in children and adolescents).
   - Actively defying or refusing to comply with rules or requests from authority figures.
   - Deliberately annoying or upsetting people.
   - Blaming others for their own mistakes or misbehavior.
3. **Vindictiveness:**
   - Spiteful or vindictive behavior, at least twice within the past six months.

It is important to note that for a diagnosis of ODD, these behaviors must cause significant impairment in social, educational, or occupational functioning, and they must not be attributable to another mental health disorder, such as a mood disorder, anxiety disorder, or a personality disorder.

The causes of ODD are believed to be a combination of genetic, environmental, and psychological factors. These can include a temperament that predisposes the child to be more challenging, family dynamics, and other social or biological factors.

Treatment for ODD often involves therapy and support both for the child and the family. Parenting training, family therapy, cognitive-behavioral therapy for the child to develop more effective coping and problem-solving skills, and educational support are common approaches. In some cases, medication may be prescribed to treat related issues, such as ADHD or mood disorders, which can co-occur with ODD.

Early intervention and treatment are important to improve outcomes for children with ODD and can help prevent the development of more serious behavioral issues in the future.

What are the symptoms of conduct disorder?

Conduct Disorder is a serious behavioral and emotional disorder that can occur in children and adolescents. It is characterized by a pattern of behavior that violates the rights of others or major societal norms or rules. The symptoms of Conduct Disorder are typically grouped into four main categories:

1. **Aggression to People and Animals:**
   - Often bullies, threatens, or intimidates others.
   - Initiates physical fights.

- Has used a weapon that can cause serious physical harm to others (e.g., a bat, brick, broken bottle, knife, gun).
- Physically cruel to people or animals.
- Steals while confronting a victim (e.g., mugging, purse snatching, extortion, armed robbery).
- Forces someone into sexual activity.

2. **Destruction of Property:**
   - Deliberately engaged in fire setting with the intention to cause damage.
   - Deliberately destroys others' property (other than by fire setting).
3. **Deceitfulness or Theft:**
   - Breaks into someone else's house, building, or car.
   - Lies to obtain goods or favors or to avoid obligations (i.e., "cons" others).
   - Steals items of nontrivial value without confronting a victim (e.g., shoplifting, but without breaking and entering).
4. **Serious Violations of Rules:**
   - Often stays out at night despite parental prohibitions, beginning before age 13 years.
   - Runs away from home overnight at least twice while living in the parental or parental surrogate home (or once without returning for a lengthy period).
   - Is often truant from school, beginning before age 13 years.

The diagnosis of Conduct Disorder is serious and is not made lightly. For a diagnosis to be considered, the behavior must be more severe than typical childhood mischief or adolescent rebelliousness. It typically involves a repetitive and persistent pattern of behavior in which the basic rights of others and major age-appropriate societal norms or rules are violated.

Children with Conduct Disorder may have trouble feeling and expressing empathy or remorse and may have difficulty forming positive relationships with others. The causes of Conduct Disorder can be a complex mix of genetic, biological, environmental, psychological, and social factors.

Treatment for Conduct Disorder may include psychotherapy, family therapy, and in some cases, medication. The goal of treatment is often to help the child learn to control and express their emotions appropriately and to improve their social skills. Early intervention can often lead to better outcomes.

What is autism and its syndrome?

Autism, formally known as Autism Spectrum Disorder (ASD), is a complex developmental disorder that affects communication, behavior, and social interaction. It is called a "spectrum" disorder because it includes a wide range of symptoms and skills. People with autism can have varying levels of functioning, from highly skilled to severely challenged.

Key characteristics of autism include:

1. **Social Communication and Interaction Challenges:**
   - Difficulties in understanding and responding to social cues such as eye contact, facial expressions, and body language.
   - Challenges in developing, maintaining, and understanding relationships. This might include difficulty in making friends or a lack of interest in social interactions.
   - Delayed speech and language skills in some, but not all, individuals with autism.
   - Difficulty in engaging in back-and-forth conversation. Some might not talk at all, while others might have fluent language but struggle with the pragmatics of language, such as taking turns in conversation or understanding sarcasm and jokes.
2. **Restricted and Repetitive Patterns of Behavior or Activities:**
   - Repetitive movements or speech patterns (such as hand-flapping, rocking, repeating words or phrases).
   - Strict adherence to routines or rituals; extreme distress at small changes in routine.
   - Highly restricted, fixated interests that are abnormal in intensity or focus.
   - Over- or under-reactivity to sensory input (such as indifference to pain/temperature, adverse response to specific sounds or textures, excessive smelling or touching of objects).

The symptoms of autism typically appear in the early developmental period, generally before age 3, although a diagnosis can sometimes be made later as social demands exceed the child's abilities.

The exact causes of autism are not fully understood, but it is believed to be caused by a combination of genetic and environmental factors. There is no "cure" for autism, but there are various treatment and education approaches that can address some of the challenges associated with the condition. Early intervention can make a significant difference in the long-term development and skills of individuals with autism.

It is important to recognize that autism is a diverse condition, and individuals with autism can have a wide range of skills, strengths, and needs. Many people with autism live full, productive lives and are an integral part of their communities.

What is the highest level of autism?

Autism Spectrum Disorder (ASD) is characterized by a wide range of symptoms and levels of impairment, and it is not typically described in terms of "levels" of high or low. However, for the purpose of diagnosis and determining the level of support needed, the Diagnostic and Statistical Manual of Mental Disorders, Fifth Edition (DSM-5), categorizes ASD into three levels based on the severity of symptoms and the amount of support required:

1. **Level 1 - "Requiring Support":**
   - Difficulty with social situations that can cause noticeable impairments without support.
   - Difficulty initiating social interactions and may appear to have decreased interest in social interactions.
   - May have inflexible behavior that interferes with functioning in one or more contexts. Resists attempts at intervention.
   - May struggle with organization and planning.
2. **Level 2 - "Requiring Substantial Support":**
   - Marked difficulties in verbal and nonverbal social communication skills.
   - Social impairments are apparent even with supports in place.
   - Limited initiation of social interactions and reduced or abnormal responses to social overtures from others.
   - Inflexibility of behavior, difficulty coping with change, or other restricted/repetitive behaviors appear frequently enough to be obvious to the casual observer and interfere with functioning in a variety of contexts.
3. **Level 3 - "Requiring Very Substantial Support":**
   - Severe difficulties in verbal and nonverbal communication.
   - Very limited initiation of social interactions and minimal response to social overtures from others.
   - Inflexibility of behavior, extreme difficulty coping with change, or other restricted/repetitive behaviors markedly interfere with functioning in all spheres. Great distress/difficulty changing focus or action.

It is important to understand that these levels are not a way to measure intelligence or potential. They are primarily used to identify the amount of support an individual needs in daily life. Additionally, an individual's level can change over time with intervention, support, and as they grow and develop. Each person with autism is unique, with their own strengths, challenges, and needs.

What are some signs of ADHD?

Attention-Deficit/Hyperactivity Disorder (ADHD) is characterized by a range of symptoms that can vary widely among individuals, but some common signs include:

1. **Inattention:** This can manifest as difficulty in focusing, making careless mistakes, failing to complete tasks, disorganization, and being easily distracted.
2. **Hyperactivity:** This often shows as fidgeting, an inability to stay seated, excessive talking, restlessness, or a feeling of being driven by a motor.
3. **Impulsivity:** This might include interrupting others, blurting out answers, difficulty waiting for one's turn, and acting without considering the consequences.
4. **Difficulty in Managing Time:** People with ADHD often struggle with time management, which can lead to missed deadlines and procrastination.
5. **Forgetfulness:** This can include forgetting daily activities, losing things frequently, and general absent-mindedness.
6. **Mood Swings:** Some individuals with ADHD experience emotional turmoil, quick temper, and mood swings.
7. **Difficulty in Following Through:** There can be a pattern of starting tasks but not finishing them, including projects, chores, or homework.

8. **Trouble Coping with Stress:** Everyday stress can seem overwhelming for someone with ADHD, leading to avoidance or withdrawal.

It is important to note that these symptoms can also occur in people without ADHD. ADHD is typically diagnosed based on a pattern of behavior observed over time and in different settings. If ADHD is suspected, a thorough evaluation by a healthcare professional is recommended.

What are signs of mild Asperger's syndrome?

Asperger's syndrome, which is now more commonly referred to as a level of Autism Spectrum Disorder (ASD) since the term was phased out in many diagnostic manuals, can manifest in various ways and to differing degrees in individuals. In cases of what might be considered 'mild' Asperger's, signs and symptoms can be subtle and may sometimes be overlooked.

1. **Social Challenges:** Difficulty in understanding and responding to social cues, leading to awkwardness in social settings. Individuals might not pick up on body language, tone of voice, or facial expressions as easily as others.
2. **Limited or Special Interests:** Intense interest in specific topics or activities, often to the exclusion of others. These interests can be pursued with great focus and detail.
3. **Preference for Routine:** A strong preference for fixed routines and schedules, and distress at changes, no matter how small.
4. **Communication Nuances:** Challenges with the subtleties of conversation, such as understanding sarcasm, humor, or idioms. Their language might be formal or pedantic.
5. **Unusual Speech Patterns:** Speaking in a monotone, with little variation in pitch or rhythm, or talking excessively about one's own interests without noticing lack of interest in others.
6. **Sensory Sensitivities:** Over- or under-sensitivity to sensory stimuli, such as light, sound, texture, or temperature. This might include discomfort with bright lights, loud noises, or certain textures.
7. **Social Anxiety and Awkwardness:** Difficulty in making friends, social anxiety, and a tendency to be withdrawn or aloof.
8. **Nonverbal Communication:** Difficulty in interpreting and using nonverbal cues like eye contact, facial expressions, and gestures.
9. **Empathy:** Challenges in understanding others' feelings or talking about their own feelings. This is not due to a lack of empathy but rather a difficulty in recognizing and responding to social/emotional cues.
10. **Detail-Oriented Thinking:** A tendency to focus on details rather than the overall picture, which can be advantageous in certain contexts.

It is important to remember that the presentation of Asperger's/ASD varies greatly from person to person. Not everyone with mild ASD will have all these symptoms, and having some of these traits does not necessarily mean a person has ASD. A professional evaluation is necessary for an accurate diagnosis. Additionally, people with mild ASD often have significant strengths, including deep knowledge in areas of interest, attention to detail, and a strong sense of fairness and justice.

Did Alan Turing have Asperger's syndrome?

The question of whether Alan Turing had Asperger's syndrome is a matter of speculation, as he was never formally diagnosed during his lifetime. Asperger's syndrome, as a distinct diagnosis, wasn't recognized until decades after Turing's death. It is important to note that making posthumous diagnoses is inherently speculative and can be problematic, as it relies on historical accounts and interpretations of behaviors rather than direct assessments.

Alan Turing was a British mathematician, logician, and cryptanalyst, best known for his work in breaking the German Enigma codes during World War II and for laying the foundations for modern computing and artificial intelligence. Accounts of his life suggest that he might have exhibited some characteristics that are often associated with Asperger's syndrome, such as social awkwardness, focused interests, and distinctive patterns of thinking. However, these traits alone do not confirm a diagnosis of Asperger's syndrome or any other condition.

Furthermore, it is essential to approach historical figures with caution when discussing possible mental health diagnoses. The understanding and criteria for such diagnoses have evolved significantly over time. Also, attributing modern diagnostic labels to historical figures can sometimes oversimplify or misinterpret their complex personalities and contributions.

In summary, while some have speculated that Alan Turing might have had traits consistent with what is now known as Autism Spectrum Disorder, there is no definitive evidence or formal diagnosis to confirm this. His legacy remains that of a brilliant and pioneering mathematician and computer scientist.

What is Antisocial Personality Disorder?

Antisocial Personality Disorder (ASPD) is a mental health condition characterized by a long-term pattern of disregarding or violating the rights of others. This disorder is part of a group of conditions called personality disorders. ASPD is more than just antisocial behaviors or attitudes; it involves a distinct set of personality traits and behaviors that are consistent over time. Key characteristics and symptoms include:

1. **Disregard for Right and Wrong:** Persistent lying or deceit to exploit others, using charm or wit to manipulate others for personal gain or personal pleasure.
2. **Deceitfulness and Manipulation:** Repeatedly lying, using aliases, or conning others for personal profit or pleasure.
3. **Impulsivity and Irresponsibility:** Tendency to make rash decisions, failure to plan ahead, chronic irresponsibility, and repeated failure to fulfil work or financial obligations.
4. **Irritability and Aggressiveness:** Often irritable and aggressive, with frequent physical fights or assaults.
5. **Reckless Disregard for Safety:** Disregard for the safety of self or others.
6. **Lack of Remorse:** Indifference to or rationalizing having hurt, mistreated, or stolen from another person.
7. **Poor or Abusive Relationships:** Consistently irresponsible, with a failure to sustain consistent work behavior or honor financial obligations.
8. **Violation of the Law:** Repeatedly performing acts that are grounds for arrest.
9. **Lack of Empathy:** Inability to understand and share the feelings of others.
10. **Egocentrism and Grandiosity:** A sense of superiority and being excessively opinionated, self-assured, or cocky.

It is important to note that a diagnosis of ASPD cannot be made until a person is at least 18 years old, and they must have had symptoms of conduct disorder before age 15. ASPD is more than just occasional antisocial behavior, which can be a part of many people's lives at one point or another. The pattern of behavior in ASPD is pervasive and persistent, significantly impairing the individual's social, work, or school functioning.

The causes of ASPD are not fully understood but are thought to be a combination of genetic and environmental factors, including childhood abuse or neglect, unstable or chaotic family life during childhood, and family history of personality disorders or other mental health disorders.

Treatment for ASPD can be challenging, as individuals with ASPD often do not seek treatment voluntarily unless required by an external circumstance, such as a court order. When treatment is sought, it typically involves psychotherapy, and there may be additional treatments for co-occurring conditions like depression or substance abuse. However, the effectiveness of treatment for ASPD can vary widely among individuals.

What is Borderline Personality Disorder?

Borderline Personality Disorder (BPD) is a complex mental health disorder characterized by a pattern of varying moods, self-image, and behavior. These symptoms often result in impulsive actions and problems in relationships with others. People with BPD may experience intense episodes of anger, depression, and anxiety that may last from a few hours to days. The key features of BPD include:

1. **Fear of Abandonment:** People with BPD are often terrified of being abandoned or left alone. Even something as innocuous as a loved one arriving home late from work or going away for the weekend may trigger intense fear. This can lead to frantic efforts to keep the other person close.
2. **Unstable Relationships:** Individuals with BPD tend to have intense, short-lived relationships. They may idealize someone one moment and then suddenly believe the person does not care enough or is cruel.
3. **Unclear or Shifting Self-Image:** A person with BPD may have a significantly distorted self-image or sense of self. They may feel good about themselves one day, but feel horribly guilty or like they don't exist at all other days.
4. **Impulsive, Self-Destructive Behaviors:** People with BPD may engage in harmful, sensation-seeking behaviors, especially when upset. This can include reckless driving, binge eating, drug or alcohol abuse, or self-harm.
5. **Self-Harm:** Suicidal behavior and deliberate self-harm are common in people with BPD. Threats of self-harm or suicidal behavior may occur in response to fear of separation or rejection.

6. **Extreme Emotional Swings:** Highly variable moods are common in BPD. Periods of intense depression, irritability, or anxiety may last only a few hours or, at most, a day.

7. **Chronic Feelings of Emptiness:** People with BPD often talk about feeling empty, as if there is a hole or a void inside them. At the extreme, they may feel as if they are "nothing" or "nobody."

8. **Explosive Anger:** Individuals with BPD may struggle with intense anger and a short temper. They may also have trouble controlling themselves once the fuse is lit—yelling, throwing things, or becoming completely consumed by rage.

9. **Feeling Suspicious or Out of Touch with Reality:** Paranoia and dissociation might occur with BPD, especially in response to stress. People with BPD may struggle with feeling suspicious or out of touch with reality.

It is important to note that BPD, like all personality disorders, is a complex and nuanced condition that varies widely in its presentation among individuals. The causes of BPD are not entirely clear but are thought to be a combination of genetic, environmental, and social factors, including a history of childhood trauma.

Treatment for BPD typically involves psychotherapy as the primary treatment, which can include dialectical behavior therapy (DBT), cognitive behavioral therapy (CBT), and other forms of talk therapy. Medication may be used to treat co-occurring disorders such as depression or anxiety. The prognosis for BPD can improve significantly with appropriate treatment, although it can be a challenging process.

What is the definition of perversion?

"Perversion" is a term that can be understood and defined in several ways, depending on the context. Broadly, it refers to a type of human behavior or action that deviates from what is considered to be normative, particularly in the context of sexual behavior. However, the usage and interpretation of this term can vary significantly across different cultures, social contexts, and historical periods. Here are some perspectives on its definition:

1. **Psychological Perspective:** In psychological contexts, perversion is often used to describe sexual behaviors or desires that are considered atypical or deviate from the norm. This can include a wide range of activities and preferences. However, it is important to note that the psychological and psychiatric communities have evolved in their understanding and classification of sexual behaviors, and many behaviors previously labeled as "perversions" are no longer classified as such in professional contexts.

2. **Moral or Ethical Perspective:** In moral or ethical discussions, perversion might be used to describe actions or behaviors that are considered morally wrong or corrupt, often with a strong emphasis on sexual morality. What constitutes a perversion in this sense can be heavily influenced by cultural, religious, and personal beliefs.

3. **Legal Perspective:** In legal terms, perversion might be used to describe sexual acts that are illegal or criminalized. This can vary widely from one jurisdiction to another and is heavily influenced by societal norms and laws.

4. **General Usage:** In everyday language, the term can be used more loosely to describe any behavior that is seen as strange, abnormal, or deviant, not necessarily limited to a sexual context.

It is important to approach the term "perversion" with caution and awareness of its context-dependent nature. What one group or culture considers a perversion may be seen as normal or acceptable in another. Additionally, the term has historically been used in ways that are stigmatizing or discriminatory, and modern understanding of human sexuality and behavior has moved towards more nuanced and less judgmental perspectives.

What can we do about perversions?

Addressing behaviors that are considered "perversions" depends largely on the context in which these behaviors are occurring and the impact they have on individuals and those around them. It is important to differentiate between behaviors that are a matter of personal preference and do not harm others, and those that are harmful or illegal. Here are some approaches based on different scenarios:

1. **When the Behavior is Consensual and Harmless:** If the behavior is among consenting adults and does not cause harm to anyone, it is generally considered a matter of personal choice. In such cases, it might not be necessary or appropriate to "do" anything about it, respecting individual freedoms and privacy.

2. **When the Behavior Causes Personal Distress:** If an individual is distressed by their own sexual preferences or behaviors, it might be helpful to seek professional help from a psychologist or psychiatrist. Therapy can provide a space to explore these feelings and behaviors in a safe,

non-judgmental environment, and can help in understanding and managing them.

3. **When the Behavior is Illegal or Harmful to Others:** If the behavior in question is illegal or involves non-consenting parties, this is a matter for legal intervention. In such cases, it is crucial to involve law enforcement and seek legal advice. It is also important for the individual to receive psychological or psychiatric evaluation and treatment.
4. **When the Behavior Affects Relationships:** If these behaviors are causing strain in personal relationships, couples therapy or individual therapy could be beneficial. A therapist can help navigate these issues in a way that respects the needs and boundaries of all parties involved.
5. **Educational and Awareness Programs:** For societal-level concerns about harmful or non-consensual behaviors, education and awareness programs can be effective. These programs can teach about consent, healthy relationships, and the importance of respecting others' boundaries.
6. **Support Groups:** For individuals struggling with their behaviors or those affected by others' behaviors, support groups can offer a community of understanding and shared experiences. These groups can provide emotional support and practical advice for coping and managing these issues.

In any case, it is important to approach this subject with sensitivity and understanding. Behaviors that deviate from the norm are not inherently wrong or harmful, and it is essential to distinguish between personal preference and behaviors that are unethical, non-consensual, or illegal. Respect for individual rights and choices, as long as they do not harm others, is a key principle in addressing issues related to human behavior and sexuality.

What is anxiety?

Anxiety is a normal and often healthy emotion. However, when a person regularly feels disproportionate levels of anxiety, it might become a medical disorder. Anxiety disorders form a category of mental health diagnoses that lead to excessive nervousness, fear, apprehension, and worry. These disorders alter how a person processes emotions and behave, also causing physical symptoms. Mild anxiety might be vague and unsettling, while severe anxiety may seriously affect day-to-day living.

Anxiety presents itself in various forms, including:

1. **Generalized Anxiety Disorder (GAD):** Characterized by chronic anxiety, exaggerated worry, and tension, even when there is little or nothing to provoke it.
2. **Panic Disorder:** Involves repeated episodes of sudden feelings of intense anxiety and fear or terror that reach a peak within minutes (panic attacks).
3. **Social Anxiety Disorder (Social Phobia):** Involves high levels of anxiety, fear, and avoidance of social situations due to feelings of embarrassment, self-consciousness, and concern about being judged or viewed negatively by others.
4. **Specific Phobias:** These are intense fears of a specific object or situation, such as spiders, heights, or flying. The level of fear is usually inappropriate to the situation and may cause the person to avoid common, everyday situations.
5. **Obsessive-Compulsive Disorder (OCD):** Involves recurrent, unwanted thoughts (obsessions) and/or repetitive behaviors (compulsions). Repetitive behaviors are often performed with the intention of preventing or reducing anxiety or preventing some dreaded event; however, these behaviors are not realistically connected to the problem they're intended to fix.
6. **Post-Traumatic Stress Disorder (PTSD):** Can develop after exposure to a terrifying event or ordeal in which grave physical harm occurred or was threatened.

Physical symptoms of anxiety may include:

- Heart palpitations
- Increased heart rate
- Rapid breathing (hyperventilation)
- Sweating
- Trembling or shaking
- Feeling weak or tired
- Difficulty concentrating
- Trouble sleeping
- Gastrointestinal problems

It is important to note that experiencing occasional anxiety is a normal part of life. However, people with anxiety disorders frequently have intense, excessive, and persistent worry and fear about everyday situations. Anxiety disorders are treatable, and a variety of treatments, including psychotherapy, medication, and lifestyle changes, can help to manage the symptoms.

What are Phobias?

Phobias are a type of anxiety disorder defined by a persistent and excessive fear of an object or situation. The phobia typically results in a rapid onset of fear and is present for more than six months. The affected person will go to great lengths to avoid the situation or object, typically to a degree greater than the actual danger posed. If the feared object or situation cannot be avoided, the individual will experience significant distress.

There are several types of phobias, which can be broadly categorized as follows:

1. **Specific Phobias (Simple Phobias):** These involve an irrational fear of a specific object or situation. Common examples include fear of spiders (arachnophobia), fear of heights (acrophobia), and fear of flying (aerophobia).
2. **Social Phobia (Social Anxiety Disorder):** This is a fear of being negatively judged or evaluated in a social or performance situation. People with social phobia feel embarrassed, self-conscious, and anxious in everyday social interactions.
3. **Agoraphobia:** This is the fear of being in situations where escape might be difficult or that help wouldn't be available if things go wrong. Many people misinterpret this as a fear of open spaces, but it can also include fear of being in crowded places, public transport, or outside of one's home alone.

The cause of phobias is not fully understood, but it is generally believed to be a combination of genetic predisposition and environmental factors. Traumatic experiences can also trigger the development of a phobia.

Symptoms of a phobia can range from mild feelings of apprehension to a full-blown panic attack. Common symptoms include:

- Rapid heartbeat
- Shortness of breath
- Trembling
- An overwhelming need to escape the situation
- Feeling dizzy or lightheaded
- Nausea or other gastrointestinal distress

Phobias are often diagnosed based on a detailed interview and criteria outlined in the Diagnostic and Statistical Manual of Mental Disorders (DSM), published by the American Psychiatric Association.

Treatment for phobias can include therapy, such as cognitive-behavioral therapy (CBT), which helps people change their thought patterns and reactions to the feared object or situation. Exposure therapy, a type of CBT, involves gradual exposure to the fear object or situation in a controlled way, to desensitize the individual to the fear. In some cases, medication can be used to manage symptoms of anxiety.

Phobias can be highly treatable, and people who receive therapy for phobias often experience good outcomes.

What is Obsessive Compulsive Disorder?

Obsessive-Compulsive Disorder (OCD) is a common, chronic, and long-lasting disorder in which a person has uncontrollable, recurring thoughts (obsessions) and behaviors (compulsions) that they feel the urge to repeat over and over. People with OCD may try to ignore or stop their obsessions, but that only increases their distress and anxiety. Ultimately, they feel driven to perform compulsive acts to try **to ease their stress.**

Key characteristics of OCD include:

1. **Obsessions:** These are repeated, persistent, and unwanted thoughts, urges, or images that cause distress or anxiety. Common obsessions include fears of germs or contamination, unwanted forbidden or taboo thoughts involving sex, religion, or harm, aggressive thoughts towards others or self, and having things symmetrical or in a perfect order.
2. **Compulsions:** These are repetitive behaviors that a person with OCD feels the urge to do in response to an obsessive thought. Common compulsions include excessive cleaning or handwashing, ordering and arranging things in a particular, precise way, repeatedly checking on things, such as repeatedly checking to see if the door is locked or that the oven is off, and compulsive counting.
3. **Recognition of Excessiveness:** People with OCD generally understand that their obsessions are not true, and their compulsive behaviors are unreasonable. Despite this recognition, they feel unable to stop themselves.
4. **Distress and Impairment:** The obsessive thoughts and compulsive behaviors cause significant distress, take up a lot of time (more than one hour a day), and interfere with daily activities, work, and social interactions.

The exact cause of OCD is unknown, but factors that may play a role include genetics, brain structure and functioning, and environmental factors, such as history of child abuse or other stress-inducing event.

OCD is typically treated with psychotherapy, medication, or a combination of the two. Cognitive Behavioral Therapy (CBT), particularly a type called Exposure and Response Prevention (ERP), is considered the most effective type of psychotherapy for OCD. Medication like selective serotonin reuptake inhibitors (SSRIs) can also help reduce the symptoms.

It is important to note that OCD is a chronic disorder, meaning it can be a lifelong condition, but treatment can help manage symptoms so that they don't rule the daily lives of individuals.

What are Panic Attacks?

Panic attacks are sudden and intense surges of fear, panic, or anxiety. They are overwhelming, and they have both emotional and physical symptoms. Many people with panic attacks may believe they are having a heart attack or they are dying or going crazy. The fear and terror that a person experiences during a panic attack are not in proportion to the true situation and may be unrelated to what is happening around them.

Key characteristics of a panic attack include:

1. **Sudden Onset:** Panic attacks typically begin suddenly, without warning. They can occur at any time — when you are driving a car, at the mall, sound asleep, or in the middle of a business meeting.
2. **Peak Intensity:** They reach their peak level of intensity in a few minutes and then the symptoms begin to lessen.
3. **Duration:** The attacks typically last for about 20 to 30 minutes, but they can vary in length from a few seconds to an hour. The symptoms can persist in a less intense form for longer.
4. **Physical Symptoms:** These can include heart palpitations or a racing heart, sweating, trembling or shaking, shortness of breath or a feeling of being smothered, choking sensation, chest pain or discomfort, nausea or abdominal distress, feeling dizzy, unsteady, lightheaded, or faint, numbness or tingling sensations, and chills or hot flashes.
5. **Emotional Symptoms:** Panic attacks are also characterized by fear of losing control or "going crazy," fear of dying, and a sense of detachment from reality or oneself (derealization or depersonalization).
6. **Recurring and Unpredictable:** Panic attacks can occur several times a day or only a few times a year.

Panic attacks can occur as part of several mental health conditions, including panic disorder, social anxiety disorder, and depression. However, not everyone who experiences panic attacks will develop panic disorder.

Treatment for panic attacks and panic disorder usually involves psychotherapy, medication, or a combination of the two. Cognitive-behavioral therapy (CBT) is one of the most effective forms of psychotherapy for panic disorder. Medications, including antidepressants and benzodiazepines, can also help manage symptoms.

Understanding and recognizing the symptoms of a panic attack can be an important step in managing and reducing the frequency of these attacks. With appropriate treatment, many people are able to reduce or eliminate their panic attacks.

What is post-traumatic stress disorder?

Post-Traumatic Stress Disorder (PTSD) is a mental health condition that is triggered by a terrifying event — either experiencing it or witnessing it. Symptoms may include flashbacks, nightmares, severe anxiety, and uncontrollable thoughts about the event. Individuals with PTSD may feel stressed or frightened even when they are not in danger.

The key features of PTSD include:

1. **Re-experiencing Symptoms:** This includes flashbacks (reliving the trauma over and over, including physical symptoms like a racing heart or sweating), nightmares, and frightening thoughts. These symptoms can cause problems in a person's everyday routine and can be triggered by words, objects, or situations that are reminders of the event.
2. **Avoidance Symptoms:** People with PTSD may try to avoid situations or people that trigger memories of the traumatic event. They may also avoid talking or thinking about the event.
3. **Arousal and Reactivity Symptoms**: These are usually constant, instead of being triggered by things that remind one of the traumatic event. They can include being easily startled, feeling tense or "on edge," having difficulty sleeping, and having angry outbursts.
4. **Cognition and Mood Symptoms:** This includes trouble remembering key features of the traumatic

event, negative thoughts about oneself or the world, distorted feelings like guilt or blame, and loss of interest in enjoyable activities.

PTSD can occur at any age, following a traumatic event such as a natural disaster, a car accident, sexual assault, war/combat, or other violent incidents. Not everyone who experiences a traumatic event will develop PTSD; it depends on a combination of factors, including the intensity and duration of the trauma, personal history, and the individual's emotional and psychological makeup.

Treatment for PTSD typically includes psychotherapy and medication. The main types of therapy include cognitive-behavioral therapy (CBT), which involves changing the thought patterns that are disturbing one's life, and exposure therapy, which helps people face and control their fear by gradually exposing them to the trauma in a safe way. Medications, such as antidepressants, can help control symptoms of depression and anxiety.

It is important to note that PTSD is not a sign of weakness, and seeking professional help is critical for improving symptoms and quality of life. With appropriate treatment, many people with PTSD can find significant relief from their symptoms and lead fulfilling lives.

What is Schizophrenia?

Schizophrenia is a serious mental disorder characterized by a profound disruption in cognition and emotion, affecting the most fundamental human attributes: language, thought, perception, affect, and sense of self. The array of symptoms, while varying widely among individuals, typically includes:

1. **Positive Symptoms:** These are psychotic behaviors not generally seen in healthy people. People with positive symptoms may "lose touch" with some aspects of reality. Symptoms include:
   - **Hallucinations:** Seeing or hearing things that don't exist. Hearing voices is the most common hallucination in schizophrenia.
   - **Delusions:** False beliefs that are not based in reality. For example, believing that some-one is plotting against you or that you are some-one famous.
   - **Thought Disorders:** Unusual or dysfunctional ways of thinking. One form is "thought blocking," where the person stops speaking abruptly in the middle of a thought.
2. **Negative Symptoms:** This refers to disruptions to normal emotions and behaviors, which might include:
   - Reduced expression of emotions through facial expression or voice tone
   - Reduced feelings of pleasure in everyday life
   - Difficulty beginning and sustaining activities
   - Reduced speaking
3. **Cognitive Symptoms:** These are subtle symptoms that may be difficult to recognize as part of the disorder and can be mistaken for other problems. Cognitive symptoms include:
   - Poor executive functioning (the ability to understand information and use it to make decisions)
   - Trouble focusing or paying attention
   - Problems with working memory (the ability to use information immediately after learning it)

Schizophrenia is believed to result from a complex interplay of genetics, brain chemistry, and environment. It affects men and women equally and appears to occur at similar rates in all ethnic groups around the world. Symptoms such as hallucinations and delusions typically start between ages 16 and 30. Men often develop symptoms at a younger age than women.

There is no cure for schizophrenia, but it is treatable. Treatments include antipsychotic medications, psychotherapy (such as cognitive behavioral therapy), psychosocial interventions, and coordinated specialty care services designed for the early stages of schizophrenia. The goals of treatment are to reduce symptoms, prevent relapses, and improve function. With effective treatment, many people with schizophrenia can lead rewarding and meaningful lives. However, they may need ongoing treatment to manage their condition.

What is evolution of psychosis?

The term "evolution of psychosis" can be interpreted in a few ways, but it generally refers to how psychotic symptoms develop and change over time, either within the course of an individual's illness or across the broader span of human history and genetics. Understanding the evolution of psychosis involves looking at both the clinical progression in individuals and the broader biological and genetic factors that contribute to its development. Here are two main perspectives on this:

1. **Clinical Progression of Psychosis in Individuals:**
   - **Prodromal Phase:** This is an early stage where changes in thoughts, feelings, and behaviors begin to emerge but are not yet fully

developed or severe enough to be classified as psychosis. Symptoms might include subtle changes in thoughts, perceptions, and behavior, such as unusual beliefs, perceptual alterations, and social withdrawal.

- **Acute Phase:** This is when the symptoms of psychosis become apparent and more severe. Hallucinations, delusions, disorganized speech, and disorganized or catatonic behavior may be present. This phase often results in the individual seeking treatment.
- **Recovery and Stabilization:** With treatment, which typically includes medication and psychotherapy, many individuals experience a reduction in symptoms. Some may recover completely, while others might have residual symptoms and may require ongoing management.
- **Chronic Phase:** In some cases, individuals may experience persistent symptoms despite treatment. This phase is characterized by long-term management of the condition.

2. **Evolutionary Perspective on the Development of Psychosis:**
   - **Genetic Factors:** Research indicates that genetic factors play a significant role in the risk of developing psychotic disorders. Studies of families, twins, and populations suggest that a combination of multiple genetic variations contributes to the development of these disorders.
   - **Evolutionary Theories:** Some theories suggest that certain traits associated with psychosis might have been advantageous in small amounts in an evolutionary context. For example, the same genetic variations that increase the risk for psychosis might also contribute to increased creativity or heightened perception, traits that could have had survival benefits.
   - **Environmental Factors:** Environmental factors, such as prenatal stress, childhood trauma, and substance use, interact with genetic predispositions to increase the risk of developing psychosis.
   - **Neurodevelopmental Perspective:** Some researchers view psychosis as the result of disruptions in normal brain development due to a combination of genetic and environmental factors. This perspective suggests that changes in brain structure and function that occur during critical developmental periods may underlie the development of psychotic disorders.

Understanding the evolution of psychosis is complex and involves an interplay of biological, psychological, and environmental factors. It is an area of active research, with ongoing studies aimed at better understanding the genetic and neurobiological underpinnings of psychotic disorders, as well as the best approaches for treatment and prevention.

What is schizophreniform psychosis?

Schizophreniform disorder is a mental health condition that is very similar to schizophrenia in terms of symptoms, but it differs in terms of duration and, sometimes, in the severity of impairment. Here are the key features of schizophreniform disorder:

1. **Duration:** The primary distinction between schizophreniform disorder and schizophrenia lies in the duration of the illness. In schizophreniform disorder, the symptoms, including hallucinations, delusions, disorganized speech, disorganized or catatonic behavior, and negative symptoms (such as diminished emotional expression), last for at least one month but less than six months. In contrast, a diagnosis of schizophrenia requires that these symptoms persist for six months or longer.
2. **Symptoms:** The symptoms of schizophreniform disorder are essentially the same as those of schizophrenia. They can include:
   - **Hallucinations:** Sensory experiences that appear real but are created by the mind (e.g., hearing voices).
   - **Delusions:** Strongly held false beliefs that are not influenced by logical reasoning or explained by a person's cultural background.
   - **Disorganized Speech:** This may manifest as incoherence or an inability to stick to one topic.
   - **Disorganized or Catatonic Behavior:** This can range from agitation to unresponsiveness.
   - **Negative Symptoms:** This includes reduced emotional expression, lack of motivation, and decreased ability to experience pleasure.
3. **Functioning:** Individuals with schizophreniform disorder may not experience as significant a drop in their ability to function in their daily lives as is

often seen in schizophrenia. However, this can vary, and some individuals may face considerable impairment.

4. **Prognosis and Transition to Schizophrenia:** In some cases, individuals initially diagnosed with schizophreniform disorder go on to develop schizophrenia. For others, the symptoms resolve after a period of less than six months, and they do not progress to schizophrenia.

5. **Treatment:** Treatment for schizophreniform disorder generally involves the same approaches used for schizophrenia, including antipsychotic medications and psychotherapy. Early treatment and support are important for improving outcomes.

6. **Diagnosis:** As with schizophrenia, the diagnosis of schizophreniform disorder is made based on a clinical assessment conducted by a mental health professional, considering the individual's symptoms, the duration of these symptoms, and the impact on functioning.

Understanding schizophreniform disorder is essential for ensuring proper diagnosis and treatment. It is considered a type of psychotic disorder and requires careful monitoring and management, especially considering the potential for it to transition into schizophrenia.

What is schizoaffective psychosis?

Schizoaffective disorder is a chronic mental health condition characterized primarily by symptoms of schizophrenia, such as hallucinations or delusions, and symptoms of a mood disorder, such as depression or mania. The disorder is defined by a combination of the symptoms of schizophrenia (including psychosis) and a mood disorder, making it distinct from both schizophrenia and mood disorders alone.

Key aspects of schizoaffective disorder include:

1. **Psychotic Symptoms:** Similar to schizophrenia, individuals with schizoaffective disorder experience psychotic symptoms, such as hallucinations (seeing or hearing things that are not there), delusions (false, fixed beliefs that are held despite evidence to the contrary), disorganized thinking, and possibly catatonic behavior.

2. **Mood Disorder Symptoms:** These can include periods of major depression or mania. The mood disorder aspect is what distinguishes schizoaffective disorder from schizophrenia.

3. **Types of Schizoaffective Disorder:**
   - Bipolar Type: This type includes episodes of mania and sometimes major depression.
   - Depressive Type: This type includes only major depressive episodes.

4. **Duration:** For a diagnosis of schizoaffective disorder, an individual must have uninterrupted illness during which there is a major mood episode (major depression or mania) concurrent with symptoms meeting the criteria for schizophrenia. Additionally, there must have been delusions or hallucinations for two or more weeks in the absence of a major mood episode.

5. **Impaired Functioning:** Schizoaffective disorder typically leads to difficulties functioning in daily life, including at work, in social situations, and with self-care.

6. **Treatment:** Treatment usually involves a combination of medications, psychotherapy, and life skills training. Medication may include antipsychotics, mood stabilizers, and anti-depressants.

7. **Course and Prognosis:** The course of schizoaffective disorder can vary greatly from person to person. Some people experience only a few episodes of mood disturbance and psychosis, while others may struggle with ongoing symptoms.

The diagnosis of schizoaffective disorder can be challenging because it includes symptoms of both schizophrenia and a mood disorder. It requires a comprehensive evaluation by a mental health professional. The overlapping symptoms with other mental health disorders can sometimes lead to misdiagnosis. Early diagnosis and treatment are important for managing symptoms effectively and improving the quality of life for individuals with schizoaffective disorder.

What is brief psychosis?

Brief Psychotic Disorder is a mental health condition characterized by sudden, short-term episodes of psychotic behavior, such as hallucinations, delusions, disorganized speech, or disorganized or catatonic behavior. The key characteristic of this disorder is its transient nature. Here are the main features of Brief Psychotic Disorder:

1. **Duration:** The duration of a Brief Psychotic Disorder is, by definition, temporary. Symptoms last for at least one day but less than one month,

and the individual fully returns to their pre-episode level of functioning.

2. **Symptoms:** The symptoms are similar to those of other psychotic disorders and can include:
   - **Delusions:** False beliefs that are not based on reality and that the person refuses to give up, even when presented with factual information.
   - **Hallucinations:** Seeing, hearing, or feeling things that are not there.
   - **Disorganized Speech:** Incoherent or nonsensical speech or switching from one topic to another.
   - **Grossly Disorganized or Catatonic Behavior:** This includes a marked decrease in reactivity to the environment or excessive and purposeless motor activity.
3. **Onset:** The onset of symptoms is typically sudden, and the disorder can occur in response to a significant stressor, such as a traumatic event or major life change, although this is not always the case. In some instances, no obvious trigger can be identified.
4. **Types:** There are three types of Brief Psychotic Disorder:
   - **With Marked Stressor(s):** When it occurs shortly after and seems to be in response to significant stressors (such as death of a loved one, major accident, etc.).
   - **Without Marked Stressor(s):** When it occurs without the presence of an obvious stressor.
   - **With Postpartum Onset:** When onset is during pregnancy or within four weeks postpartum.
5. **Diagnosis:** Diagnosis is based on the presence of one or more of the above symptoms. It is important for a healthcare professional to rule out other potential causes, such as substance abuse or a medical condition, and to distinguish it from other mental health disorders.
6. **Treatment:** Treatment often involves a combination of medication (such as anti-psychotics) and psychotherapy. The focus is on relieving symptoms and ensuring the safety of the individual and others.
7. **Prognosis:** The prognosis for Brief Psychotic Disorder is generally good, as the disorder is temporary. However, some individuals may go on to develop other psychotic disorders like schizophrenia or schizoaffective disorder.

Understanding Brief Psychotic Disorder is important for effective treatment and support, as well as for distinguishing it from other, more chronic psychotic disorders.

What is Bipolar Disorder?

Bipolar Disorder, formerly known as manic-depressive illness, is a mental health condition characterized by extreme mood swings that include emotional highs (mania or hypomania) and lows (depression). These mood swings can affect sleep, energy, activity, judgment, behavior, and the ability to think clearly.

The key features of Bipolar Disorder include:

1. **Manic Episodes:** A manic episode is a period of abnormally elevated, expansive, or irritable mood and persistently increased goal-directed activity or energy lasting at least one week. Symptoms may include:
   - Inflated self-esteem or grandiosity
   - Decreased need for sleep (e.g., feeling rested after only a few hours of sleep)
   - More talkative than usual or pressure to keep talking
   - Flight of ideas or subjective experience that thoughts are racing
   - Distractibility
   - Increase in goal-directed activity (either socially, at work or school, or sexually) or psychomotor agitation
   - Excessive involvement in activities that have a high potential for painful consequences (e.g., engaging in unrestrained buying sprees, sexual indiscretions, or foolish business investments)
2. **Hypomanic Episodes:** These are similar to manic episodes but less severe and do not cause significant impairment in social or occupational functioning or require hospitalization. They last at least four consecutive days.
3. **Depressive Episodes:** These involve symptoms such as persistent feelings of sadness, emptiness, or hopelessness, loss of interest or pleasure in most activities, significant weight loss

or gain, insomnia or hypersomnia, fatigue or loss of energy, feelings of worthlessness or excessive or inappropriate guilt, diminished ability to think or concentrate, and recurrent thoughts of death or suicide.

4. **Types of Bipolar Disorder:**
   - **Bipolar I Disorder:** Defined by manic or mixed episodes that last at least seven days, or by manic symptoms that are so severe that immediate hospital care is needed. Depressive episodes usually occur as well, typically lasting at least two weeks.
   - **Bipolar II Disorder:** Defined by a pattern of depressive episodes and hypomanic episodes, but not the full-blown manic episodes described above.
   - **Cyclothymic Disorder (Cyclothymia):** Defined by periods of hypomanic symptoms as well as periods of depressive symptoms lasting for at least two years (one year in children and adolescents); however, the symptoms do not meet the diagnostic requirements for a hypomanic episode and a depressive episode.

The exact cause of bipolar disorder is unknown, but a combination of genetics, environment, and altered brain structure and chemistry may play a role.

Treatment usually includes a combination of medications and psychotherapy. Medications may include mood stabilizers, antipsychotic medications, and, in some cases, antidepressants. Psychotherapy, such as cognitive behavioral therapy and family-focused therapy, is also important for managing the disorder.

It is a lifelong condition, but with effective treatment, people with bipolar disorder can lead healthy and productive lives. Managing symptoms and preventing complications begins with proper diagnosis and treatment, including medications and therapy. Regular follow-up with a mental health professional is crucial for maintaining stability and quality of life.

What is Depression?

Depression, also known as major depressive disorder or clinical depression, is a common and serious medical illness that negatively affects how you feel, the way you think, and how you act. It is more than just a bout of the blues; depression is a persistent problem, not a passing one. It involves episodes during which the symptoms last for at least two weeks. Depression can lead to a variety of emotional and physical problems and can decrease a person's ability to function at work and at home.

Key features of depression include:

1. **Persistent Sad, Anxious, or "Empty" Mood:** Feeling down is a common symptom of depression. Some people may feel hopeless or pessimistic.
2. **Loss of Interest or Pleasure in Activities Once Enjoyed:** This includes loss of interest in hobbies, sports, sex, or other activities that used to be enjoyable.
3. **Changes in Appetite:** Weight loss or gain unrelated to dieting can be a sign of depression.
4. **Sleep Disturbances:** This can include insomnia or sleeping too much.
5. **Restlessness or Irritability:** This may manifest as an inability to sit still or a feeling of being "on edge."
6. **Fatigue or Loss of Energy:** Everyday tasks can feel exhausting or overwhelming.
7. **Feeling Worthless or Guilty:** Fixating on past failures or blaming oneself when things aren't going right.
8. **Difficulty Thinking, Concentrating, or Making Decisions:** This can include trouble focusing, making decisions, or remembering things.
9. **Recurrent Thoughts of Death or Suicide, or Suicide Attempts:** Depression is often associated with thoughts of death, self-harm, or suicide.

The causes of depression are complex and not entirely understood, but it is believed to be due to a combination of genetic, biological, environmental, and psychological factors. Depression can happen at any age, but often begins in adulthood.

Depression is typically treated with medications, psychotherapy, or a combination of the two. Antidepressants can help modify one's brain chemistry. Psychotherapies such as cognitive-behavioral therapy (CBT) and interpersonal therapy (IPT) are also effective forms of treatment. Lifestyle changes, such as regular exercise, adequate sleep, and maintaining social support, can also help to manage symptoms.

It is important to recognize that depression is not a sign of personal weakness or a condition that can be willed or wished away. People with depression cannot merely "pull themselves together" and get better. Proper treatment is often crucial for recovery.

What is the evolution of depression?

The "evolution of depression" refers to how our understanding of depression has developed over time, both in terms of its causes and treatments, and from an evolutionary perspective, why depressive traits might have persisted in the human population. This concept can be explored through several lenses:

1. **Historical Perspective on Depression:**
   - Ancient times saw depression as a result of spiritual or demonic possession. Treatments ranged from spiritual rituals to drastic measures like trepanation (drilling a hole in the skull to release evil spirits).
   - In the era of Hippocrates (around 400 BC), depression (then known as "melancholia") was thought to be caused by an imbalance of the body's four humors. Treatment focused on rebalancing these humors.
   - The 19th and early 20th centuries brought a more scientific understanding, with depression being recognized as a psychiatric disorder. Treatments, however, were still primitive, ranging from institutionalization to early forms of electroconvulsive therapy.
2. **Evolutionary Theories of Depression:**
   - The "Psychosocial Stress" model suggests that depression may have evolved as a response to unavoidable stresses, helping individuals conserve energy and avoid conflict.
   - The "Social Navigation" or "Analytical Rumination" hypothesis posits that depression is an adaptive response for deeply analyzing complex life problems, promoting a focus on problem-solving.
   - "Attachment Theory" views depression as a method of eliciting care and support from others in a social group during times of need.
3. **Biological and Genetic Research Evolution:**
   - Modern research has delved into the genetic and neurochemical aspects of depression, identifying links with neurotransmitters like serotonin, norepinephrine, and dopamine.
   - The role of genetics in depression has been highlighted, but it is clear that there is no single "depression gene." Instead, it is thought to result from complex interactions among multiple genes and environmental factors.
4. **Development in Treatment:**
   - The 20th century saw significant advancements with the development of antidepressants like MAOIs, tricyclics, and SSRIs.
   - Psychotherapy methods, including cognitive-behavioral therapy, have been increasingly refined.
   - Recent years have seen the exploration of treatments like transcranial magnetic stimulation (TMS) and ketamine infusions.
5. **Cultural and Societal Understanding:**
   - There has been a growing recognition of the role of societal factors such as stress, lifestyle, and social inequality in depression.
   - Awareness and destigmatization efforts have increased, emphasizing mental health as a crucial component of overall health.

The evolution of depression as a concept reflects not only advances in medical and psychological sciences but also changes in social attitudes and philosophical understandings of what it means to be human. It is a field that continues to grow and evolve, as researchers seek to better understand and treat this complex and widespread condition.

What is mania?

Mania is a state of abnormally elevated arousal, affect, and energy level, or "a heightened state of euphoria, energy, and irritability," often occurring in people with bipolar disorder, though it can also be seen in other conditions. Mania is the "high" or "up" part of the mood swing in bipolar disorder and is characterized by a distinct period of an overly happy or outgoing mood, or an irritable mood, along with other symptoms.

Key features of mania include:

1. **Elevated Mood:** This is often characterized by feelings of euphoria, extreme optimism, and an increase in self-esteem. People in a manic state frequently report feeling an intense sense of well-being or feeling "on top of the world."
2. **Increased Energy and Activity Levels:** There is often a noticeable increase in energy and a reduced need for sleep. Individuals may feel restlessly driven and are often involved in many projects at once.
3. **Racing Thoughts and Rapid Speech:** Thoughts may race, and individuals often speak quickly and

excitedly, jumping from one idea to another. This can lead to disjointed or incoherent speech.

4. **Impulsiveness and Poor Judgment:** During manic episodes, individuals may show poor judgment and impulsivity, engaging in risky behaviors, such as excessive spending, reckless sexual activity, or unwise business investments.

5. **Irritability or Agitation:** Some individuals experience irritability and agitation rather than an elevated mood, especially if their goals are thwarted or if they are criticized.

6. **Decreased Need for Sleep:** People experiencing mania often feel rested after very few hours of sleep.

7. **Distractibility:** Easily distracted by irrelevant things, having trouble focusing on a single task.

8. **Grandiosity:** Overinflated sense of self-esteem or grandiosity, potentially leading to unrealistic beliefs in one's abilities or powers.

9. **Psychosis:** In severe cases, manic episodes can also include symptoms of psychosis, such as delusions (false beliefs) and hallucinations (seeing or hearing things that aren't there).

Mania can vary in severity and may require hospitalization if the symptoms are extreme or if the individual is at risk of harming themselves or others. In the context of bipolar disorder, mania is typically followed by periods of depression, though not always immediately.

Treatment for mania often includes a combination of mood stabilizers, antipsychotic medications, and psychotherapy. It is essential for individuals experiencing mania to get proper treatment, as the impulsivity and poor judgment associated with manic episodes can lead to dangerous behaviors and consequences.

What is evolution of mania?

The term "evolution of mania" can be interpreted in a couple of ways: the progression of a manic episode in an individual over time or the historical and scientific understanding of mania throughout history.

1. **Clinical Progression of Mania in Individuals:**
   - **Early Stages:** The onset of a manic episode can begin with a period of heightened energy, creativity, and elevated mood. Individuals may feel more sociable, talkative, and confident.
   - **Increasing Symptoms:** As the episode progresses, these symptoms can intensify to the point of causing problems. Sleep becomes less necessary, judgment becomes impaired, and behavior more erratic. Speech may become rapid and difficult for others to follow.
   - **Full-Blown Mania:** In the peak of a manic episode, individuals might experience grandiose delusions, engage in risky behaviors, and have a greatly reduced sense of personal danger or consequence. Hallucinations and delusions might occur in severe cases.
   - **Resolution:** Manic episodes typically do not last forever and will eventually diminish. This can happen naturally or as a result of treatment. Post-mania, individuals often feel exhausted and may have a period of depression or reflection on their actions during the episode.

2. **Historical and Scientific Understanding of Mania:**
   - **Ancient and Medieval Times:** In ancient times, mania was often viewed through a supernatural lens or as a divine punishment. Hippocrates and other ancient physicians, however, began to suggest biological and physiological causes.
   - **Renaissance to 18th Century:** There was gradual recognition of mania as a medical and psychological condition. Descriptions of manic symptoms started to appear in medical literature.
   - **19th and Early 20th Century:** The modern conceptualization of mania began to take shape. Emil Kraepelin, a German psychiatrist, distinguished bipolar disorder (then termed "manic-depressive insanity") from schizophrenia.
   - **Contemporary Understanding:** Today, mania is understood as a component of bipolar disorder, characterized by specific diagnostic criteria. Research focuses on understanding its biological basis, including genetic, neurochemical, and structural brain differences, and its effective management through medication and psychotherapy.

The evolution of the concept of mania reflects broader changes in the fields of psychiatry and neurology. From being seen as a mystical or supernatural phenomenon, it has come to be understood as a complex psychiatric condition with biological, psychological, and environmental factors.

What is Eating Disorders?

Eating disorders are complex mental health conditions characterized by severe and persistent disturbances in eating behaviors and associated distressing thoughts and emotions. They can have serious impacts on physical health, emotional well-being, and overall functioning. The most common eating disorders are:

1. **Anorexia Nervosa:** This disorder is characterized by an intense fear of gaining weight and a distorted body image leading to severe restriction of food intake and often extreme thinness. Individuals with anorexia nervosa typically weigh themselves repeatedly, severely restrict the amount and types of food they eat, and may exercise excessively.
2. **Bulimia Nervosa:** Bulimia involves recurrent episodes of binge eating followed by compensatory behaviors such as vomiting, fasting, excessive exercise, or misuse of laxatives, diuretics, or enemas. Binge eating involves eating large amounts of food in a specific period and feeling a lack of control over eating during the episode.
3. **Binge Eating Disorder:** Similar to bulimia nervosa, binge eating disorder features episodes of eating large quantities of food to the point of discomfort. However, there is no regular use of compensatory behaviors as in bulimia. This can lead to weight gain and is often associated with feelings of shame and guilt.
4. **Avoidant/Restrictive Food Intake Disorder (ARFID):** Unlike anorexia, ARFID does not involve distress about body shape or size, or fears of being fat, but it does involve limitations in the amount or types of food eaten. This can lead to significant weight loss or nutritional deficiencies.
5. **Other Specified Feeding or Eating Disorders (OSFED):** This category includes eating disorders that do not meet the full criteria for any of the above disorders but still cause significant distress or impairment.

Eating disorders can affect individuals of any age, race, gender, or background. While they are most commonly identified in adolescents and young adults, particularly females, they can also affect older adults, men, and younger children.

The causes of eating disorders are complex and multifactorial, involving a range of biological, psychological, and sociocultural factors. Genetics, personality traits, cultural ideals around body image, and environmental stressors can all play a role.

Treatment typically involves a comprehensive approach including psychological therapy, nutritional education and counseling, and medical monitoring. Psychotherapies like cognitive-behavioral therapy (CBT) are commonly used. In severe cases, hospitalization may be necessary to address critical health issues.

It is important to seek treatment early for eating disorders as they can lead to serious health problems, including heart conditions, digestive problems, bone loss, and in severe cases, death. With proper treatment, people with eating disorders can recover and regain their health.

What does amnesia tell us about memory?

Amnesia, a condition characterized by memory loss, provides valuable insights into the complexities of human memory. Studying amnesia helps scientists understand how memory works, how different types of memory are stored and retrieved, and the brain structures involved in these processes. Key insights from amnesia about memory include:

1. **Different Types of Memory:** Amnesia often affects certain types of memory while leaving others intact, revealing the different memory systems in the brain. For example, people with amnesia might struggle with forming new long-term memories (anterograde amnesia) but retain skills and knowledge (procedural memory) learned before the onset of amnesia.
2. **Role of Brain Structures in Memory:** Amnesia has been crucial in identifying the parts of the brain involved in memory. For instance, damage to the hippocampus, a structure in the medial temporal lobe, is commonly associated with difficulties in forming new memories. This underscores the hippocampus's role in converting short-term memories into long-term ones.
3. **Memory Consolidation:** Amnesia demonstrates the process of memory consolidation – the way short-term memories become stabilized into long-term memory. Disruption in this process, often seen in amnesiac patients, can prevent the formation of new long-term memories.
4. **Implicit vs. Explicit Memory:** Research on amnesia has helped distinguish between implicit (unconscious) and explicit (conscious) memory. Individuals with amnesia may not recall specific events (explicit memory) but can often learn new skills (implicit memory), suggesting that these types of memory involve different brain systems.

5. **Temporal Gradient of Memory Loss (Ribot's Law):** In some cases, amnesia affects recent memories more severely than older ones, known as retrograde amnesia. This pattern supports the idea that memories undergo a process over time that makes them more resistant to disruption.

6. **Emotional Memories:** Studies of amnesia have also shed light on the role of the amygdala and other structures in the formation and retrieval of emotional memories. Emotional memories are often better preserved than non-emotional ones in people with amnesia.

7. **Neuroplasticity and Recovery:** Observations of patients recovering from amnesia have contributed to understanding the brain's plasticity. The brain can sometimes compensate for damaged areas by reorganizing and forming new connections, allowing partial recovery of memory.

8. **Role of Sleep in Memory:** Research involving amnesia suggests a role for sleep in memory consolidation. Sleep disturbances can exacerbate memory problems, while healthy sleep patterns can help consolidate memories and aid recovery in some forms of amnesia.

In summary, amnesia is a window into the inner workings of memory, illustrating its complexity and the intricate interplay of different brain regions. It highlights the fact that memory is not a single, unified system but a complex integration of different processes and structures within the brain.

How do you get amnesia?

Amnesia, the loss of memories, can occur due to a variety of causes. It is important to note that amnesia usually involves problems with memory encoding, storage, retrieval, or a combination of these. Some common causes include:

1. **Brain Injury:** Traumatic brain injuries (TBI), such as those from accidents, falls, or sports injuries, can cause amnesia. The severity of the memory loss often correlates with the severity of the injury.

2. **Stroke:** A stroke can disrupt blood supply to the brain and damage areas critical for memory processing, leading to amnesia.

3. **Alcohol Abuse:** Excessive alcohol consumption can lead to Wernicke-Korsakoff syndrome, a chronic memory disorder caused by severe thiamine (vitamin B1) deficiency.

4. **Dementia:** Conditions like Alzheimer's disease and other forms of dementia can lead to progressive memory loss (amnesia) as part of their symptomatology.

5. **Seizures:** Certain types of seizures, particularly those originating in the temporal lobe, can cause amnesia.

6. **Brain Surgery or Infections:** Surgery on the brain, infections like encephalitis or meningitis, and tumors can affect areas of the brain responsible for memory.

7. **Psychological Trauma:** In rare cases, severe emotional distress can lead to a type of amnesia known as dissociative amnesia, where a person may forget important personal information and events, usually about traumatic or stressful experiences.

8. **Medications:** Certain medications, particularly sedatives, can impair memory functioning and potentially lead to forms of amnesia.

9. **Electroconvulsive Therapy (ECT):** ECT, used for severe depression and other mental health disorders, can cause short-term memory loss.

10. **Lack of Oxygen to the Brain:** Situations where the brain's oxygen supply is compromised (such as in heart attacks, respiratory distress, or carbon monoxide poisoning) can result in amnesia.

The nature and extent of amnesia depend on the cause and the region of the brain that is affected. For instance, damage to the hippocampus, a part of the brain essential for forming new memories, can lead to difficulties in creating new long-term memories (anterograde amnesia), while damage to other parts of the brain might affect existing memories (retrograde amnesia).

Treatment and prognosis for amnesia vary based on the underlying cause. Some types of amnesia, such as those caused by a mild brain injury or a temporary lack of oxygen, may resolve over time. Other types, especially when due to progressive conditions like Alzheimer's disease, may be irreversible. Management typically involves strategies to support memory and coping mechanisms, and addressing the underlying cause, if treatable.

What to do for amnesia?

Managing and treating amnesia involves a combination of strategies, therapies, and support, depending on the type and cause of the amnesia. Here are some general approaches:

1. **Medical Treatment:** If the amnesia is caused by a medical condition (like a brain injury, stroke, alcohol abuse, or an infection), treating that underlying condition is crucial. This might involve medication, surgery, or other medical interventions.

2. **Cognitive Rehabilitation:** For some people with amnesia, especially those who have suffered a brain injury, cognitive rehabilitation can help. This type of therapy involves a range of activities and exercises designed to improve memory, attention, and other cognitive functions.

3. **Occupational Therapy:** Occupational therapists can help individuals relearn necessary everyday skills and use compensatory strategies to cope with memory loss. This can include learning how to use electronic organizers, notebooks, or calendars to keep track of daily activities.

4. **Psychological Support:** Psychological counseling can help individuals and their families to cope with the emotional impact of living with amnesia. Therapy can also address any co-existing mental health issues, such as depression or anxiety.

5. **Memory Training:** This can involve teaching techniques for organizing information so it is easier to remember and using memory aids like mnemonics.

6. **Environmental Adjustments:** Simplifying a living space with clear labeling of items, maintaining a regular routine, and minimizing the need for remembering complex sequences of tasks can help.

7. **Family and Social Support:** Support from family and friends is vital. They can help with day-to-day tasks, provide emotional support, and assist with memory cues and reminders.

8. **Safety Measures:** For those with severe memory problems, it is important to implement safety measures to prevent wandering, accidents, or injuries. This might include staying with a companion when going out or using GPS devices for location tracking.

9. **Nutrition and Lifestyle:** Healthy lifestyle choices, such as a balanced diet, regular exercise, and adequate sleep, may help improve overall brain health.

10. **Avoid Alcohol and Drugs:** Avoid substances that can negatively affect memory and cognitive function.

11. **Regular Medical Check-ups:** Ongoing medical evaluation is important to monitor the condition and make adjustments to the treatment plan as needed.

It is important to note that some types of amnesia may resolve over time, while others may be permanent. The approach to managing amnesia must be personalized to the individual's specific needs and circumstances. In all cases, the support of a multidisciplinary team including medical professionals, therapists, and support from family and friends is crucial for the best outcome.

What are signs of dissociative identity disorder?

Dissociative Identity Disorder (DID), formerly known as Multiple Personality Disorder, is a complex psychological condition characterized by the presence of two or more distinct personality states or identities within a single individual. These different identities may have their own names, ages, histories, and characteristics, including distinct manners of talking and writing. DID is often a result of severe trauma during early childhood, usually extreme, repetitive physical, sexual, or emotional abuse. Key signs and symptoms include:

1. **Multiple Identities or Personality States:** The individual experiences two or more distinct identities or personality states, each with its own enduring pattern of perceiving, relating to, and thinking about the environment and self.

2. **Amnesia:** There are gaps in memory about everyday events, personal information, and/or traumatic events. This amnesia is more than simple forgetfulness and can be quite extensive, involving lost time, confused life history, and forgetting important personal information.

3. **Time Loss:** Experiencing chunks of time lost, finding oneself in places without remembering how one got there, or finding oneself in the middle of doing something without remembering the start of the action.

4. **Trance-like States:** Periods of blanking out or staring, during which responsiveness to external stimuli is decreased.

5. **Alterations in Sense of Self:** A sense of being detached from oneself; observing one's actions, feelings, thoughts, and body as if they belong to someone else (depersonalization).

6. **Variations in Skills and Preferences:** Different identities may have different abilities, including knowledge of foreign languages, artistic talent, or handwriting styles. Preferences in food, clothes, and activities can also change.
7. **Fluctuations in Relationships and Attitudes:** Sudden changes in attitudes towards people, for instance, going from being close to someone to not recognizing them or feeling suddenly uncomfortable around them.
8. **Distinct Physical Characteristics:** Different identities may exhibit different physical characteristics, such as differences in voice, posture, or facial expressions. There might also be a variation in medical conditions such as allergies or vision acuity.
9. **Psychological Distress and Impairment:** Symptoms cause significant distress and impairment in social, occupational, or other areas of functioning.
10. **Other Symptoms:** Headaches, time distortion, trance-like states, auditory or visual hallucinations, and self-injurious behaviors can also be associated with DID.

It is important to note that DID is a controversial and often misunderstood condition. Its diagnosis is complex and should only be made by a qualified mental health professional through a comprehensive evaluation. DID is often comorbid with other psychiatric disorders, including depression, anxiety, and PTSD, and effective treatment usually involves long-term psychotherapy. The goal of therapy is to integrate the separate identities into one primary identity and to address the trauma that led to the development of DID.

How is amnesia diagnosed?

Diagnosing amnesia typically involves a comprehensive evaluation that includes a detailed medical history, physical and neurological examinations, and cognitive testing. The process is designed to assess memory loss, identify its possible causes, and rule out other conditions. Here is a closer look at the typical steps involved in diagnosing amnesia:

1. **Medical History:** The doctor will ask about the patient's memory loss, including when it started, how it has progressed, and any factors that could have contributed to it, such as head injuries, recent surgeries, alcohol use, or family history of neurological conditions.
2. **Physical Examination:** A general physical examination can help rule out other potential causes of memory loss, like an infection or nutritional deficiency.
3. **Neurological Exam:** This exam tests reflexes, sensory function, balance, and other aspects of the brain and nervous system.
4. **Cognitive Tests:** These tests assess memory, problem-solving skills, math skills, language abilities, and other intellectual functions. They help determine the extent of memory loss and which areas of memory are affected.
5. **Laboratory Tests:** Blood tests can detect physical problems that can affect memory, such as thyroid dysfunction or vitamin deficiencies.
6. **Brain Imaging:** Imaging tests such as magnetic resonance imaging (MRI) or computed tomography (CT) scans can detect brain abnormalities that might be causing memory problems. These could include brain tumors, strokes, or damage from head trauma.
7. **Psychiatric Evaluation:** This can help determine whether depression, anxiety, or another mental health condition is contributing to the symptoms.
8. **Neuropsychological Testing:** This comprehensive assessment of cognitive skills can be particularly helpful. It might be used to determine the extent of memory impairment, what kind of help the patient needs, how well they can handle daily life activities, and whether they can safely operate a vehicle.

There is no one test that confirms amnesia. Instead, diagnosis is typically made based on the pattern of symptoms and by ruling out other conditions that could cause similar symptoms. In cases where the cause of the amnesia is not clear, the diagnosis may need to be revisited over time as new symptoms appear or current symptoms evolve.

What is delirium?

Delirium is a serious disturbance in mental abilities that results in confused thinking and reduced awareness of the environment. It is a rapid-onset, acute, and usually reversible condition that is quite common, particularly among older adults, hospitalized patients, and those with serious, chronic, or terminal illnesses. Delirium represents a significant change from the individual's baseline level of cognitive function and is often temporary.

Key characteristics of delirium include:

1. **Altered Level of Consciousness:** This can range from hyperalertness to drowsiness or stupor. The level of consciousness may fluctuate throughout the day.
2. **Reduced Awareness and Attention:** Difficulty focusing, maintaining, or shifting attention is a core feature. There might be an inability to stay on task or follow conversations.
3. **Disorganized Thinking:** This manifests as rambling or irrelevant speech, unclear or illogical flow of ideas, or confusion about time and place.
4. **Memory Deficits:** Short-term memory loss is common, though long-term memory may remain intact.
5. **Disorientation:** The person may not know where they are, the time or date, or even their own identity in severe cases.
6. **Perceptual Disturbances:** These can include hallucinations (often visual) or delusions, which can be distressing for the individual.
7. **Behavioral Changes:** There may be rapid mood swings, restlessness, agitation, or a decrease in responsiveness.
8. **Sleep Disturbances:** This includes insomnia or, conversely, excessive sleepiness, as well as a disturbed sleep-wake cycle.

The causes of delirium are numerous and can include infections, medication side effects or withdrawal, metabolic imbalances (like low sodium or low calcium), dehydration, alcohol or drug intoxication, lack of sleep, surgery, and severe physical illness, among others. In many cases, delirium is multifactorial, meaning it results from a combination of factors.

Diagnosis involves a medical assessment that includes a review of medications, medical history, neurological exam, and sometimes blood tests or brain imaging to identify or rule out possible causes.

Treatment of delirium focuses on addressing the underlying cause(s) and may include medication adjustments, rehydration, treating infections, or addressing metabolic imbalances. Supportive care is also important, including ensuring a safe environment, aiding orientation and communication, and involving family and caregivers.

Early recognition and treatment of delirium can significantly improve outcomes, but if left untreated, it can lead to serious complications, including a decline in long-term cognitive function.

What is delirium tremens (DT)?

Delirium Tremens (DTs) is a severe form of alcohol withdrawal that involves sudden and severe mental or nervous system changes. It is a potentially life-threatening condition and is considered a medical emergency. Delirium tremens most commonly occurs in individuals who have a history of heavy alcohol use for prolonged periods (years) and suddenly stop or significantly reduce their alcohol consumption. It typically appears 48 to 96 hours after the last drink, but it can occur up to 10 days after drinking stops.

Key features of delirium tremens include:

1. **Severe Confusion and Disorientation:** This is a hallmark of DTs and can be severe enough to significantly impair a person's ability to function normally.
2. **Tremors:** The "tremens" in the name refers to the shaking (tremors) commonly experienced, particularly in the hands.
3. **Hallucinations:** Individuals may experience visual, auditory, or tactile hallucinations. Visual hallucinations can be particularly vivid and frightening.
4. **Agitation and Irritability:** These symptoms are common and can fluctuate in intensity.
5. **Seizures:** Grand mal seizures are a dangerous symptom of DTs and typically occur within the first 48 hours after the last drink.
6. **Changes in Mental Function:** This can include memory loss, confusion, and difficulty concentrating or paying attention.
7. **Autonomic Hyperactivity:** This includes symptoms like rapid heart rate, high blood pressure, fever, and excessive sweating.
8. **Sleep Disturbances:** Difficulty sleeping or nightmares are common.
9. **Sensitivity to Light, Sound, and Touch:** Individuals may have an exaggerated response to sensory stimuli.

The risk of DTs increases with a history of repeated episodes of alcohol withdrawal, older age, and the presence of concurrent medical or psychiatric conditions.

Treatment for delirium tremens typically requires hospitalization and may include:

- **Benzodiazepines:** These are the first-line treatment for DTs and help reduce withdrawal symptoms.
- **Fluid Replacement and Nutritional Support:** Replenishing fluids, vitamins (especially thiamine), and nutrients is crucial.
- **Treatment of Co-occurring Medical Issues:** Any other medical problems that arise or are present need to be treated.
- **Monitoring and Support:** Continuous monitoring to ensure the patient's safety and to manage complications is vital.

Without treatment, DTs can lead to significant complications, including respiratory failure, cardiac arrhythmias, aspiration pneumonia, and even death. With appropriate medical treatment, however, the prognosis improves significantly.

What causes DT's in alcoholics?

Delirium Tremens (DTs) in alcoholics is primarily caused by a sudden withdrawal from heavy and prolonged alcohol use. Alcohol has a depressive effect on the brain and, over time, the chronic use of alcohol causes the brain to adapt to its presence. When alcohol is suddenly removed or significantly reduced, the brain remains in a hyperactive, or hyperaroused, state, leading to the symptoms of withdrawal, which can be severe in the case of DTs. Several factors contribute to the development of DTs:

1. **Neurochemical Imbalance:** Chronic alcohol use disrupts the balance of neurotransmitters in the brain, particularly gamma-aminobutyric acid (GABA), which has inhibitory effects, and glutamate, which has excitatory effects. Alcohol enhances the inhibitory effects of GABA and suppresses the excitatory effects of glutamate. When alcohol use is suddenly stopped, there is a relative deficiency of GABA's inhibitory effects and an excess of glutamate's excitatory effects, leading to symptoms of hyperarousal and excitability.
2. **Chronic Heavy Alcohol Use:** DTs typically occur in individuals who have a history of heavy alcohol use over a period of years. The risk increases with the duration and intensity of alcohol abuse.
3. **Previous Withdrawal Episodes:** Repeated episodes of alcohol withdrawal can alter neuronal activity and make subsequent withdrawals more severe, a phenomenon known as kindling.
4. **Nutritional Deficiencies:** Chronic alcoholism often leads to poor nutrition and deficiencies in key vitamins, especially thiamine (vitamin B1), which is critical for brain function. These deficiencies can exacerbate withdrawal symptoms and contribute to the severity of DTs.
5. **Physical Health:** Poor overall physical health, liver disease, and co-existing medical conditions can increase the risk and severity of DTs.
6. **Genetic Factors:** There may be a genetic predisposition that makes some individuals more susceptible to alcohol withdrawal syndromes, including DTs.
7. **Age and General Health:** Older adults and those with underlying health conditions may be at higher risk for severe withdrawal symptoms.
8. **Abrupt Cessation or Reduction of Alcohol:** DTs is most likely to occur when a person who is dependent on alcohol either stops drinking entirely or significantly reduces their alcohol intake too quickly.

DTs is a serious and potentially life-threatening condition. It is crucial for individuals at risk of DTs to seek medical assistance when attempting to quit or reduce alcohol use, as withdrawal should be managed under professional medical supervision. Medical treatment typically involves the use of benzodiazepines, which can help to safely manage the symptoms of withdrawal, along with supportive care and treatment of any nutritional deficiencies.

What causes delirium after surgery?

Delirium after surgery, often referred to as postoperative delirium, can be caused by a variety of factors. These include:

1. **Anesthetic Agents:** Some anesthetic drugs can contribute to the development of delirium, especially in elderly patients or those with pre-existing cognitive impairments.
2. **Age:** Older adults are at higher risk for postoperative delirium, possibly due to decreased physiological reserve and the presence of other medical conditions.
3. **Pre-existing Cognitive Impairment:** Patients with dementia, Alzheimer's disease, or other forms of cognitive decline are more susceptible to delirium.
4. **Type and Duration of Surgery:** Longer and more complex surgeries, particularly cardiac and major

orthopedic procedures, are associated with a higher risk of delirium.

5. **Postoperative pain and pain management:** Inadequately controlled pain, as well as certain pain medications, can contribute to the development of delirium.
6. **Electrolyte imbalances and dehydration:** These conditions can occur during or after surgery and can affect brain function.
7. **Infection:** Postoperative infections, including pneumonia and urinary tract infections, can lead to delirium, especially in older adults.
8. **Environmental factors:** Being in an unfamiliar environment, such as a hospital, especially with altered sleep patterns and sensory input, can contribute to delirium.
9. **Psychological factors:** Stress, anxiety, and depression related to surgery can also play a role.
10. **Other medical conditions:** Pre-existing or newly developed conditions such as heart failure, stroke, or respiratory problems can increase the risk.

It is important to note that delirium is often multifactorial, meaning that it is usually caused by a combination of these factors rather than a single cause. Prevention and management of postoperative delirium involve addressing as many of these factors as possible, both before and after surgery.

What is dementia?

Dementia is a broad term used to describe a decline in cognitive function severe enough to interfere with daily life. It is not a specific disease but rather a general term that encompasses a wide range of specific medical conditions, including Alzheimer's disease. The symptoms of dementia can vary greatly, but at least two of the following core mental functions must be significantly impaired to be considered dementia:

1. **Memory:** This is often one of the first signs of dementia, where the individual may forget information they have recently learned, important dates or events, or ask for the same information over and over.
2. **Communication and Language:** A person with dementia may have difficulty following or joining a conversation. They may stop in the middle of a conversation and have no idea how to continue, or they may repeat themselves.
3. **Ability to Focus and Pay Attention:** Concentration can be affected, making it difficult to focus on tasks.
4. **Reasoning and Judgment:** There may be changes in judgment or decision-making. For example, a person with dementia may make poor decisions in social interactions or give away large sums of money when it is out of character for them.
5. **Visual Perception:** Problems with visual and spatial abilities can also occur, such as difficulty reading, judging distance, and determining color or contrast, potentially causing problems with driving.

Different types of dementia are associated with particular types of brain cell damage in particular regions of the brain. For example, in Alzheimer's disease, high levels of certain proteins inside and outside brain cells make it hard for brain cells to stay healthy and to communicate with each other. The brain region called the hippocampus is the center of learning and memory in the brain, and the brain cells in this region are often the first to be damaged.

It is important to note that dementia is more common as people grow older, but it is not a normal part of aging. Many people live into their 90s and beyond without any signs of dementia. The cause of dementia depends on the underlying disease. In some cases, dementia may be reversible, especially when caused by factors such as medication side effects, depression, vitamin deficiencies, or thyroid problems. However, most forms of dementia are progressive and incurable. Early diagnosis and intervention strategies are improving dramatically, and treatment can help manage symptoms in some cases.

How is delirium different from dementia?

Delirium and dementia are both conditions that affect mental function, but they have distinct differences in terms of their onset, duration, and underlying causes:

1. **Onset:**
   - Delirium typically develops over a short period, often hours to a few days. It represents a sudden change from the person's baseline level of cognitive function.
   - Dementia, on the other hand, develops gradually over months to years. The changes in cognition are slow and progressive.
2. **Duration:**
   - Delirium is usually a temporary condition. The

symptoms can fluctuate throughout the day, and it often resolves with proper treatment of the underlying cause.

- Dementia is generally a chronic and progressive condition. Although the rate of progression can vary, the cognitive decline is typically irreversible.

3. **Symptoms:**

- Delirium is primarily characterized by confusion, disorientation, and attention deficits. Hallucinations and delusions are common, and there may be rapid shifts in mood and behavior.
- Dementia mainly involves memory loss, especially difficulty with short-term memory. Other symptoms include problems with language, problem-solving, and other cognitive skills necessary for daily life.

4. **Causes:**

- Delirium can be triggered by a variety of factors, such as medication side effects, infections, dehydration, substance intoxication or withdrawal, and acute medical illnesses.
- Dementia is caused by damage to brain cells, which can be due to diseases like Alzheimer's, vascular dementia, Lewy body dementia, or frontotemporal dementia.

5. **Consciousness:**

- Delirium often affects consciousness. People with delirium may have periods of inattention, distraction, or even stupor.
- Dementia does not typically affect the level of consciousness. People with dementia are usually alert, barring complications or co-occurring illnesses.

6. **Reversibility:**

- Delirium is often reversible if the underlying cause is identified and treated promptly.
- Dementia is typically not reversible. Some forms of dementia may have medications available that can help slow the progression or manage symptoms, but these do not cure the condition.

In clinical practice, it can be challenging to distinguish between delirium and dementia, especially since patients with dementia are at higher risk of developing delirium. Sometimes, they may coexist, which complicates the diagnosis and management. Understanding these differences is crucial for proper treatment and care.

What is addiction?

Addiction is a complex condition, often referred to as a substance use disorder in medical terms. It is characterized by compulsive engagement in rewarding stimuli, despite adverse consequences. Here are key aspects of addiction:

1. **Compulsive Behavior:** Addiction involves engaging in a behavior or using a substance to the point where it becomes a compulsive action. The individual feels an overwhelming need to continue the behavior or use the substance.
2. **Physical and Psychological Dependence:** Over time, a person may develop a physical dependence on a substance, meaning their body has adapted to its presence and will experience withdrawal symptoms without it. Psychological dependence involves emotional or mental reliance on a substance or behavior, often used as a coping mechanism for stress or other emotional states.
3. **Tolerance:** With continued use, tolerance can develop, meaning the individual needs more of the substance to achieve the same effect.
4. **Withdrawal Symptoms:** Stopping the substance or behavior often leads to withdrawal symptoms, which can be physical (like nausea, shaking, or sweating) and psychological (like irritability, anxiety, or depression).
5. **Continued Use Despite Negative Consequences:** People with addiction will continue to use the substance or engage in the behavior despite experiencing significant negative consequences, such as health problems, financial issues, or strained relationships.
6. **Changes in Brain Function:** Addiction can cause changes in areas of the brain involved in reward, motivation, learning, judgment, and memory. These changes can last long after the immediate effects of the substance wear off.

Addiction is not limited to substances like alcohol, nicotine, or illicit drugs. Behaviors, such as gambling, can also be addictive. The causes of addiction are complex and multifaceted, including genetic, environmental, and psychological factors.

Treatment for addiction typically involves a combination of therapy, medication, lifestyle changes, and support groups. The goal of treatment is to help the individual stop using the substance or engaging in the behavior, manage withdrawal symptoms, and develop healthier coping mechanisms. Recovery from addiction is a lifelong process with challenges, but with proper support and treatment, individuals can overcome addiction and lead productive lives.

What is the most common addiction?

As of my last update in April 2023, the most common addiction worldwide is typically related to nicotine, due to the widespread use of tobacco products. Nicotine addiction is prevalent because tobacco is legally available in most countries, and its use is often socially accepted or even encouraged in certain cultures. Other common addictions include:

1. **Alcohol:** Alcohol use disorder is another widespread addiction. Due to its legal status and cultural acceptance in many societies, alcohol is readily available and frequently abused.
2. **Prescription Drugs:** Opioids, sedatives, and anxiolytics prescribed for pain, anxiety, or sleep disorders can be highly addictive. The misuse of these drugs has led to significant health crises in several countries, notably in the United States.
3. **Illicit Drugs:** Substances such as cocaine, heroin, and methamphetamine are also common sources of addiction. These drugs are illegal in most jurisdictions but are abused for their psychoactive effects.
4. **Cannabis:** While cannabis is the most widely used illicit drug globally, its addiction rates are generally lower compared to substances like alcohol or opioids. However, its increased legalization and changing societal attitudes may impact its use and potentially its rates of addiction.
5. **Behavioral Addictions:** Addictions to behaviors such as gambling, internet use, or sex are increasingly recognized. While they don't involve substance abuse, they share similar patterns of compulsive behavior and negative impact on life.

It is important to note that the prevalence of specific addictions can vary significantly by region, culture, and socioeconomic factors. Additionally, the growing awareness and changing legal statuses of substances (like cannabis) can also influence patterns of addiction over time.

What is the most addictive drug?

The concept of the "most addictive drug" can be subjective and varies depending on the criteria used to define addiction. However, certain substances are commonly recognized for their high potential for addiction due to their powerful effects on the brain and body. Some of the most addictive drugs include:

1. **Heroin:** Often considered one of the most addictive substances, heroin, an opioid, is known for creating a rapid sense of euphoria by acting on the brain's reward system. It also leads to a high degree of physical dependence and severe withdrawal symptoms.
2. **Cocaine and Crack Cocaine:** Cocaine, especially in its freebase form known as crack cocaine, is highly addictive. It stimulates the brain's reward pathways and can create a powerful, but short-lived, euphoric effect, leading to repeated use and increased risk of addiction.
3. **Methamphetamine:** Known for its powerful stimulant effects, methamphetamine can create a strong sense of euphoria, increased energy, and alertness. It also significantly alters the brain's dopamine system, which can lead to rapid development of addiction.
4. **Nicotine:** Found in tobacco products, nicotine is one of the most commonly used addictive substances. It is considered highly addictive due to its widespread availability and the rapidity with which it affects the brain.
5. **Alcohol:** Despite being legal in many parts of the world, alcohol has a high potential for addiction. It alters the brain's reward system and can lead to physical dependence and withdrawal symptoms.
6. **Benzodiazepines:** Used to treat anxiety and insomnia, benzodiazepines can be highly addictive, especially when used over a long period or misused. They cause physical dependence and have potentially severe withdrawal symptoms.
7. **Opioid Painkillers:** Prescription opioids like oxycodone and fentanyl are highly addictive. They produce significant euphoria and pain relief, but they also carry a high risk of addiction and overdose.

The addictiveness of a drug can depend on various factors, including how quickly it affects the brain, the intensity of the pleasure it produces, how long its effects last, and the severity of withdrawal symptoms. Additionally, individual factors such as genetics, personal history, and the presence of mental health disorders also play a significant role in addiction risk.

What is alcohol addiction?

Alcohol addiction, also known as alcoholism or alcohol use disorder (AUD), is a chronic, often progressive medical condition characterized by an inability to control or stop alcohol use despite adverse social, occupational, or health consequences. It encompasses a range of behaviors and symptoms, indicating that a person's drinking habits are problematic and potentially harmful. Key aspects of alcohol addiction include:

1. **Craving or Strong Urge to Drink:** Feeling a strong, often irresistible urge to consume alcohol.
2. **Loss of Control:** Inability to limit drinking in terms of both frequency and quantity.
3. **Physical Dependence:** Experiencing withdrawal symptoms when not drinking, such as sweating, shaking, nausea, and anxiety.
4. **Tolerance:** Needing to drink increasingly larger amounts of alcohol to feel its effects.
5. **Continued Use Despite Problems:** Continuing to drink alcohol even though it is causing physical health problems, mental health issues like anxiety or depression, or problems in relationships, work, or other areas of life.
6. **Neglect of Other Activities:** Spending less time on activities that used to be important (hobbies, socializing, work) due to alcohol use.
7. **Drinking in Risky Situations:** Using alcohol in situations where it is hazardous, like drinking and driving or operating machinery.

The causes of alcohol addiction are multifactorial and can include genetic predisposition, environmental factors, psychological issues, and social influences. Often, it is a combination of these factors. The effects of alcohol addiction can be far-reaching, impacting almost every organ in the body and leading to a variety of health issues, including liver disease, cardiovascular problems, neurological damage, and increased risk for certain cancers.

Alcohol addiction also has significant psychological, social, and economic impacts, both for the individual and their wider community. It can strain relationships, cause work-related issues, and lead to financial problems.

Treatment for alcohol addiction is multi-faceted and can include detoxification (especially for those with physical dependence), behavioral therapies, medication, and support groups. The goal of treatment is to help the individual stop using alcohol, manage withdrawal symptoms and cravings, and address any underlying psychological or social issues that may contribute to their addiction. Recovery is a long-term process and often requires ongoing support and management.

What is the difference between dependence and alcohol abuse?

Dependence and alcohol abuse are related but distinct concepts when discussing alcohol use disorders. Understanding the difference between them is important for recognizing and treating these conditions effectively.

1. **Alcohol Dependence:**
   - **Definition:** Alcohol dependence is a physical or physiological state in which the body becomes accustomed to the presence of alcohol and adapts to its effects. It is often a component of addiction.
   - **Characteristics:**
     - o **Tolerance:** Needing increasing amounts of alcohol to achieve the same effect.
     - o **Withdrawal Symptoms:** Experiencing physical and psychological symptoms (like nausea, sweating, shaking, and anxiety) when alcohol use is reduced or stopped.
     - o **Compulsion to Drink:** A strong or uncontrollable desire to consume alcohol.
   - **Consequence:** Dependence primarily refers to the physical and psychological aspects of alcohol use and can lead to significant health problems and disruptions in daily functioning.
2. **Alcohol Abuse:**
   - **Definition:** Alcohol abuse, often considered a pattern of drinking, refers to the misuse of alcohol in a way that is harmful or in which it causes detrimental effects on a person's life.
   - **Characteristics:**
     - o **Harmful Use:** Drinking in a way that is damaging to health, both physical and mental.
     - o **Neglect of Responsibilities:** Failing to fulfill work, school, or home responsibilities due to drinking.

  - o **Risky Behavior:** Engaging in potentially dangerous activities while drinking, like driving under the influence.
  - o **Legal and Social Problems:** Experiencing legal issues, such as arrests for behavior related to alcohol use, or having social and relationship problems.
- **Consequence:** Alcohol abuse focuses more on the behavioral aspect and the impact of drinking on various areas of life, rather than the physical dependence.

It is possible for someone to abuse alcohol without being dependent on it. For example, a person may engage in binge drinking (a form of alcohol abuse) on weekends without showing signs of dependence like tolerance or withdrawal. Conversely, someone can be dependent on alcohol (needing it to function or avoid withdrawal symptoms) without necessarily abusing it in a socially or legally problematic way.

Both alcohol dependence and abuse are serious conditions that can lead to long-term health problems and other negative outcomes. They may require different approaches to treatment, with dependence often needing medical management for withdrawal and abuse potentially focusing more on behavioral interventions and lifestyle changes.

What is pain?

Pain is a complex and subjective experience that involves sensory and emotional components. It is a signal in the nervous system that something may be wrong. Pain is not just a physical sensation but also influenced by attitudes, beliefs, personality, and social factors, and can affect emotional and mental wellbeing. Here are some key aspects of pain:

1. **Types of Pain:**
   - Acute Pain: Usually a sharp sensation, acute pain starts suddenly and is often caused by something specific. It acts as an alert to disease or a threat to the body and typically lasts for a short time.
   - Chronic Pain: This type of pain lasts for a longer period, often persisting for months or even longer. Chronic pain can result from an ongoing cause, such as arthritis, or can be the result of nerve damage or other factors, even after the initial injury or illness has healed.
2. **Causes of Pain:**
   - Pain can arise from tissue damage (nociceptive pain), such as cuts or burns, or from nerve damage or dysfunction (neuropathic pain).
   - It can also be psychogenic, meaning it is related to psychological factors.
3. **Physiological Response:** When you experience pain, signals are transmitted through the nervous system to the brain, where the pain is interpreted and perceived.
4. **Purpose of Pain:** In its basic form, pain is a critical mechanism that helps protect the body. It prompts the individual to react and take action to prevent further injury.
5. **Variability:** Pain is highly subjective and can vary greatly from person to person. Factors such as mood, genetic makeup, and previous experiences can influence how an individual perceives pain.
6. **Management:** Pain management can be complex and may involve medications (like analgesics and anti-inflammatories), physical therapy, psychological approaches (like cognitive-behavioral therapy), and lifestyle changes (such as exercise and relaxation techniques).

Understanding pain is crucial for effective treatment and management. Since pain is a personal experience, effective pain management often requires a holistic approach that addresses both the physical and emotional aspects of pain.

What is evolutionary aspect of pain?

The evolutionary aspect of pain is deeply rooted in its role as a critical survival mechanism. From an evolutionary perspective, pain serves several important functions:

1. **Protection from Injury:** Pain acts as a warning signal that alerts an organism to potential or actual damage to its tissues. This immediate sensation of pain prompts protective reflexes, like withdrawing a hand from a hot surface, helping to prevent more severe injuries.
2. **Promotes Healing:** After an injury, pain typically leads to a behavior change, such as reduced use of an injured part (like limping to reduce pressure on a wounded leg). This involuntary or voluntary reduction in activity helps ensure that the injured area is protected from further damage and can heal properly.
3. **Avoidance Learning:** Painful experiences are powerful teachers. The unpleasant nature of pain creates a strong memory association with the harmful stimuli or circumstances that caused it.

This learned avoidance helps organisms steer clear of similar threats in the future, enhancing survival.

4. **Indication of Disease or Internal Disorders:** Pain is not always the result of external injuries. It can also signal internal problems, such as diseases or infections, prompting the individual to seek help or treatment.

5. **Social Cohesion and Empathy:** In social species, like humans, witnessing pain in others can foster empathy, cooperation, and social bonding. The ability to perceive and respond to pain in others can lead to behaviors that benefit group survival, such as caring for the injured.

6. **Natural Selection and Adaptation:** Throughout evolution, individuals who could effectively respond to pain by avoiding or minimizing injuries and diseases were more likely to survive and reproduce. This natural selection process has led to the development and refinement of pain systems in various species.

In summary, pain is a crucial biological mechanism that has evolved to protect organisms from harm, promote healing, facilitate learning to avoid danger, signal internal disorders, and in some species, reinforce social bonds. Its role in survival and adaptation makes it a fundamental aspect of the evolutionary process.

What is chronic fatigue syndrome?

Chronic Fatigue Syndrome (CFS), also known as Myalgic Encephalomyelitis (ME), is a complex and long-term illness characterized by extreme fatigue that cannot be fully explained by an underlying medical condition. The fatigue worsens with physical or mental activity but does not improve with rest. The cause of CFS is still not completely understood, and there is no single test to diagnose it. Here are some key aspects of Chronic Fatigue Syndrome:

1. **Symptoms:** The primary symptom of CFS is persistent and unexplained fatigue. Other common symptoms include:
   - Sleep problems.
   - Muscle or joint pain.
   - Headaches.
   - Sore throat or sore lymph nodes that are not swollen.
   - Cognitive difficulties, often described as "brain fog," involving problems with memory, concentration, and processing information.
   - Physical or mental exertion causing exhaustion (post-exertional malaise) that lasts more than 24 hours.
   - Dizziness or nausea.

2. **Diagnosis:** There is no specific test for CFS. Diagnosis is usually made based on symptoms and after ruling out other potential causes of fatigue, such as sleep disorders, mental health issues, and other medical conditions that cause similar symptoms.

3. **Causes:** The exact cause of CFS is unknown. Potential triggers have been identified, including viral infections, psychological stress, immune dysfunction, and hormonal imbalances. Some people may have a genetic predisposition to the disorder.

4. **Treatment:** Treatment of CFS focuses on symptom relief and includes a combination of:
   - Cognitive-behavioral therapy (CBT) to help manage symptoms.
   - Graded exercise therapy, which involves slowly increasing the duration and intensity of physical activity.
   - Medications to address pain, sleep disturbances, and other specific symptoms.
   - Lifestyle changes, like pacing activities and stress management.

5. **Prognosis:** The course of CFS varies widely. Some people gradually improve and may recover fully, while others continue to experience symptoms for years. Early diagnosis and a comprehensive approach to management can improve the chances of improvement.

6. **Controversy and Awareness:** CFS/ME has been a subject of much debate and controversy, partly due to the lack of clear diagnostic criteria and unknown etiology. Increased awareness and understanding have led to more recognition of CFS/ME as a legitimate and disabling condition.

CFS/ME is often misunderstood and can be debilitating for those who suffer from it. Ongoing research is crucial for better understanding, diagnosing, treating, and ultimately finding a cure for this challenging condition.

Is chronic fatigue and fibromyalgia the same thing?

Chronic Fatigue Syndrome (CFS) and Fibromyalgia are distinct conditions, but they share some similarities, which can sometimes lead to confusion or misdiagnosis. Here is a comparison to highlight their differences and similarities:

Chronic Fatigue Syndrome (CFS):

- **Primary Symptom:** Extreme fatigue that significantly interferes with daily activities and is not relieved by rest.
- **Other Symptoms:** Post-exertional malaise (worsening of symptoms after physical or mental exertion), muscle and joint pain, headaches, sleep disturbances, and problems with memory and concentration.
- **Cause:** The exact cause is unknown, but it may be triggered by viral infections, immune dysfunction, and hormonal imbalances.
- **Diagnosis:** Based on symptoms, after ruling out other causes of fatigue. There are no specific tests for CFS.

Fibromyalgia:

- **Primary Symptom:** Widespread musculoskeletal pain accompanied by fatigue, sleep, memory, and mood issues.
- **Other Symptoms:** Tender points on the body, headaches, irritable bowel syndrome, anxiety, and depression.
- **Cause:** The exact cause is unclear but may involve genetic factors, infections, physical or emotional trauma, and abnormalities in pain perception.
- **Diagnosis:** Based on a history of widespread pain lasting more than three months and the presence of other typical symptoms. There are no definitive tests for fibromyalgia.

Similarities:

- Both conditions are characterized by fatigue and pain.
- Neither has a clear, identifiable cause or a definitive diagnostic test.
- Both conditions are more common in women.
- Management of both often involves a combination of medication, exercise, stress reduction, and cognitive-behavioral therapy.

Differences:

- The primary complaint in CFS is persistent and debilitating fatigue, while in fibromyalgia, it is chronic pain.
- Fibromyalgia is often identified by specific tender points on the body, which is not a feature of CFS.
- The nature and extent of fatigue differ between the two conditions.

While they are distinct conditions, it is not uncommon for a person to suffer from both CFS and fibromyalgia simultaneously, which can complicate diagnosis and treatment. In both cases, an individualized approach to management and treatment is essential.

What is chronic pain?

Chronic pain is a persistent pain that lasts for weeks, months, or even years. It differs from acute pain, which is a normal sensation triggered in the nervous system to alert you to possible injury and the need to take care of yourself. Chronic pain persists long past the time of the initial injury or the usual course of an illness. Here are some key aspects of chronic pain:

1. **Duration:** Chronic pain is typically defined as pain that lasts more than 3 to 6 months, or beyond the normal healing time for an injury.
2. **Causes:** It can arise from a variety of causes, including ongoing health conditions (like arthritis or cancer), injuries that have healed but left pain pathways altered, nerve damage, and sometimes the cause of chronic pain remains unknown.
3. **Types:** It can manifest in various forms, such as headaches, joint pain, pain from injury, back pain, tendinitis, sinus pain, carpal tunnel syndrome, and pain affecting specific parts of the body, like the shoulders, pelvis, and neck.
4. **Impact on Quality of Life:** Chronic pain can lead to decreased mobility, difficulty sleeping, changes in mood (including symptoms of depression and anxiety), a decrease in appetite, and an overall reduced quality of life.
5. **Physical Changes:** Prolonged pain can cause changes in the nervous system that make the body more sensitive to pain. This phenomenon, known as "central sensitization," can make even mild or normal stimuli painful.
6. **Treatment:** Managing chronic pain often requires a multifaceted approach. This can include medications (pain relievers, anti-inflammatory drugs, antidepressants, anticonvulsants), physical therapy, exercise, acupuncture, local electrical stimulation, brain stimulation, psychological therapy, and sometimes surgery.

7. **Psychological Aspect:** Because of the ongoing nature of chronic pain, it can have significant psychological impacts. Treatment often involves addressing the emotional aspect of pain, which can include strategies like cognitive-behavioral therapy (CBT) to help manage the psychological effects of chronic pain.

Chronic pain is a complex and challenging condition to treat because it is influenced by many factors, including the person's physical health, environment, and psychological state. Effective management often requires a combination of therapies and a tailored approach to each individual's situation.

What is headache?

A headache is a pain or discomfort in the head, scalp, or neck. It is one of the most common forms of pain and can range from a mild, temporary condition to a symptom of a more serious disorder. Headaches can vary greatly in terms of their intensity, frequency, and duration. There are several types of headaches, each with its own set of causes, symptoms, and treatment methods. The most common types of headaches include:

1. **Tension Headaches:** The most common type of headache among adults and teenagers. Tension headaches are often described as a feeling of a tight band around the head, with a constant, dull ache on both sides. They are usually caused by muscle tension in the head and neck, but the exact cause is often unknown.

2. **Migraines:** Migraines are often characterized by a throbbing or pulsing pain on one side of the head. They can be accompanied by other symptoms like sensitivity to light and sound, nausea, and vomiting. Migraines can last for hours to days, and the pain can be so severe that it interferes with daily activities.

3. **Cluster Headaches:** These are severe headaches that occur in clusters or patterns, typically around one eye or one side of the head. They can be extremely painful, often described as a burning or piercing sensation. Cluster headaches are rare and the exact cause is unknown, though they may be related to the body's biological clock.

4. **Sinus Headaches:** Associated with sinusitis, these headaches are felt in the forehead, cheeks, and bridge of the nose. They are usually accompanied by other sinus symptoms, such as a runny nose, fever, and facial swelling.

5. **Secondary Headaches:** These are headaches that are caused by another medical condition, such as a sinus infection, neck injuries, brain tumors, or high blood pressure.

The treatment of headaches depends on the type and frequency of the headaches as well as the underlying cause. Common treatments include pain relievers, lifestyle changes such as stress management and improved sleep habits, and, for more severe cases like migraines and cluster headaches, prescription medications or other medical treatments.

Preventive measures can also be effective in reducing the frequency and severity of headaches. These may include regular exercise, staying hydrated, maintaining a regular sleep schedule, eating balanced meals, and avoiding known headache triggers. For chronic or severe headaches, consulting a healthcare provider is recommended to determine the best course of treatment.

What is the most common type of headache?

The most common type of headache is the tension headache. Tension headaches are widespread and can affect anyone, although they are more prevalent in adults and adolescents. These headaches are often described as a constant dull, aching sensation on both sides of the head or a sensation of tightness or pressure across the forehead or on the sides and back of the head. Some people also experience tenderness on their scalp, neck, and shoulder muscles.

Unlike migraines, tension headaches typically do not cause nausea or vomiting, and they do not usually worsen with physical activity. While they can be bothersome, tension headaches generally do not disrupt daily activities as severely as migraines can.

The exact cause of tension headaches is not completely understood, but several factors are believed to contribute to their occurrence, including stress, muscle strain, and poor posture. They can also be triggered by environmental and lifestyle factors such as eye strain, lack of sleep, poor posture, stress, and anxiety.

Most tension headaches can be effectively treated with over-the-counter pain relievers like acetaminophen or ibuprofen, as well as lifestyle modifications to reduce stress and improve posture. For those who experience chronic tension headaches, healthcare professionals may recommend preventative measures, relaxation techniques, and sometimes prescription medications.

What is the difference between migraine and tension headache?

Migraine and tension headaches are two of the most common types of headaches, but they have distinct characteristics and symptoms:

Tension Headaches

- **Description:** Often described as a constant, dull ache on both sides of the head. It feels like a tight band or pressure around the head.
- **Pain Intensity:** Generally mild to moderate.
- **Associated Symptoms:** Rarely cause symptoms beyond the headache itself. There is no nausea or vomiting, and they don't typically worsen with routine physical activity.
- **Duration:** Can last from 30 minutes to a week.
- **Triggers:** Often related to stress, muscle strain, or posture.
- **Treatment:** Usually managed with over-the-counter pain relievers, stress management, and relaxation techniques.

Migraines

- **Description:** Characterized by a throbbing or pulsing pain, often on one side of the head.
- **Pain Intensity:** Tends to be moderate to severe.
- **Associated Symptoms:** May include nausea or vomiting, sensitivity to light and sound, and sometimes visual disturbances known as "aura" (like flashes of light, blind spots, or other vision changes).
- **Duration:** Last anywhere from 4 hours to 3 days.
- Triggers: Can include hormonal changes, certain foods and drinks, stress, sensory stimuli, changes in wake-sleep pattern, physical factors, changes in the environment, and medications.
- **Treatment:** Might require specific medication prescribed by a doctor, such as triptans, ergotamine, or preventive medications. Lifestyle changes and avoiding triggers are also important.

Key Differences

1. **Pain Characteristics:** Tension headaches are usually described as a feeling of pressure or tightness, often like a band around the head, whereas migraines are typically a pulsing or throbbing pain.
2. **Pain Location:** Tension headaches generally affect both sides of the head, while migraines are often felt on just one side.
3. **Severity and Impact:** Migraines are usually more severe and can be debilitating, significantly impacting a person's ability to carry out daily activities.
4. **Associated Symptoms:** Migraines are often accompanied by other symptoms like nausea, sensitivity to light/sound, and aura, which are not typically seen in tension headaches.
5. **Triggers and Causes:** Both can have different triggers and underlying causes.

Understanding these differences is crucial for effective treatment and management. If someone experiences frequent or severe headaches of any type, it is important to consult a healthcare provider for a proper diagnosis and treatment plan.

What is epilepsy?

Epilepsy is a chronic neurological disorder characterized by recurrent, unprovoked seizures. These seizures are episodes of disturbed brain activity that cause changes in attention or behavior. Epilepsy is one of the most common conditions affecting the brain, and it can affect people of all ages. Here are some key aspects of epilepsy:

1. **Seizures:** The hallmark of epilepsy is recurrent seizures. Seizures are bursts of electrical activity in the brain that temporarily affect how it works. They can manifest in various ways, from brief lapses of attention or muscle jerks to severe and prolonged convulsions. Seizures can also be subtle, leading to periods of confusion, feelings of fear or dread, or unusual sensations.
2. **Types of Seizures:** There are several types of seizures, broadly categorized as focal (starting in one part of the brain) or generalized (affecting both sides of the brain). Focal seizures can be with or without loss of consciousness, while generalized seizures include absence seizures (brief loss of awareness, often in children), tonic-clonic seizures (convulsions with muscle rigidity and jerking), and others.
3. **Causes:** Epilepsy can have various causes. It may be genetic or result from brain conditions such as stroke, tumor, or traumatic brain injury. In many cases, the cause remains unknown.
4. **Diagnosis:** Diagnosing epilepsy involves ruling out other conditions that might cause seizures, such as fainting or a high fever in children (febrile seizures). It typically includes a neurological examination and diagnostic tests like an Electroencephalogram (EEG) to look for abnormal

brain waves, or brain imaging (like MRI) to detect structural abnormalities.

5. **Treatment:** Treatment usually focuses on controlling seizures with medication. Most people with epilepsy can achieve good seizure control with anti-epileptic drugs (AEDs). In some cases where medication is ineffective, other treatments might include surgery, nerve stimulation, or dietary changes.
6. **Living with Epilepsy:** With proper treatment, many people with epilepsy can lead normal lives, although they may need to avoid certain activities to prevent injury during seizures. In some cases, children may outgrow epilepsy, while adults may see an improvement or even a cessation of seizure activity.
7. **Social and Emotional Impact:** Epilepsy can have significant social and emotional impacts, including challenges related to education, employment, driving, and social relationships. Stigma and misunderstanding about epilepsy are also common.

It is important for individuals with epilepsy to work closely with a healthcare provider to manage their condition effectively, including adjusting treatment plans as needed and addressing any associated psychological and social challenges.

How would you know if you have epilepsy?

Recognizing epilepsy involves identifying a pattern of recurrent, unprovoked seizures. Since seizures are the primary symptom of epilepsy, their presence, especially more than one unprovoked seizure, is a key indicator. However, because other conditions can cause seizure-like symptoms, a thorough evaluation by a healthcare professional is necessary for an accurate diagnosis. Here are some steps and signs that can help in identifying epilepsy:

1. **Observation of Seizure Symptoms:**
   - **Generalized Seizures:** These might include convulsions with muscle rigidity (tonic) and jerking (clonic), loss of consciousness, or absence seizures (brief lapses in awareness, often in children).
   - **Focal Seizures:** These may involve altered consciousness, unusual sensations, involuntary jerking of a body part, changes in emotions or sensations, or other symptoms depending on the part of the brain involved.
2. **Frequency and Pattern of Seizures:** More than one unprovoked seizure, typically over a period, may suggest epilepsy. Unprovoked means that the seizures occur without an immediate cause, such as high fever, acute head injury, or drug withdrawal.
3. **Medical History and Examination:** A thorough medical history, including any history of head injuries, infections, or family history of seizures, is important.
4. **Diagnostic Tests:**
   - **Electroencephalogram (EEG):** An EEG records the electrical activity of the brain and can detect abnormal patterns indicative of epilepsy.
   - **Brain Imaging:** MRI or CT scans can identify structural changes in the brain that might be causing seizures.
5. **Ruling Out Other Conditions:** Conditions such as fainting, transient ischemic attacks, migraines, sleep disorders, or panic attacks can sometimes mimic seizures, so it is important to rule these out.
6. **Consultation with a Neurologist:** A neurologist, particularly one specializing in epilepsy, is often involved in making a definitive diagnosis.
7. **Response to Medications:** Sometimes, the diagnosis is further supported by a positive response to anti-seizure medications.

If you suspect that you or someone else may have epilepsy, it is important to seek medical advice. Documenting what happens before, during, and after the seizures can be very helpful for healthcare professionals. This information, combined with medical testing, plays a crucial role in determining whether the seizures are due to epilepsy or another condition.

What are the main types of seizures?

Seizures, which are the primary symptom of epilepsy, come in various types. These types are generally classified based on how and where they begin in the brain. The two main categories are focal seizures (also known as partial seizures) and generalized seizures:

Focal Seizures

These start in one area of the brain. They are further classified into:

1. **Focal Aware Seizures (formerly known as simple partial seizures):**
   - Awareness is maintained.
   - May involve twitching, changes in sensation, dizziness, or other symptoms.
2. **Focal Impaired Awareness Seizures (formerly known as complex partial seizures):**
   - Consciousness or awareness is impaired or lost.
   - Might include unusual behaviors like unresponsiveness, chewing, or walking in circles.
3. **Focal to Bilateral Tonic-Clonic Seizures:**
   - Start in one part of the brain and then spread to both sides.
   - Often begin as a focal seizure with or without impaired awareness and then evolve into a generalized tonic-clonic seizure.

Generalized Seizures

These affect both sides of the brain from the start and are further categorized into several types:

1. **Absence Seizures (formerly known as petit mal seizures):**
   - Brief, lasting only a few seconds.
   - Characterized by a lapse in awareness, staring, and subtle body movements like eyelid fluttering.
2. **Tonic-Clonic Seizures (formerly known as grand mal seizures):**
   - The most dramatic type of epileptic seizure.
   - Include a tonic phase (stiffening of the body) and a clonic phase (rhythmic jerking of the limbs).
   - Often associated with a cry or moan, loss of consciousness, and postictal confusion.
3. **Tonic Seizures:**
   - Involve sudden stiffening of the muscles.
   - Usually affect muscles in the back, arms, and legs and may cause a fall.
4. **Clonic Seizures:**
   - Characterized by rhythmic jerking movements of the arms and legs.
5. **Myoclonic Seizures:**
   - Brief, shock-like jerks of a muscle or a group of muscles.
6. **Atonic Seizures (also known as drop seizures):**
   - Lead to a loss of muscle control, which may cause the person to suddenly collapse or fall down.

It is important to note that seizures are complex, and a person may experience different types at different times. The type of seizure can influence both the treatment approach and the overall management of the condition. Accurate diagnosis of the seizure type, often requiring observation and testing in a medical setting, is essential for effective treatment.

What are tonic clonic seizures?

Tonic-clonic seizures, formerly known as grand mal seizures, are a type of generalized seizure that affects the entire brain. They are one of the most recognizable types of seizures and consist of two stages: the tonic phase and the clonic phase. Here is a detailed look at each stage:

1. **Tonic Phase:**
   - **Duration:** This initial phase typically lasts about 10 to 20 seconds.
   - **Symptoms:** The muscles of the person experiencing the seizure suddenly become rigid. If standing, they often lose consciousness and fall to the ground. The rigidity can cause a cry or moan due to air being forced past the vocal cords.
   - **Breathing:** Breathing may become irregular or stop briefly, leading to a bluish coloration of the skin (cyanosis).
2. **Clonic Phase:**
   - **Duration:** This phase usually lasts for one to three minutes.
   - **Symptoms:** Following the tonic phase, the muscles begin to contract and relax rapidly, leading to convulsive, rhythmic jerking movements. The person may bite their tongue or inside of their cheek, and there may be loss of bladder or bowel control.
   - **Aftermath:** After the clonic phase subsides, the individual typically enters a postictal state, characterized by confusion, drowsiness, headache, and sometimes temporary weakness or paralysis.

Tonic-clonic seizures can be very distressing to witness, but it is important to remain calm and ensure the person's safety:

- **During the Seizure:** Place the person gently on their side to help keep the airway clear and place something soft under their head. Do not try to restrain them or put anything in their mouth.
- **After the Seizure:** Once the seizure has ended, check for injuries and provide comfort and reassurance as consciousness returns.

Tonic-clonic seizures are commonly associated with epilepsy, but they can also occur in people with no history of epilepsy due to various triggers like high fever, severe head injury, or certain medical conditions. It is important for anyone experiencing a tonic-clonic seizure for the first time, or having a significant change in their seizure pattern, to seek medical evaluation. In individuals diagnosed with epilepsy, these seizures are typically managed with anti-epileptic drugs (AEDs) and lifestyle modifications to reduce triggers.

What is a tonic seizure?

A tonic seizure is a type of generalized seizure characterized by the sudden stiffening of muscles. These seizures are more commonly seen in people with certain types of epilepsy, such as Lennox-Gastaut syndrome, which is a severe form of childhood-onset epilepsy, but they can occur in adults as well. Key features of tonic seizures include:

1. **Muscle Stiffening:** During a tonic seizure, the muscles, particularly those in the back, arms, and legs, suddenly become stiff. This stiffening can cause the person to fall to the ground if they are standing when the seizure begins.
2. **Consciousness:** The person may lose consciousness or have significantly altered awareness during the seizure.
3. **Duration:** Tonic seizures are typically brief, usually lasting less than 20 seconds.
4. **Post-Seizure Effects:** After the seizure, the individual might experience confusion or fatigue, although the postictal state is generally not as pronounced as it is with tonic-clonic seizures.
5. **Safety Concerns:** Due to the sudden muscle stiffening and potential for falls, tonic seizures can pose a risk of injury. Precautions to ensure a safe environment are important for individuals prone to these types of seizures.
6. **Diagnosis and Monitoring:** Tonic seizures are diagnosed through a combination of medical history, description of the seizures, and diagnostic tests like an electroencephalogram (EEG). In some cases, video EEG monitoring may be used to capture and analyze the seizure.
7. **Treatment:** Management typically involves the use of anti-epileptic drugs (AEDs). The choice of medication depends on the individual's overall health, the frequency and severity of the seizures, and any other types of seizures they experience.

Understanding and recognizing tonic seizures are important for proper management and treatment, especially since they can be a part of more complex epilepsy syndromes in children. As with all types of epilepsy, a comprehensive approach that may include medication, lifestyle changes, and sometimes dietary interventions is essential for managing tonic seizures effectively.

How long does a tonic seizure last?

Tonic seizures are generally brief, typically lasting less than 20 seconds. During a tonic seizure, the muscles in the body, particularly the back, arms, and legs, suddenly become rigid and tense. Due to their short duration and the specific muscle groups they affect, tonic seizures can often cause the person experiencing them to fall, especially if they are standing when the seizure begins.

It is important to note that the duration of seizures can vary from person to person, and in some cases, tonic seizures might last slightly longer. However, they are usually one of the shorter types of seizures.

After the seizure, individuals might experience a short period of confusion or disorientation, but this postictal state is typically less severe and shorter than that following tonic-clonic seizures.

If someone experiences a tonic seizure for the first time, or if there is a significant change in their seizure pattern, it is crucial to seek medical advice for an accurate diagnosis and appropriate management. For those with known seizure disorders, ensuring a safe environment to minimize the risk of injury during a seizure is essential.

What are myoclonic seizures?

Myoclonic seizures are a type of seizure characterized by brief, shock-like jerks of a muscle or a group of muscles. They are a feature of many types of epilepsy syndromes, including juvenile myoclonic epilepsy, which often begins in adolescence. Here are some key aspects of myoclonic seizures:

1. **Sudden Muscle Contractions:** During a myoclonic seizure, the person experiences sudden, brief involuntary muscle jerks. These can be single or multiple and can occur in a series.
2. **Body Parts Affected:** The jerks typically involve the arms and legs, but any part of the body can be affected. In some instances, the jerks are forceful enough to cause the person to drop objects or fall.
3. **Consciousness:** Unlike many other seizure types, consciousness is usually not impaired during myoclonic seizures, although they can occur in conjunction with other types of seizures that do affect awareness.
4. **Duration:** Myoclonic seizures are very brief, usually lasting only a second or two.
5. **Frequency:** These seizures can happen sporadically, in clusters, or at regular intervals.
6. **Causes:** They can be seen in various epilepsy syndromes and can also be triggered by external factors in some cases, like sleep deprivation, stress, or flashing lights.
7. **Age of Onset:** Myoclonic seizures commonly begin in childhood or adolescence, especially in cases of juvenile myoclonic epilepsy, but they can occur at any age depending on the underlying cause.
8. **Diagnosis:** They are diagnosed based on the clinical description of the seizure. An Electroencephalogram (EEG) can help confirm the diagnosis, showing specific patterns of brain activity associated with this type of seizure.
9. **Treatment:** Myoclonic seizures are typically treated with anti-epileptic drugs. The choice of medication depends on the individual's overall health and the type of epilepsy they have.
10. **Impact on Daily Life:** While myoclonic seizures are generally brief and not dangerous by themselves, they can be disruptive to daily life, especially if they occur frequently or result in falls or dropping items.

If someone experiences myoclonic jerks, especially frequently or in patterns, it is important to seek medical evaluation to determine the cause and appropriate treatment.

What causes juvenile myoclonic epilepsy?

Juvenile Myoclonic Epilepsy (JME) is a type of epilepsy that typically begins in adolescence and is characterized by myoclonic jerks (quick, involuntary muscle twitches), usually in the morning. The exact cause of JME is not entirely understood, but it is believed to involve a combination of genetic and environmental factors:

1. **Genetic Factors:**
   - JME has a strong genetic component. It is often seen in multiple members of the same family, suggesting a hereditary predisposition.
   - Specific genes have been associated with JME, but it is likely that multiple genetic factors contribute to the condition. These genes are thought to affect the regulation of neurotransmitters in the brain, particularly GABA, a neurotransmitter that inhibits brain activity and helps prevent seizures.
2. **Neurotransmitter Imbalance:**
   - Imbalances in brain neurotransmitters, especially the balance between excitatory and inhibitory neurotransmitters like glutamate and GABA, are believed to play a role in JME.
3. **Brain Structure and Function:**
   - While most individuals with JME have normal brain structures, as seen on MRI scans, some studies suggest there may be subtle differences in the way their brains are wired or function.
4. **Triggers:**
   - Certain triggers can precipitate seizures in individuals with JME. These include sleep deprivation, stress, alcohol consumption, flickering lights (like from video games or television screens), and sometimes caffeine.
5. **Age of Onset:**
   - JME typically begins in adolescence, with most individuals experiencing their first seizures between the ages of 12 and 18. This onset during the teenage years suggests that brain development during this period may play a role.
6. **Hormonal Factors:**
   - Hormonal changes during puberty might influence the onset and pattern of seizures in JME, though this relationship is not fully understood.

It is important to note that while there is a genetic predisposition, not everyone who carries a genetic mutation associated with JME will develop the condition. Lifestyle factors and seizure management, including regular sleep patterns, avoiding alcohol, and taking prescribed medication, are important for individuals with JME.

What is benign childhood epilepsy?

Benign childhood epilepsy, more formally known as Benign Childhood Epilepsy with Centrotemporal Spikes (BCECTS), also known as Rolandic epilepsy, is a common epilepsy syndrome in children. It is considered "benign" because most children outgrow it and it typically does not cause any cognitive or neurological deficits. Here are some key aspects of this condition:

1. **Age of Onset:** BCECTS usually begins in children between the ages of 3 and 13, with the peak incidence around 7-8 years of age.
2. **Seizure Characteristics:**
   - The seizures in BCECTS are typically focal (affecting only one part of the brain), often occurring during sleep or upon waking.
   - Common symptoms include twitching, numbness, or tingling in the face or tongue, which can affect speech. The child may also experience twitching or weakness in one side of the body.
   - Seizures are generally brief and tend to occur infrequently.
3. **EEG Findings:**
   - The electroencephalogram (EEG) of children with BCECTS shows characteristic patterns, known as centrotemporal spikes, which are crucial for diagnosis.
4. **Prognosis:**
   - The prognosis for BCECTS is excellent. Most children outgrow the condition by adolescence, and it typically does not affect cognitive development or learning abilities.
   - The seizures usually respond well to medication, but in many cases, treatment with anti-epileptic drugs (AEDs) is not necessary unless the seizures are frequent or particularly bothersome.
5. **Management:**
   - Management primarily focuses on monitoring the child, providing reassurance to the family, and treatment with AEDs if seizures are frequent or severe.
   - Since the seizures often occur during sleep, they may not significantly impact the child's daily life.
6. **Cause:**
   - The exact cause of BCECTS is not clear, but there appears to be a genetic component, as it can sometimes be seen in multiple family members.

Benign childhood epilepsy with centrotemporal spikes is an example of an epilepsy syndrome where the term "benign" is used to indicate a good prognosis. It is important for parents and caregivers to understand that while the condition is termed "epilepsy," its impact is typically limited, and the long-term outlook for children with BCECTS is very positive.

What is absence seizure?

An absence seizure, formerly known as a petit mal seizure, is a type of seizure that is common in children, but can also occur in adults. It is characterized by brief episodes of staring and subtle body movements. These seizures are a feature of several forms of epilepsy, particularly childhood and juvenile absence epilepsy. Key aspects of absence seizures include:

1. **Brief Loss of Consciousness:** The individual typically experiences a sudden, brief lapse in awareness, which might appear as a blank stare. They become unresponsive to external stimuli during this time.
2. **Subtle Movements:** Absence seizures may be accompanied by subtle movements such as eyelid fluttering, lip smacking, or slight hand movements.
3. **Duration:** These seizures are very brief, usually lasting just a few seconds.
4. **Frequency:** Absence seizures can occur multiple times a day and are sometimes so brief that they go unnoticed.
5. **Onset:** They most commonly begin in childhood, typically between the ages of 4 and 14, with a peak onset around 5 to 6 years of age.
6. **Lack of Postictal Symptoms:** Unlike other types of seizures, absence seizures usually don't have a postictal phase (the period following the end of a seizure). The individual typically resumes their previous activity without any confusion or other residual effects.

7. **Diagnosis:** Diagnosis often involves observing the seizure characteristics and conducting an electroencephalogram (EEG). During an EEG, a typical absence seizure shows a pattern of 3 Hz spike-and-wave discharges.
8. **Treatment:** Absence seizures are generally well-controlled with anti-seizure medications. Ethosuximide, valproic acid, and lamotrigine are commonly used.
9. **Impact on Daily Life:** While individual seizures are brief and not dangerous, their frequency can impact learning, attention, and daily activities, particularly in children. It is important for teachers and caregivers to recognize these seizures, as they can often be mistaken for daydreaming or inattention.
10. **Prognosis:** Many children with absence seizures outgrow them by their teenage years, though some may go on to develop other types of seizures.

It is important for absence seizures to be diagnosed and treated appropriately, as their high frequency can significantly impact a child's life, particularly in educational and social settings. With proper management, most children with absence epilepsy do well and lead normal lives.

What is a simple partial seizure?

A simple partial seizure, now more commonly referred to as a "focal onset aware seizure" in medical terminology, is a type of seizure that originates in one area of the brain and does not impair consciousness. Individuals experiencing this kind of seizure remain awake and aware throughout the episode. These seizures can manifest in a variety of ways, depending on the function of the affected part of the brain. Here are key aspects of simple partial (focal onset aware) seizures:

1. **Awareness and Memory:** During a simple partial seizure, the person's awareness and memory are typically unaffected. They are usually fully conscious and can remember the seizure event.
2. **Motor Symptoms:** These can include jerking or stiffening of a part of the body, like an arm or a leg, and can spread to other parts in a pattern known as Jacksonian march.
3. **Sensory Symptoms:** The individual might experience unusual sensations, such as tingling, dizziness, or seeing flashing lights. They might also experience auditory, olfactory, or gustatory hallucinations (hearing, smelling, or tasting things that aren't there).
4. **Autonomic Symptoms:** These are changes related to the part of the nervous system that controls automatic functions of the body, such as heart rate and digestion. Examples include changes in heart rate, skin flushing, or pupil dilation.
5. **Psychic Symptoms:** These include changes in emotion (sudden fear, joy, or anger), déjà vu (a feeling of familiarity), or jamais vu (a feeling of unfamiliarity). They can also involve cognitive distortions such as difficulty speaking or understanding language.
6. **Duration:** Simple partial seizures are typically short, usually lasting less than 2 minutes.
7. **Post-Seizure:** After the seizure, there may be temporary weakness or sensory changes in the area affected by the seizure, but there are usually no other post-seizure (postictal) symptoms like confusion, which are common in other types of seizures.
8. **Diagnosis and Treatment:** Diagnosis often involves a detailed medical history and diagnostic tests like an electroencephalogram (EEG) and brain imaging. Treatment depends on the frequency and severity of the seizures and may include anti-epileptic drugs.

It is important to accurately diagnose and manage simple partial seizures, as they can sometimes progress to more complex seizures involving loss of consciousness. If someone experiences recurrent episodes that could be simple partial seizures, they should seek medical evaluation for appropriate diagnosis and treatment.

What is complex partial seizure?

A complex partial seizure, now more commonly referred to as a "focal onset impaired awareness seizure" in medical terminology, is a type of seizure that starts in one area of the brain and is accompanied by a loss of awareness or altered consciousness. These seizures can affect a person's ability to interact with their surroundings and may cause confusion. Here are the key aspects of complex partial (focal onset impaired awareness) seizures:

1. **Altered Consciousness:** During the seizure, the person's awareness and responsiveness are impaired. They may not respond to external stimuli, and they might appear dazed or confused.

2. **Automatisms:** These are repetitive, automatic movements that can occur during the seizure, such as lip smacking, chewing, fidgeting, walking in circles, or performing simple tasks.

3. **Memory Impairment:** The individual often does not remember the events that occurred during the seizure and may have only a vague recollection of the moments leading up to it.

4. **Onset:** The seizure may begin with a simple partial seizure (focal onset aware seizure), where the person is aware, and then progress to impaired awareness.

5. **Duration:** These seizures usually last between one and two minutes.

6. **Post-Seizure (Postictal) State:** After the seizure, the person often experiences a period of confusion, fatigue, and disorientation that can last several minutes to hours.

7. **Aura:** Some individuals may experience an aura (a particular sensation or feeling) before the seizure, which can serve as a warning sign. An aura is actually a simple partial seizure that occurs before the loss of awareness.

8. **Diagnosis and Treatment:** Diagnosing complex partial seizures involves a neurological examination, an electroencephalogram (EEG), and sometimes brain imaging like MRI. Treatment typically includes anti-epileptic drugs, and in some cases, surgery or other therapies may be considered.

9. **Impact on Daily Life:** Because of their unpredictable nature and the impairment of consciousness, these seizures can significantly impact daily life, including the ability to work, drive, and perform other activities safely.

10. **Potential Progression:** In some cases, a complex partial seizure may evolve into a generalized seizure, affecting the entire brain and leading to a loss of consciousness and convulsions.

It is important for individuals experiencing symptoms of complex partial seizures to seek medical evaluation and treatment, as effective management can greatly improve quality of life and reduce the risk of injury during seizures.

What are the signs of a partial seizure?

Partial seizures, now referred to as focal onset seizures in medical terminology, begin in one specific area of the brain and can manifest with a variety of symptoms, depending on the part of the brain involved. Focal seizures are categorized into two types: Focal Onset Aware Seizures (formerly known as simple partial seizures) and Focal Onset Impaired Awareness Seizures (formerly known as complex partial seizures). Here are common signs of each:

Signs of Focal Onset Aware Seizures (Simple Partial Seizures)

1. **Motor Symptoms:** Jerking or twitching of a specific body part, such as an arm or leg.

2. **Sensory Symptoms:** Changes in vision, hearing, smell, taste, or touch, like seeing flashing lights, hearing ringing, or a strange taste or smell.

3. **Autonomic Symptoms:** Changes in autonomic functions, such as heart rate, flushing, or gastrointestinal sensations.

4. **Psychic Symptoms:** Altered mental states, including feelings of déjà vu, fear, anxiety, or euphoria; cognitive disturbances like difficulty speaking or understanding language may also occur.

Signs of Focal Onset Impaired Awareness Seizures (Complex Partial Seizures)

1. **Altered Awareness:** Reduced awareness of surroundings, leading to a dazed or confused state.

2. **Automatisms:** Repetitive, involuntary movements like lip smacking, chewing, hand rubbing, or walking in circles.

3. **Unusual Behaviors:** Performing complex activities without full awareness, such as undressing or fumbling.

4. **Memory Gaps:** No recollection of the seizure episode, often with confusion or disorientation afterward.

5. **Emotional Changes:** Sudden fear, anxiety, or other emotional responses not appropriate to the context.

Both types of focal seizures can sometimes progress to bilateral tonic-clonic seizures, which affect both sides of the brain and are characterized by loss of consciousness and convulsions.

It is important to note that symptoms can vary significantly from person to person, and an individual may experience different symptoms in different seizures. Diagnosis of focal seizures typically involves a detailed medical history, observation of symptoms, and diagnostic tests like an electroencephalogram (EEG) or brain imaging.

If someone is experiencing symptoms suggestive of focal seizures, it is important to consult a healthcare professional for proper diagnosis and management. This is crucial not only for treatment but also for safety, as uncontrolled seizures can lead to injury and impact quality of life.

What is frontal lobe related seizures?

Frontal lobe seizures are a type of focal seizure that originates in the frontal lobe of the brain. The frontal lobe is the largest of the brain's four main lobes and is involved in important functions like voluntary movement, language, and executive functions. Seizures that begin in this part of the brain can have various symptoms and characteristics:

1. **Motor Symptoms:** Given the frontal lobe's role in controlling movement, these seizures often involve motor symptoms. This can include rhythmic muscle contractions, jerking movements (often in the arms or legs), and sometimes bizarre, complex movements that may appear planned or coordinated.
2. **Brief Duration:** Frontal lobe seizures tend to be brief, often lasting less than 30 seconds.
3. **Night-time Occurrence:** They commonly occur during sleep and may be mistaken for sleep disorders or nocturnal disturbances.
4. **Frequency:** These seizures can occur in clusters, with several seizures happening one after another, and they can be frequent.
5. **Sudden Onset and End:** They often start and stop suddenly.
6. **Altered Consciousness:** While consciousness may be preserved in some frontal lobe seizures, others may involve altered awareness or responsiveness.
7. **Speech and Vocalization:** Some individuals may scream, laugh, or cry out involuntarily during a seizure.
8. **Autonomic Symptoms:** These can include sweating, flushing, or changes in heart rate.
9. **Distinguishing from Other Seizures:** Frontal lobe seizures can sometimes be difficult to distinguish from other types of seizures, particularly temporal lobe seizures, because of the diversity of symptoms. However, the brief duration, frequency, and motor symptoms can be key differentiators.
10. **Diagnosis:** Diagnosing frontal lobe seizures typically involves capturing the seizures on an electroencephalogram (EEG), although it can be challenging due to the brief nature of the seizures and the fact that frontal lobe seizure activity may not always show up clearly on an EEG.
11. **Treatment:** Treatment usually involves anti-epileptic drugs. In some cases, surgery may be considered, especially if the seizures are resistant to medication.

Frontal lobe seizures are unique due to the frontal lobe's complex role in controlling behavior, movement, and personality. This complexity often leads to varied and sometimes unusual seizure manifestations. If frontal lobe epilepsy is suspected, a thorough evaluation by a neurologist or an epilepsy specialist is crucial for accurate diagnosis and effective treatment.

What are subtypes of frontal lobe seizures?

Frontal lobe seizures, originating from the frontal lobe of the brain, encompass a diverse range of subtypes due to the frontal lobe's involvement in various functions like movement, emotion, and behavior. These subtypes can be categorized based on the specific region of the frontal lobe affected and the nature of the seizure manifestations. Some of the common subtypes include:

1. **Motor Seizures:**
   - Characterized by motor symptoms such as jerking, stiffening, or rhythmic movements.
   - Can involve specific body parts (localized) or more generalized movements.
2. **Jacksonian March Seizures:**
   - Start in one area (such as a finger or toe) and spread to other parts of the body on the same side.
   - The progression of movement reflects the sequential activation of motor areas in the frontal lobe.
3. **Supplementary Motor Area (SMA) Seizures:**
   - Originating from the supplementary motor area, these seizures may involve abrupt cessation of activity, tonic posturing, or complex automatisms.
   - Can be mistaken for complex partial seizures originating in the temporal lobe.

4. **Cingulate Seizures:**
   - Originate in the cingulate gyrus.
   - May include complex emotional or experiential symptoms, such as fear, laughter, or a sense of impending doom.
5. **Frontal Operculum Seizures:**
   - Can affect speech (if occurring on the dominant hemisphere) and cause atypical vocalizations.
   - May also involve facial movements or swallowing automatisms.
6. **Dorsolateral Frontal Cortex Seizures:**
   - Might involve complex motor activities that can appear planned or purposeful.
   - Patients might walk around, perform repetitive movements, or exhibit bicycling motions.
7. **Orbitofrontal Cortex Seizures:**
   - Can include unusual behaviors or sensations, such as olfactory hallucinations (smelling odors that are not there).
   - May involve complex emotional responses.
8. **Frontopolar Seizures:**
   - These seizures may manifest with autonomic symptoms, such as changes in heart rate or blood pressure, and altered consciousness.

The symptoms and clinical manifestations of frontal lobe seizures can vary significantly, making them sometimes challenging to diagnose. In some cases, the behaviors exhibited during these seizures can be mistaken for psychiatric disorders or other medical conditions.

Diagnosis often requires detailed observation, patient history, and specialized tests like video EEG monitoring. Treatment typically involves anti-epileptic medications, and in drug-resistant cases, surgical interventions may be considered.

Because of the complex nature of frontal lobe seizures and the potential for varied manifestations, management by a neurologist or an epilepsy specialist is essential for accurate diagnosis and effective treatment.

What is temporal lobe related seizure?

Temporal lobe seizures, originating from the brain's temporal lobe, are a common type of focal (or partial) seizure. The temporal lobe, located on the sides of the brain just above the ears, is responsible for processing sensory input, including sound and smell, as well as playing a key role in forming memories. These seizures can manifest in various ways:

1. **Sensory Symptoms:** Given the temporal lobe's role in sensory processing, these seizures may involve unusual sensations such as smelling odors that aren't present (olfactory hallucinations) or experiencing strange tastes.
2. **Auditory Symptoms:** Some people may hear sounds, music, or voices that aren't there (auditory hallucinations).
3. **Visual Disturbances:** This can include seeing shapes, lights, or other visual illusions.
4. **Gustatory Hallucinations:** Experiencing unusual tastes.
5. **Memory or Emotional Disturbances:** Experiencing feelings of déjà vu (a feeling of familiarity), jamais vu (a feeling of unfamiliarity), fear, or euphoria. Some may have memory flashbacks or feel as though they are in a dream.
6. **Complex Automatisms:** These are repetitive, automatic movements such as lip smacking, chewing, swallowing, or fidgeting with clothes or objects. The person may appear dazed and unresponsive to others.
7. **Altered Consciousness:** In complex temporal lobe seizures, consciousness may be impaired. The person might be unable to respond to external stimuli and have no memory of the seizure.
8. **Postictal Phase:** After the seizure, the individual may experience confusion, fatigue, and may not remember what happened during the seizure.
9. **Duration:** Temporal lobe seizures typically last between 30 seconds and 2 minutes.

Temporal lobe seizures can be challenging to diagnose because their symptoms can be subtle and are sometimes mistaken for psychiatric disorders or other medical conditions. The diagnosis usually involves a neurological examination, an electroencephalogram (EEG), and sometimes brain imaging like an MRI.

Treatment typically includes anti-epileptic drugs, and in cases where medication is not effective, surgery might be an option. Lifestyle modifications and managing triggers such as stress and lack of sleep are also important aspects of treatment.

It is essential for individuals who experience symptoms suggestive of temporal lobe seizures to seek a thorough evaluation by a healthcare professional for appropriate diagnosis and management.

What are subtypes of temporal lobe related seizures?

Temporal lobe seizures, stemming from the brain's temporal lobe, encompass a variety of subtypes, each with distinct characteristics. The temporal lobe plays a crucial role in processing sensory information, emotions, and memory, leading to diverse seizure manifestations. Here are some common subtypes:

1. **Simple Focal Seizures (Focal Onset Aware Seizures):**
   - The individual remains conscious and aware.
   - May include auditory or visual hallucinations, olfactory or gustatory experiences, vertigo, or complex memory phenomena like déjà vu or jamais vu.
   - Motor symptoms might include discrete movements in the face or hand.
2. **Complex Focal Seizures (Focal Onset Impaired Awareness Seizures):**
   - Consciousness or awareness is impaired.
   - May involve automatisms such as lip smacking, picking at clothes, or fumbling movements.
   - Behavioral arrest (stopping all activity) is common.
   - The person may appear confused or dazed.
3. **Focal to Bilateral Tonic-Clonic Seizures:**
   - Begins in the temporal lobe and then spreads to both sides of the brain.
   - Initially may have focal onset aware or impaired awareness features, followed by the tonic-clonic activity (stiffening and jerking of the limbs).
4. **Auditory Seizures:**
   - Manifest as hearing sounds or voices that are not present.
   - Might include distortions of sounds or changes in the perception of volumes.
5. **Gustatory Seizures:**
   - Involve abnormal taste sensations.
6. **Olfactory Seizures:**
   - Characterized by smelling odors that are not actually present.
7. **Psychic Seizures:**
   - Involve alterations in emotions or psychological experiences, such as sudden fear, happiness, or feelings of familiarity or unfamiliarity.
8. **Autonomic Seizures:**
   - Affect autonomic functions like heart rate, flushing, or gastrointestinal sensations.

Temporal lobe seizures can vary widely in their presentation and impact on the individual. Accurate diagnosis typically involves a comprehensive evaluation, including a detailed medical history, observation of symptoms, and diagnostic tests such as an electroencephalogram (EEG) and brain imaging. Treatment usually involves anti-epileptic medications, and in some cases, surgical intervention may be considered, especially for drug-resistant temporal lobe epilepsy.

Given the complexity of temporal lobe seizures, individuals experiencing these symptoms should seek evaluation and management by a healthcare professional, preferably a neurologist or an epilepsy specialist.

What is parietal lobe related seizures?

Parietal lobe seizures originate in the parietal lobe of the brain, which is located near the top and center of the brain. This lobe is responsible for processing sensory information from various parts of the body, spatial and visual perception, and integrating sensory input to form a single perception (cognition). Seizures originating in this area can have distinct characteristics:

1. **Somatic Sensory or Somatosensory Symptoms:** One of the most common features of parietal lobe seizures is unusual sensations. This could include feelings of tingling, numbness, or a sensation of electric shock in specific parts of the body. These sensations may move or spread to other parts of the body.
2. **Distorted Perception of Size and Shape:** Individuals may experience altered perceptions, such as feeling that a part of the body is distorted in size (dysmorphopsia).
3. **Visual Symptoms:** While the primary visual processing areas are in the occipital lobe, the parietal lobe's role in integrating visual information can lead to visual illusions or difficulties in spatial perception during a seizure.

4. **Difficulty with Spatial and Body Awareness:** There might be an impaired ability to understand and interpret spatial relationships or an altered sense of one's own body.

5. **Complex Sensory Illusions:** In some cases, complex illusions such as feeling detached from one's body or experiencing visual hallucinations can occur.

6. **Language and Speech Disturbances:** If the seizure affects the dominant hemisphere (usually the left hemisphere in right-handed individuals), there can be problems with language and speech.

7. **Motor Symptoms:** Although less common, there might be involuntary motor movements, particularly if the seizure spreads to the motor cortex.

8. **Duration and Frequency:** The duration of parietal lobe seizures can vary, and they may occur infrequently or in clusters.

9. **Postictal Symptoms:** After the seizure, there might be residual sensory disturbances or weakness.

10. **Diagnosis:** Diagnosing parietal lobe seizures involves capturing the seizure on an electro-encephalogram (EEG) and often includes brain imaging like MRI to look for structural abnormalities.

11. **Treatment:** Treatment typically involves anti-epileptic medications. The choice of medication and treatment approach depends on the individual's seizure type, frequency, and overall health.

Given the diverse and sometimes subtle symptoms of parietal lobe seizures, they can be challenging to recognize and diagnose. It is important for individuals experiencing symptoms suggestive of parietal lobe seizures to seek evaluation and treatment from a healthcare professional.

What are subtypes of parietal lobe related seizures?

Parietal lobe seizures originate in the parietal region of the brain, which is key in processing sensory information and spatial orientation. Due to the diverse functions of the parietal lobe, seizures originating from this area can manifest in various subtypes, each with its unique characteristics:

1. **Somatosensory Seizures:**
   - Characterized by abnormal sensations, such as tingling, numbness, or a feeling of electricity in a specific body part.
   - These sensations often start in one area and may spread to other parts of the body.

2. **Visuospatial Seizures:**
   - May involve difficulties in perceiving the relationship between objects in space.
   - Can cause illusions of altered spatial orientation or visual distortions, such as objects appearing closer or farther away than they are.

3. **Language Seizures (if involving the dominant hemisphere, typically the left):**
   - Can result in difficulties with speech or language comprehension during the seizure.
   - These are less common and usually occur if the seizure spreads from the parietal to the temporal lobe.

4. **Motor Symptoms:**
   - Although the parietal lobe is not primarily responsible for motor control, seizures here may cause involuntary movements if they spread to adjacent motor areas.
   - Movement symptoms might include jerking or twitching of a limb.

5. **Complex Sensory Seizures:**
   - May cause more complex sensory experiences, such as feelings of body distortion or out-of-body experiences.
   - These seizures can be difficult to describe and are often overlooked or misdiagnosed.

6. **Autonomic Seizures:**
   - Can include changes in autonomic functions, like sweating, flushing, or changes in heart rate, though these are less common.

7. **Cognitive or Emotional Seizures:**
   - In some cases, seizures might affect cognitive or emotional processes, leading to confusion, fear, or euphoria during the seizure.

Parietal lobe seizures are often challenging to diagnose due to their varied and sometimes subtle manifestations. Accurate diagnosis typically involves a comprehensive evaluation, including detailed medical history, observation of symptoms, and diagnostic tests like an electroencephalogram (EEG) and brain imaging. Treatment typically involves anti-epileptic medications, and the choice of treatment depends on the individual's overall health, seizure type, and frequency.

Due to the complex nature of parietal lobe seizures, individuals experiencing these symptoms should seek evaluation and management by a healthcare professional.

What is occipital lobe related seizures?

Occipital lobe seizures originate from the occipital lobe, the region of the brain located at the back of the head. This lobe is primarily responsible for processing visual information. Given its function, seizures originating in this area often have visual symptoms. Here are some key features of occipital lobe seizures:

1. **Visual Hallucinations or Illusions:** Individuals may experience visual disturbances, such as seeing flashing lights, spots, or patterns. Some may see objects or colors that are not there, or their vision may be distorted with objects appearing larger (macropsia) or smaller (micropsia) than they actually are.
2. **Eye Movement Abnormalities:** There might be involuntary eye movements, difficulty in controlling eye movements, or a sensation that the eyes are rolling.
3. **Rapid Onset of Symptoms:** Occipital seizures typically begin suddenly and can be brief, often lasting just a few seconds to a few minutes.
4. **Headache or Migraine:** These seizures can be followed by a headache, which may be migraine-like. For some individuals, the seizure itself can be triggered by a migraine.
5. **Spread to Other Brain Areas:** The seizure activity can spread to adjacent areas of the brain, leading to other symptoms like muscle twitching or tingling sensations in the limbs (if it spreads to the parietal lobe) or altered consciousness (if it spreads to the temporal lobe).
6. **Motor Symptoms:** If the seizure spreads to the frontal lobe, it may result in tonic or clonic movements of the limbs.
7. **Nausea and Vomiting:** These symptoms can sometimes accompany the seizures, particularly in children.
8. **Postictal Symptoms:** After the seizure, individuals may experience temporary vision loss or impairment, headache, or confusion.

Diagnosing occipital lobe seizures involves a detailed medical history, neurological examination, and diagnostic tests like an electroencephalogram (EEG) and brain imaging (MRI). The EEG may not always capture the seizure activity in the occipital lobe, making diagnosis challenging.

Treatment typically involves anti-epileptic medications. The choice of treatment is based on factors like the individual's overall health, the frequency and severity of the seizures, and any underlying conditions.

Occipital lobe seizures are unique due to their visual symptoms, and their management requires careful evaluation and monitoring by healthcare professionals, often including a neurologist or an epilepsy specialist.

What are subtypes of occipital lobe related seizure?

Occipital lobe seizures originate from the occipital lobe of the brain, which is primarily responsible for visual processing. Due to this specific function, the subtypes of occipital lobe seizures are mainly characterized by visual disturbances. Here are some common subtypes:

1. **Elementary Visual Hallucinations:**
   - These involve simple, unformed visual hallucinations, such as flashes of light, spots, or geometric patterns.
   - The hallucinations can appear in various colors and might move around.
2. **Complex Visual Hallucinations:**
   - Involves more elaborate visual experiences, such as seeing scenes, people, or objects that are not actually present.
   - These hallucinations are less common than elementary visual hallucinations.
3. **Ictal Blindness:**
   - Temporary blindness or loss of vision during the seizure.
   - This can be a frightening experience, but vision typically returns to normal after the seizure ends.
4. **Eye Movement Abnormalities:**
   - Involuntary movements of the eyes, such as rapid blinking or eye fluttering.
   - The individual might also experience the sensation of the eyes moving or rolling upwards.
5. **Visual Field Deficits:**
   - Loss or impairment of part of the field of vision.

- This can include phenomena like tunnel vision or blind spots.

6. **Migraine-like Symptoms:**
   - Headaches, often severe and similar to migraines, may accompany or follow occipital seizures.
   - Nausea and sensitivity to light (photophobia) can also occur.

7. **Spread to Other Brain Regions:**
   - Seizure activity may spread to adjacent areas of the brain, leading to additional symptoms such as tingling or numbness (if it spreads to the parietal lobe), or even convulsive movements (if it spreads to the frontal lobe).

8. **Postictal Symptoms:**
   - Following the seizure, individuals may experience residual effects such as headache, confusion, or continued visual disturbances.

Diagnosis of occipital lobe seizures often involves capturing the seizures on an electroencephalogram (EEG) and brain imaging like MRI. However, occipital lobe seizures can sometimes be challenging to diagnose due to their visual symptoms being mistaken for other conditions, such as migraines or psychiatric disorders.

Treatment typically involves anti-epileptic drugs, and the approach depends on the individual's seizure type, frequency, and overall health. Managing occipital lobe seizures effectively requires a comprehensive approach that may involve neurologists or epilepsy specialists.

What are pre - seizure symptoms?

Pre-seizure symptoms, often referred to as "aura" or " prodrome," are sensations or changes in behavior that precede a seizure. They are considered a warning sign that a seizure may soon occur. It is important to note that not everyone with epilepsy experiences auras, and the nature of these pre-seizure symptoms can vary widely depending on the individual and the type of epilepsy they have. Here are some common pre-seizure symptoms:

1. **Sensory Changes:**
   - Visual changes such as flashing lights, blurred vision, or patterns.
   - Auditory sensations like hearing buzzing, ringing, or a specific sound.
   - Altered sense of smell or taste, often experiencing unusual or unpleasant odors or flavors.
   - Tingling sensations or feelings of numbness in part of the body.

2. **Emotional Changes:**
   - Sudden feelings of fear, anxiety, or a sense of impending doom.
   - Experiences of joy, euphoria, or other intense emotions without an apparent cause.

3. **Cognitive Changes:**
   - Déjà vu (feeling that something currently happening has been experienced before).
   - Jamais vu (feeling of unfamiliarity with a familiar situation).
   - Confusion or difficulty concentrating.

4. **Gastrointestinal Sensations:**
   - Nausea or a rising sensation in the stomach, similar to the "butterflies" one might feel in a nervous situation.

5. **Physical Symptoms:**
   - Dizziness or light-headedness.
   - Headache or a feeling of pressure in the head.
   - Fatigue or a general sense of feeling unwell.

6. **Behavioral Changes:**
   - Restlessness, irritability, or a change in mood.
   - Acting out of character or performing repetitive movements.

Auras are actually focal seizures (focal onset aware seizures) that occur before a larger seizure, especially in the case of focal to bilateral tonic-clonic seizures. They can last from a few seconds to a couple of minutes and provide an opportunity for the person to get to a safe place or position to prevent injury during the impending seizure.

Recognizing these pre-seizure symptoms can be crucial for individuals with epilepsy to manage their condition effectively. It allows them to take precautionary measures, such as sitting or lying down, moving away from potentially dangerous areas, or notifying someone nearby for assistance. Documenting these symptoms can also provide valuable information to healthcare providers for better management of the condition.

What are the most common symptoms of mild seizures?

Mild seizures, which can encompass various types of focal (partial) seizures, may present with subtle symptoms that can sometimes go unnoticed or be mistaken for other health issues. The specific symptoms largely depend on the area of the brain where the seizure activity occurs. Here are some of the most common symptoms associated with mild seizures:

1. **Sensory Changes:**
   - Unusual sensations such as tingling, numbness, or a feeling of electric shock, particularly in one part of the body.
   - Visual disturbances like seeing flashing lights, spots, or patterns.
   - Auditory changes, such as hearing a ringing or buzzing noise.
2. **Motor Symptoms:**
   - Subtle, involuntary movements like twitching of a muscle or a group of muscles, often confined to one part of the body.
   - Slight jerking movements that may not be very pronounced.
3. **Autonomic Symptoms:**
   - Changes in autonomic functions, such as abnormal sweating, flushing, or changes in heart rate.
   - Gastrointestinal sensations like nausea or a feeling of "butterflies" in the stomach.
4. **Cognitive or Emotional Changes:**
   - Brief episodes of confusion or memory lapses.
   - Sudden and unexplained feelings of fear, anxiety, or joy.
   - Experiences of déjà vu or jamais vu (a feeling of familiarity or unfamiliarity).
5. **Behavioral Symptoms:**
   - Staring spells, during which the person is unresponsive and may not remember the episode afterward.
   - Brief lapses in consciousness or "spacing out."
6. **Olfactory or Gustatory Changes:**
   - Smelling odors that aren't present (olfactory hallucinations).
   - Experiencing a strange or unpleasant taste (gustatory hallucinations).
7. **Speech Disturbances:**
   - Difficulty speaking or understanding language.
   - Stuttering or pausing during speech without an apparent reason.

It is important to recognize that these symptoms can be easily overlooked or attributed to other causes, such as fatigue, stress, or even daydreaming. However, if they occur repeatedly or in a pattern, it is advisable to consult a healthcare professional for evaluation. Mild seizures, even if not immediately disruptive, can be a sign of an underlying neurological condition that requires attention and management.

What is pre-seizure behavior?

Pre-seizure behavior, also known as preictal behavior, refers to changes in mood, sensations, or actions that occur before the onset of a seizure. These changes can vary greatly among individuals and depend on the type of epilepsy and seizures they experience. Recognizing pre-seizure behavior is important for some people with epilepsy as it can serve as a warning sign, allowing them to take precautions to prevent injury during the seizure. Common pre-seizure behaviors include:

1. **Aura:** Often considered a part of the seizure itself, an aura is a sensory or experiential symptom that precedes a seizure. It can manifest as a specific smell, taste, visual disturbance, sound, or a feeling of déjà vu or jamais vu.
2. **Mood Changes:** Some individuals may experience sudden and unexplained shifts in mood before a seizure, such as irritability, anxiety, depression, or a sense of unease.
3. **Cognitive Changes:** Difficulty in concentrating, confusion, or a feeling of being 'spaced out' or detached from surroundings can precede a seizure.
4. **Physical Sensations:** Unusual sensations such as headaches, nausea, dizziness, or general malaise might occur before a seizure.
5. **Fatigue or Drowsiness:** Feeling unusually tired or sleepy can be a pre-seizure symptom for some individuals.
6. **Restlessness:** Some people may feel restless, agitated, or have an unexplained sense of impending doom.
7. **Altered Perception:** Changes in perception, such as visual or auditory hallucinations or altered sense of space, can occur.

8. **Repetitive or Unusual Behavior:** Engaging in repetitive movements or behaviors that are not typical for the individual may be a pre-seizure sign.

It is important to note that not everyone with epilepsy experiences noticeable pre-seizure symptoms. For those who do, these symptoms can vary from one seizure to another. Documenting these symptoms and discussing them with a healthcare provider can be crucial for managing epilepsy effectively. This information can help in understanding the patterns of seizures, identifying triggers, and taking appropriate safety measures.

What medicines cause seizures?

Several medications and substances can potentially increase the risk of seizures or provoke them in susceptible individuals. Some common examples include:

1. **Antidepressants:** Certain antidepressants, especially bupropion and tricyclic antidepressants can lower the seizure threshold.
2. **Antipsychotics:** Some antipsychotic drugs, particularly clozapine, have been associated with an increased risk of seizures.
3. **Stimulants:** Medications like amphetamines and methylphenidate, used for attention deficit hyperactivity disorder (ADHD), can provoke seizures, especially in high doses or in susceptible individuals.
4. **Theophylline:** Used for asthma and other breathing disorders, high doses of theophylline can cause seizures.
5. **Illegal Drugs:** Substances such as cocaine, amphetamines, and ecstasy (MDMA) can provoke seizures.
6. **Alcohol:** Heavy alcohol use, especially during withdrawal, can lead to seizures.
7. **Certain Antibiotics:** Some antibiotics, like penicillin and quinolones, might lower the seizure threshold.
8. **Withdrawal from Sedative Drugs:** Withdrawal from drugs like benzodiazepines and barbiturates can cause seizures.
9. **Over-the-Counter Medications:** Some over-the-counter medications, particularly those containing stimulants like pseudoephedrine, can increase seizure risk in susceptible individuals.

It is important to note that the risk of seizures depends on various factors, including the dose of the medication, individual susceptibility, and whether the person has a pre-existing seizure disorder. Always consult healthcare providers for personalized advice and before starting or stopping any medication.

What is aging?

Aging refers to the biological process of growing older in a deleterious sense. It is a complex phenomenon that involves a gradual decline in physical, cognitive, and reproductive functions, accompanied by an increased susceptibility to disease and a higher risk of death. The process of aging is influenced by a combination of genetic, environmental, and lifestyle factors.

Key aspects of aging include:

1. **Cellular Aging:** Over time, cells accumulate damage due to environmental factors and the body's metabolic processes. This damage can lead to a decrease in cellular function and an increased likelihood of cell death. Telomere shortening, a critical aspect of cellular aging, occurs as cells divide and the protective caps at the ends of chromosomes get progressively shorter.
2. **Molecular Damage:** Aging is associated with the accumulation of various types of molecular damage, including DNA mutations, protein misfolding, and lipid peroxidation. These damages can disrupt cellular and organ function.
3. **Metabolic Changes:** As people age, their metabolism typically slows down, leading to changes in energy balance and nutrient utilization. This can affect body weight and composition, and can increase the risk of metabolic disorders.
4. **Hormonal Changes:** Aging is associated with changes in hormone levels, such as decreases in growth hormone, sex hormones, and melatonin, which can affect a wide range of bodily functions.
5. **Decline in Physiological Functions:** There is a gradual decline in the function of various organs and tissues, such as the heart, lungs, brain, and muscles, which can affect overall health and vitality.
6. **Increased Risk of Diseases:** With aging, the risk of various diseases, including heart disease, cancer, Alzheimer's disease, and osteoporosis, increases significantly.

7. **Immune System Changes:** Aging affects the immune system, leading to a reduced ability to fight off infections and an increased risk of autoimmune diseases.
8. **Psychological and Cognitive Changes:** Aging can be accompanied by changes in cognitive function, such as memory and processing speed, as well as emotional and psychological adjustments.

Aging is a natural part of life, and while it cannot be stopped, its effects can be managed through a healthy lifestyle, including a balanced diet, regular exercise, mental stimulation, and social engagement. Research in gerontology continues to explore the mechanisms of aging and potential strategies to promote healthy aging.

What is it like living with mental disorders for patients, relatives and caregivers?

Living with a mental disorder can be challenging not only for the individual experiencing it but also for their relatives and caregivers. The experience varies greatly depending on the type of mental disorder, its severity, the support systems in place, and individual coping mechanisms. Here is an overview of the impact on patients, relatives, and caregivers:

For Patients:

1. **Daily Challenges:** Depending on the disorder, patients may face difficulties in managing emotions, thoughts, and behaviors. This can impact daily activities, work, and relationships.
2. **Stigma and Misunderstanding:** Many people with mental disorders face stigma and misunderstandings about their conditions, which can lead to feelings of shame, isolation, and low self-esteem.
3. **Treatment and Management:** Ongoing treatment, which may include medication and therapy, can be essential but also challenging. Side effects of medications and the emotional work of therapy can be taxing.
4. **Impact on Relationships:** Mental disorders can strain relationships with family, friends, and colleagues, especially if others do not understand the condition or how to support the person.
5. **Fluctuating Symptoms:** Many mental disorders have periods of remission and exacerbation, making life unpredictable and planning difficult.

For Relatives:

1. **Emotional Stress:** Watching a loved one struggle with a mental disorder can be emotionally stressful. Relatives may feel helpless, frustrated, or saddened by the changes in their loved one.
2. **Financial and Social Impact:** There can be financial implications due to medical costs or lost income, as well as social impacts such as changing dynamics in friendships and family relationships.
3. **Educational Needs:** Relatives often need to educate themselves about the disorder to provide appropriate support and understand the patient's experiences and needs.
4. **Balancing Care with Personal Needs:** Relatives may struggle to balance the care of their loved one with their own personal needs, leading to potential burnout or neglect of their own health.

For Caregivers:

1. **High Responsibility:** Professional caregivers may carry the responsibility for the patient's safety and well-being, which can be particularly challenging in cases of severe mental illness.
2. **Emotional Involvement:** While trained to maintain professional boundaries, caregivers can become emotionally involved and affected by their patients' struggles and successes.
3. **Risk of Burnout:** The demanding nature of caregiving, especially in mental health, can lead to burnout, characterized by exhaustion, reduced effectiveness, and sometimes cynicism.
4. **Requirement for Continuous Learning:** Mental health care is a constantly evolving field, requiring caregivers to continually update their knowledge and skills.
5. **Rewarding Experiences:** Despite the challenges, many caregivers find their work deeply rewarding as they help individuals manage their mental disorders and improve their quality of life.

Overall, living with or caring for someone with a mental disorder requires understanding, patience, and resilience. Access to resources, community support, and effective treatment strategies can significantly improve the experience and outcomes for everyone involved.

What does it mean to live with anxiety and depression?

Living with anxiety and depression is a complex and deeply personal experience, varying significantly from one person to another. These mental health conditions can profoundly impact an individual's daily life, relationships, and overall well-being. Here is a general overview of what it might mean to live with anxiety and depression:

Living with Anxiety:

1. **Persistent Worry and Fear:** Individuals often experience constant, uncontrollable worry about everyday matters. This worry is often disproportionate to the actual likelihood or impact of the feared event.
2. **Physical Symptoms:** Anxiety can manifest physically, with symptoms like heart palpitations, sweating, trembling, dizziness, or shortness of breath, which can be distressing and debilitating.
3. **Avoidance and Overthinking:** People with anxiety may avoid situations or places that trigger their anxiety. They might overthink decisions and possible scenarios, leading to indecision or inaction.
4. **Impact on Social Life:** Social interactions can be challenging, with fears of judgment or embarrassment leading to avoidance of social gatherings, which can lead to feelings of isolation.
5. **Sleep Disturbances:** Anxiety can disrupt sleep patterns, leading to difficulties in falling asleep, staying asleep, or restless sleep.

Living with Depression:

1. **Persistent Sadness and Hopelessness:** A prevailing feeling of sadness, emptiness, or hopelessness that does not go away can dominate daily life, making even routine tasks feel overwhelming.
2. **Loss of Interest or Pleasure:** Activities that were once enjoyable may no longer bring pleasure, leading to disengagement from hobbies, social activities, or relationships.
3. **Changes in Appetite and Sleep:** Significant changes in sleep patterns and appetite are common, with some experiencing insomnia or oversleeping, and either loss of appetite or overeating.
4. **Fatigue and Lack of Energy:** Constant fatigue and a decrease in energy levels can make everyday activities, like getting out of bed or going to work, feel insurmountable.
5. **Feelings of Worthlessness or Guilt:** Individuals may experience harsh self-criticism, feelings of unworthiness, or disproportionate guilt over past events.

Co-Occurrence of Anxiety and Depression:

Many people experience symptoms of both anxiety and depression, which can complicate diagnosis and treatment. The combination of these conditions can be particularly challenging, as they can exacerbate each other. For example, the persistent worry of anxiety can lead to the hopelessness of depression, and the fatigue of depression can make it harder to manage anxiety.

Overall Impact:

- **Daily Functioning:** Both conditions can impair one's ability to work, study, engage in social relationships, and perform daily tasks.
- **Physical Health:** There is a strong connection between mental and physical health. Chronic anxiety and depression can increase the risk of other health problems like heart disease, diabetes, and chronic pain.
- **Relationships:** Maintaining relationships can be difficult, as these conditions can strain communication, intimacy, and social engagement.
- **Coping Strategies:** People develop various coping mechanisms, some healthy (like seeking therapy or practicing mindfulness) and some potentially harmful (like substance abuse).

Living with anxiety and depression often requires a combination of treatments, including therapy, medication, lifestyle changes, and support from loved ones. It is a journey of ups and downs, and what works for one person may not work for another. The key is often to seek professional help and to build a supportive network that understands and respects the challenges these conditions bring.

What it is like living with depression?

Living with depression can be an intensely challenging and often debilitating experience, significantly impacting every aspect of a person's life. It is important to note that depression manifests differently in different individuals, and what one person experiences may not be the same as another. Here are some common aspects of living with depression:

Emotional Symptoms:

1. **Persistent Sadness or Emptiness:** A deep, unshakeable feeling of sadness, emptiness, or hopelessness that is more than just feeling "down" and does not go away.
2. **Lack of Interest or Pleasure:** Losing interest in activities, hobbies, and things that used to bring joy or pleasure, including social activities and possibly relationships.
3. **Feelings of Worthlessness or Guilt:** Harsh self-criticism, feelings of inadequacy, and unwarranted guilt over minor issues or past events.
4. **Irritability or Frustration:** Even over small matters, which can be quite different from the person's usual behavior.
5. **Suicidal Thoughts or Behaviors:** Thoughts of death or suicide are not uncommon in severe cases of depression.

Physical Symptoms:

1. **Changes in Sleep Patterns:** This can include insomnia, difficulty falling or staying asleep, or oversleeping (hypersomnia).
2. **Appetite or Weight Changes:** Significant weight loss or gain due to a decrease or increase in appetite.
3. **Fatigue and Lack of Energy:** Feeling tired nearly all the time, even after sleeping or resting.
4. **Physical Pain:** Unexplained physical symptoms like back pain, headaches, and muscle aches.

Cognitive and Behavioral Symptoms:

1. **Difficulty Concentrating or Making Decisions:** Trouble focusing, making decisions, or remembering things.
2. **Social Withdrawal:** Avoiding social gatherings, losing interest in maintaining relationships, and preferring to be alone.
3. **Reduced Productivity:** Decreased effectiveness at work or school, often due to lack of concentration, energy, and motivation.
4. **Neglecting Responsibilities and Self-Care:** Difficulty in performing daily tasks, neglecting personal hygiene, and a lack of motivation to engage in routine activities.

Overall Impact:

- **Quality of Life:** Depression can significantly reduce the quality of life, making everyday tasks and activities feel overwhelming or meaningless.
- **Strain on Relationships:** It can strain relationships with friends, family, and colleagues, especially if they don't understand the condition.
- **Risk of Comorbidities:** People with depression often have other mental health conditions, like anxiety, or physical health issues, which can complicate treatment and recovery.
- **Stigma and Misunderstanding:** Stigma surrounding mental health can make people reluctant to seek help or discuss their experiences openly.

Coping and Management:

- **Professional Help:** Seeking therapy and, in some cases, medication, is often crucial in managing depression.
- **Support Systems:** Having a strong support network of friends, family, or support groups can provide emotional comfort and practical help.
- **Lifestyle Changes:** Regular exercise, a healthy diet, good sleep hygiene, and mindfulness practices can help manage symptoms.
- **Continuous Effort:** Living with depression often requires ongoing effort and strategies to manage symptoms and prevent relapses.

It is important to recognize that depression is a real and serious medical condition. It is not a sign of weakness or something that can be overcome through willpower alone. Effective treatment can make a significant difference, but the journey may take time and patience.

How to live with obsessive compulsive neurotic patient?

Living with someone who has Obsessive-Compulsive Disorder (OCD) can be challenging and requires understanding, patience, and a supportive approach. OCD is characterized by uncontrollable, recurring thoughts (obsessions) and behaviors (compulsions) that the person feels the urge to repeat over and over. Here are some guidelines on how to live with and support someone with OCD:

Understand the Disorder

1. **Educate Yourself:** Learn about OCD to understand what your loved one is experiencing.

   Recognize that obsessions and compulsions are not logical, but they are incredibly real and distressing to the person experiencing them.

2. **Recognize the Symptoms:** Understanding their specific symptoms can help you empathize with their struggles.

Provide Support Without Enabling

1. **Be Patient and Compassionate:** Show empathy and understanding. Avoid judgment or dismissiveness about their fears and compulsions.
2. **Avoid Enabling:** While it is tempting to help them complete their compulsions, this can reinforce the behavior. Instead, encourage them to resist their compulsions and practice coping strategies.
3. **Encourage Treatment:** Support them in seeking professional help like therapy (especially Exposure and Response Prevention Therapy) and medication.

Communication is Key

1. **Open and Honest Dialogue:** Maintain open lines of communication. Discuss how their OCD affects both your lives and work together to find solutions.
2. **Use "I" Statements:** When discussing your concerns, focus on your own feelings (e.g., "I feel worried when I see you struggling") rather than making accusatory statements.
3. **Be a Team:** Work together against OCD, not against each other. Make it clear that you are on their side.

Set Boundaries

1. **Personal Boundaries:** It is important to set limits on what you are willing to do in relation to their compulsions.
2. **Family Boundaries:** If you live in a family setting, it is crucial to agree on boundaries and rules that everyone understands and respects.

Self-Care for Yourself

1. **Take Care of Your Own Needs:** Living with someone who has OCD can be draining. Make sure you are looking after your own mental and physical health.
2. **Seek Support:** Consider joining a support group for families of people with OCD, or seeking your own therapy to learn coping strategies.

Create a Supportive Environment

1. **Routine and Structure:** A stable routine can be helpful for people with OCD.
2. **Minimize Stress:** High-stress situations can exacerbate symptoms, so try to create a calm and predictable home environment.

Be Patient with Progress

1. **Celebrate Small Victories:** Recovery from OCD is a gradual process. Celebrate small steps and progress, no matter how minor they may seem.
2. **Understand Relapses:** Be prepared for and understanding of potential relapses. They are a normal part of the recovery process.

Remember, every individual with OCD is unique, and what works for one person may not work for another. It is important to approach each situation with flexibility and understanding. Encouraging and supporting your loved one to adhere to their treatment plan is one of the most helpful things you can do.

How to live with bipolar disorder?

Living with bipolar disorder, a mental health condition characterized by extreme mood swings that include emotional highs (mania or hypomania) and lows (depression), presents unique challenges. However, with effective management, people with bipolar disorder can lead healthy and productive lives. Here are some strategies for individuals living with bipolar disorder and for their loved ones or caregivers:

For Individuals with Bipolar Disorder:

1. **Adhere to Treatment:** Consistently follow your treatment plan, including medications and psychotherapy. Regular consultations with mental health professionals are crucial.
2. **Monitor Mood Changes:** Be aware of your mood swings and triggers. Keeping a mood diary can help you and your healthcare provider notice patterns and triggers in your mood changes.
3. **Establish a Routine:** Try to maintain a regular schedule for sleeping, eating, and physical activity. A routine can help manage mood swings.
4. **Avoid Alcohol and Drugs:** Substance abuse can worsen bipolar disorder symptoms and make treatment less effective.
5. **Learn About Your Condition:** Educating yourself about bipolar disorder can empower you to understand your symptoms and treatment options.

6. **Practice Stress Management:** Engage in stress-reducing activities like meditation, yoga, or deep breathing exercises.
7. **Stay Physically Active:** Regular exercise can help manage symptoms like depression and anxiety.
8. **Build a Support System:** Surround yourself with supportive family members and friends. Consider joining a support group for people with bipolar disorder.
9. **Have a Plan for Manic Episodes:** Develop a plan with your healthcare provider and family for what to do if you start experiencing mania or hypomania.

For Loved Ones and Caregivers:

1. **Educate Yourself:** Learn about bipolar disorder to better understand the challenges and behaviors associated with the condition.
2. **Be Patient:** Understand that mood swings are a part of the disorder and not a reflection of the person's character.
3. **Offer Support:** Be supportive and encouraging, especially during mood episodes.
4. **Communicate Openly:** Keep the lines of communication open and discuss how you can be helpful.
5. **Recognize Warning Signs:** Be aware of the signs of both manic and depressive episodes. Encourage your loved one to seek help if you notice these signs worsening.
6. **Encourage Treatment:** Support your loved one in adhering to their treatment plan.
7. **Take Care of Yourself:** Supporting someone with bipolar disorder can be challenging. Ensure you also take time for your own mental health and seek support if needed.
8. **Set Boundaries:** Establish clear boundaries for your own well-being. It is important to maintain a balance between supporting your loved one and taking care of yourself.
9. **Plan for Emergencies:** Have a plan in place for how to respond in case of a crisis or emergency situation related to their bipolar disorder.

Remember:

Bipolar disorder is a lifelong condition, but it can be managed effectively with a combination of medication, therapy, lifestyle changes, and support. Both individuals with bipolar disorder and their loved ones should focus on open communication and building a strong support network to manage the condition effectively.

How to support a loved one with schizophrenia?

Supporting a loved one with schizophrenia, a chronic and often debilitating mental health disorder characterized by hallucinations, delusions, and disordered thinking and behavior, requires patience, understanding, and a commitment to their long-term well-being. Here are some strategies to provide support:

Educate Yourself About Schizophrenia

1. **Understand the Disorder:** Learn about schizophrenia, its symptoms, and its impact. This understanding can help you empathize with your loved one's experiences.
2. **Know the Myths vs. Facts:** There are many misconceptions about schizophrenia. Understanding the truth can help you better support your loved one.

Provide Emotional Support

1. **Be Patient and Understanding:** Recognize that your loved one may have difficulty expressing emotions or participating in social activities.
2. **Listen and Communicate Effectively:** Offer a listening ear and speak calmly and clearly. Avoid arguing about their delusions.
3. **Respect Their Experiences:** Acknowledge their feelings and experiences without judgment, even if they seem out of touch with reality.

Encourage Treatment and Support Their Care

1. **Encourage Professional Help:** Gently suggest seeking professional help if they have not already done so. Offer to help find a healthcare provider or attend appointments with them.
2. **Support Medication Management:** Help them manage their medications, ensuring they take them as prescribed.
3. **Be Aware of Side Effects:** Understand the side effects of their medication and help them address these with their doctor.

Help with Daily Life

1. **Assist with Daily Tasks:** Offer help with everyday tasks that can be overwhelming for them, like grocery shopping or housekeeping.
2. **Encourage Routine:** A predictable routine can provide a sense of stability and security.

Look for Warning Signs of Relapse

1. **Monitor for Changes:** Be aware of any signs that their condition might be worsening, like increased withdrawal or changes in mood or behavior.
2. **Have a Crisis Plan:** Know what to do in case of a crisis, including who to contact and where to go.

Take Care of Yourself

1. **Seek Support for Yourself:** It is crucial to look after your own mental health. Consider joining support groups for families of people with schizophrenia.
2. **Set Boundaries:** Establish personal boundaries for what you can and cannot do, and stick to them.

Foster Independence and Empowerment

1. **Encourage Independence:** Encourage them to be as independent as possible, which can help boost their confidence and sense of self-worth.
2. **Focus on Strengths and Abilities:** Emphasize their strengths and encourage them to pursue interests and activities they enjoy.

Maintain Hope and Positivity

1. **Stay Hopeful:** Encourage optimism about the future and the management of schizophrenia.
2. **Celebrate Progress:** Acknowledge and celebrate any progress or accomplishments, no matter how small.

Remember, each person with schizophrenia experiences the condition differently, so tailor your support to his or her specific needs and circumstances. It is a challenging journey, but with appropriate treatment and support, many individuals with schizophrenia can lead fulfilling lives.

How to live with personality disorder?

Living with a personality disorder can be challenging both for the individual affected and for those around them. Personality disorders are characterized by enduring patterns of behavior, cognition, and inner experience that deviate markedly from the expectations of the individual's culture. These patterns are inflexible and pervasive across many personal and social situations, leading to significant distress or impairment in social, occupational, or other areas of functioning.

Here are some strategies for individuals living with a personality disorder and for their loved ones or caregivers:

For Individuals with a Personality Disorder:

1. **Seek Professional Help:** Engage with a mental health professional experienced in treating personality disorders. Therapy can be highly effective in managing symptoms and improving quality of life.
2. **Stick to Treatment Plans:** Consistently follow through with therapy sessions and any prescribed medication. Treatment for personality disorders often requires long-term commitment.
3. **Self-Awareness and Reflection:** Work on becoming more aware of your thoughts, feelings, and behaviors, and how they affect your life and relationships.
4. **Develop Coping Skills:** Learn and practice coping strategies to manage emotions, reduce impulsive behaviors, and improve relationships. Techniques can include mindfulness, stress reduction, and emotion regulation skills.
5. **Build a Support System:** Cultivate relationships with understanding friends and family. Consider joining a support group for people with similar challenges.
6. **Educate Yourself:** Learn about your disorder to better understand yourself and explain your condition to others.
7. **Lifestyle Changes:** Regular exercise, a healthy diet, adequate sleep, and avoiding drugs and alcohol can help manage symptoms.

For Loved Ones and Caregivers:

1. **Educate Yourself:** Understanding the nature of personality disorders is crucial in providing support. It helps in developing empathy and realistic expectations.
2. **Encourage Treatment:** Support your loved one in seeking and adhering to professional treatment. Be patient, as progress can be slow.

3. **Effective Communication:** Learn and practice ways of communicating that reduce conflict and misunderstandings. Avoid judgmental or confrontational language.
4. **Set Boundaries:** Establish clear and consistent boundaries. It is important for your well-being and helps the person with the personality disorder understand acceptable behaviors.
5. **Offer Emotional Support:** Be a stable and understanding presence. Acknowledge their feelings and experiences without enabling unhealthy behaviors.
6. **Take Care of Yourself:** Living with or caring for someone with a personality disorder can be stressful. Ensure you have your own support system and consider seeking therapy for yourself.
7. **Avoid Personalizing Behaviors:** Recognize that the challenging behaviors are part of the disorder and not directed at you personally.
8. **Plan for Crisis:** Have a plan for how to handle potential crises, including who to contact and what actions to take if the person becomes a danger to themselves or others.

General Tips:

- **Patience and Understanding:** Managing a personality disorder is a long-term process with ups and downs.
- **Focus on Strengths:** Encourage and celebrate positive traits and accomplishments.
- **Regular Routine:** A structured and predictable routine can be beneficial.

It is important to remember that personality disorders are complex and require a nuanced approach to treatment and support. With the right help and strategies, individuals with personality disorders can lead fulfilling lives.

How to live with an alcoholic?

Living with an alcoholic can be an emotionally taxing and challenging situation. It often involves navigating a complex mix of emotions and behaviors while trying to support your loved one. Here are some strategies and considerations for living with an alcoholic:

Understand the Nature of Alcoholism

1. **Educate Yourself:** Recognize that alcoholism is a disease characterized by a physical and psychological dependence on alcohol.
2. **Know the Signs:** Be aware of the signs of alcohol abuse and alcoholism so you can better understand your loved one's struggles.

Support Your Loved One

1. **Encourage Treatment:** Gently encourage them to seek professional help. This could be medical treatment, counseling, or joining a recovery program like Alcoholics Anonymous.
2. **Avoid Enabling:** Avoid behaviors that enable their addiction, like covering up for them or providing them with alcohol.
3. **Express Concern in a Non-Confrontational Way:** Share your concerns with empathy and without judgment. Use "I" statements to express how their drinking affects you.

Take Care of Yourself

1. **Set Boundaries:** Establish clear boundaries for what you will and will not accept. Stick to these boundaries to protect your well-being.
2. **Seek Support:** Consider joining a support group like Al-Anon, where you can meet others who are in similar situations and learn from their experiences.
3. **Manage Stress:** Take time for yourself and engage in activities that help you relax and de-stress.

Create a Safe Environment

1. **Remove Alcohol:** Keep your home environment alcohol-free to reduce temptation.
2. **Plan for Safety:** Have a plan for how to keep yourself and others safe, especially in situations where the alcoholic's behavior becomes dangerous or abusive.

Avoid Certain Behaviors

1. **Don't Argue When They're Drunk:** Trying to reason with someone who is intoxicated is usually futile and can escalate to conflict.
2. **Don't Blame Yourself:** Remember, you are not responsible for their drinking behavior.
3. **Don't Expect Immediate Change:** Recovery is a process that can take time.

Focus on Positive Actions

1. **Encourage Healthy Habits:** Promote activities that support sobriety, such as exercise, hobbies, or joining support groups.
2. **Celebrate Small Successes:** Acknowledge positive steps, no matter how small they may seem.

Prepare for Difficult Decisions

1. **Consider Interventions:** In some cases, staging an intervention with the help of a professional may be necessary.
2. **Be Prepared to Make Tough Choices:** There may come a point where you need to consider distancing yourself or your family from the situation for everyone's safety and well-being.

Understand That Relapse Can Be Part of the Process

1. **Know the Signs of Relapse:** Being aware of the signs can help in taking early action.
2. **Offer Support, Not Judgment:** If a relapse occurs, offer support to get back on track rather than expressing disappointment or judgment.

Living with an alcoholic often requires a balance between supporting your loved one and maintaining your own health and well-being. It is a challenging journey, but with the right support and boundaries, it is possible to manage. Remember, professional help is crucial both for the individual with alcoholism and for their family members.

When should a person be considered an alcoholic?

Determining when someone should be considered an alcoholic, now more commonly referred to as having an Alcohol Use Disorder (AUD), involves evaluating various factors related to their drinking habits and the impact of these habits on their life. AUD is a medical condition characterized by an impaired ability to stop or control alcohol use despite adverse social, occupational, or health consequences. It ranges from mild to severe, and the criteria for diagnosis are outlined in the Diagnostic and Statistical Manual of Mental Disorders (DSM-5), published by the American Psychiatric Association.

Here are key indicators that someone might be experiencing Alcohol Use Disorder:

1. **Uncontrolled Drinking:** Drinking more or for a longer time than intended, or having a persistent desire or unsuccessful efforts to cut down or control alcohol use.
2. **Preoccupation with Alcohol:** Spending a lot of time obtaining, using, or recovering from the effects of alcohol.
3. **Cravings:** Experiencing strong cravings or urges to drink alcohol.
4. **Impact on Responsibilities:** Recurrent alcohol use resulting in a failure to fulfill major role obligations at work, school, or home.
5. **Social and Interpersonal Problems:** Continued alcohol use despite having persistent or recurrent social or interpersonal problems caused or exacerbated by the effects of alcohol.
6. **Withdrawal Activities:** Giving up or reducing important social, occupational, or recreational activities because of alcohol use.
7. **Hazardous Situations:** Recurrent alcohol use in situations where it is physically hazardous (e.g., driving, operating machinery).
8. **Tolerance:** A need for markedly increased amounts of alcohol to achieve intoxication or desired effect, or a markedly diminished effect with continued use of the same amount of alcohol.
9. **Withdrawal Symptoms:** The characteristic withdrawal syndrome for alcohol, or using alcohol (or a closely related substance) to relieve or avoid withdrawal symptoms.
10. **Continued Use Despite Knowledge of Harm:** Continued alcohol use despite having a persistent or recurrent physical or psychological problem that is likely to have been caused or exacerbated by alcohol.
11. **Physical or Psychological Harm:** Experiencing physical or psychological harm as a result of alcohol use.

It is important to note that these criteria are intended to be used as guidelines by qualified professionals. If you or someone you know is exhibiting these signs, it is important to seek help from a healthcare provider who can make an appropriate diagnosis and recommend treatment options. Early intervention can be key in managing AUD effectively.

How must a relative trying to deal with an addict, act?

Dealing with a loved one who is struggling with addiction is a challenging and often heart-wrenching experience. It requires a balance of support, understanding, and setting boundaries. Here are some strategies relatives can use:

Educate Yourself About Addiction

1. **Understand the Nature of Addiction:** Recognize that addiction is a complex brain disorder, not a moral failing or a matter of willpower.
2. **Learn About the Recovery Process:** Familiarize yourself with what the recovery process entails, including the potential for relapse.

Provide Support Without Enabling

1. **Encourage Treatment:** Gently encourage your loved one to seek professional help. Offer to help find treatment options or to accompany them to appointments.
2. **Avoid Enabling Behaviors:** Do not cover up or make excuses for their behaviors, and avoid giving them money that could be used for substances.
3. **Express Love and Concern:** Let them know you care about them and are concerned for their well-being, but be clear that you do not support their addictive behaviors.

Communicate Effectively

1. **Use "I" Statements:** Express your feelings and concerns without blaming or shaming. For example, say, "I feel worried when I see you drinking so much," instead of "You are always drinking and ruining everything."
2. **Be Honest and Direct:** Be honest about the impact their addiction has on you and your family, but do so with compassion.

Set Boundaries

1. **Establish Clear Boundaries:** Determine what behaviors you will not tolerate and what consequences will be if those boundaries are crossed.
2. **Be Consistent:** Stick to the boundaries you set. Consistency is key in helping your loved one understand the seriousness of their situation.

Take Care of Yourself

1. **Seek Support for Yourself:** Join support groups like Al-Anon or Nar-Anon, where you can share experiences and learn from others who are in similar situations.
2. **Practice Self-Care:** Take time for yourself and engage in activities that help you relax and recharge.

Prepare for Difficult Decisions

1. **Consider Interventions:** Sometimes, staging an intervention with the help of a professional may be necessary.
2. **Be Prepared for Tough Choices:** You may need to make difficult decisions, like not bailing them out of legal troubles or refusing to let them stay in your home if they're using.

Stay Hopeful Yet Realistic

1. **Acknowledge Small Victories:** Celebrate progress, no matter how small, such as attending a therapy session or a day without substance use.
2. **Understand That Relapse Can Be Part of the Process:** Relapse does not mean failure; it is often a step in the journey to recovery.

Protect Yourself and Your Family

1. **Safety First:** If the situation becomes dangerous, prioritize the safety of yourself and other family members.
2. **Limit Financial Support:** Don't provide financial assistance that could enable their habit.

Seek Professional Advice

1. **Consult a Therapist:** Consider seeking advice from a therapist or counselor experienced in addiction issues for guidance on how to handle specific situations.

Remember, while you can offer support and encourage your loved one to get help, ultimately, the decision to change and seek recovery must come from them. It is a difficult journey, but with the right support and boundaries, it is possible for both you and your loved one to navigate through it.

What treatment are available for an addict?

Treatment for addiction, often termed substance use disorder, varies depending on the type of addiction, the individual's circumstances, and the severity of the disorder. The goal of treatment is to help the individual stop using the substance, maintain a drug-free lifestyle, and achieve productive functioning in the family, at work, and in society. Here is an overview of the commonly available treatments:

1. Detoxification

- **Medically Assisted Detox:** Helps people safely withdraw from drugs or alcohol until the substances are no longer present in their system. This is often the first step in treatment programs and may be accompanied by medication to help alleviate withdrawal symptoms.

2. Medication

- **Maintenance Therapy:** Especially for opioid, alcohol, and nicotine addiction, medications can help reduce cravings and withdrawal symptoms.
- **Treatment of Co-Occurring Disorders:** Medications may also be prescribed for co-occurring mental health conditions like depression or anxiety.

3. Behavioral Therapies

- **Cognitive-Behavioral Therapy (CBT):** Helps individuals identify and change thinking and behavior patterns related to substance use, develop coping skills, and learn to manage triggers and stress.
- **Motivational Interviewing**: Focuses on the individual's readiness to change their behavior and enter treatment.
- **Contingency Management:** Uses positive reinforcement such as rewards or privileges to encourage sobriety.

4. Rehabilitation Programs

- **Inpatient Programs:** Provide intensive treatment in a live-in facility. Programs typically include medical and psychological care.
- **Outpatient Programs:** Allow individuals to live at home while receiving treatment. The intensity and frequency of therapy can vary.

5. Support Groups and Peer Support

- **12-Step Programs (like Alcoholics Anonymous and Narcotics Anonymous):** Offer a framework for recovery and ongoing peer support.
- **Non-12-Step Programs:** Such as SMART Recovery, offer an alternative to the traditional 12-step approach.

6. Dual Diagnosis Treatment

- For individuals with a co-occurring mental health disorder, integrated treatment that addresses both conditions simultaneously is crucial.

7. Family and Couples Therapy

- Addresses issues in the family system that may contribute to substance use and improves family dynamics and communication.

8. Holistic Therapies

- Approaches like yoga, meditation, acupuncture, and art therapy can complement traditional treatments by reducing stress and improving mental well-being.

9. Aftercare and Relapse Prevention

- Ongoing support and counseling to prevent relapse, which may include sober living arrangements, continued therapy, and support group participation.

10. Lifestyle Changes

- Encouraging healthy habits, such as regular exercise, proper nutrition, and adequate sleep, which are important components of a comprehensive treatment plan.

It is important to note that treatment should be individualized and often requires a combination of therapies and services. The effectiveness of treatment depends on the nature of the addiction, the individual's personal circumstances and history, and their level of engagement and commitment to recovery. Early intervention and a willingness to seek and adhere to treatment significantly improve outcomes.

What is biofeedback?

Biofeedback is a technique that teaches people to control physiological functions that are typically involuntary, such as heart rate, muscle tension, blood pressure, skin temperature, and brainwave patterns. It is based on the concept of "mind over matter," where individuals learn to use information (feedback) provided by biofeedback devices to gain control over these autonomic bodily functions.

How Biofeedback Works:

1. **Sensors:** Small sensors or electrodes are attached to the body. These sensors measure specific physiological parameters like heart rate, muscle tension, skin conductivity, respiratory rate, or brain activity.
2. **Feedback:** The sensors are connected to a machine or computer that provides real-time, easy-to-understand feedback about these physiological states. This feedback is often displayed through visual (like a graph on a monitor) or auditory signals.

3. **Training and Practice:** Under the guidance of a trained biofeedback therapist, the individual learns to recognize and control their physiological responses. This involves understanding how to interpret the feedback and using techniques like relaxation, guided imagery, or mindfulness to influence these bodily functions.
4. **Application:** Over time, individuals learn to control these functions without the need for biofeedback equipment, applying these skills in everyday situations to manage or alleviate symptoms.

Types of Biofeedback:

- **Electromyography (EMG):** Measures muscle activity and tension.
- **Thermal Biofeedback:** Measures skin temperature.
- **Neurofeedback (or EEG Biofeedback):** Focuses on brainwave patterns.
- **Heart Rate Variability (HRV):** Measures the variations in heart rate.
- **Galvanic Skin Response (GSR):** Measures the sweat gland activity, which is reflective of arousal or stress.

Uses of Biofeedback:

Biofeedback is used for a variety of health problems, especially those related to stress or chronic pain. Common applications include:

- **Stress and Anxiety:** Helps in recognizing and controlling physiological signs of stress.
- **Chronic Pain:** Assists in identifying and reducing muscle tension that contributes to pain.
- **Migraine and Tension Headaches:** Teaches control of blood flow and muscle tension to alleviate headaches.
- **High Blood Pressure:** Can aid in learning relaxation techniques to help control blood pressure.
- **Urinary Incontinence:** Helps in strengthening pelvic floor muscles.
- **ADHD and Other Neurological Conditions:** Neurofeedback can be used to improve focus and attention.

Benefits of Biofeedback:

- **Non-Invasive:** It is a non-invasive method of treatment.
- **Self-Control and Empowerment:** Provides a sense of control over health and well-being.
- **Complementary:** Can be used alongside other traditional treatments.
- **Reduces the Need for Medication:** In some cases, biofeedback can reduce the dependence on medications.

Finding a Practitioner:

Biofeedback should be performed by a trained therapist. When seeking biofeedback therapy, it is important to look for a certified professional who has experience in treating your specific condition.

In summary, biofeedback is a valuable tool in the realm of mind-body therapies, offering a way for individuals to take a more active role in their own health care, especially in the management of stress-related and psychophysiological disorders.

What can be the etiology of anxiety and its management?

The etiology (or cause) of anxiety is multifaceted, often involving a combination of biological, psychological, and environmental factors. Understanding these factors can help in developing effective management strategies.

Etiology of Anxiety

1. **Genetic Factors:** Anxiety disorders can run in families, suggesting a genetic component. However, having a family member with an anxiety disorder does not guarantee that someone will develop one.
2. **Brain Chemistry: Imbalances** in neurotransmitters, chemicals in the brain that relay messages between neurons, can contribute to anxiety disorders.
3. **Personality Traits:** Certain personality traits, like being prone to shyness or nervousness, can increase the risk of developing anxiety disorders.
4. **Life Experiences:** Traumatic life events, such as abuse, the death of a loved one, or being involved in a major accident, can trigger anxiety disorders. Chronic stress, including work stress or ongoing financial pressures, can also play a role.
5. **Developmental Factors:** Experiences during childhood and adolescence, such as parental overprotection or exposure to adverse experiences, can influence the development of anxiety disorders.

6. **Physical Health Conditions:** Certain physical health conditions, like thyroid problems or heart arrhythmias, can produce or exacerbate anxiety symptoms.

7. **Substance Use:** Abuse of or withdrawal from alcohol, drugs, or certain medications can lead to or worsen anxiety.

Management of Anxiety

1. **Psychotherapy:** Cognitive-Behavioral Therapy (CBT) is particularly effective for anxiety disorders. It helps individuals identify and challenge negative thought patterns and behaviors and replace them with more constructive ones.

2. **Medication:** Antidepressants, such as SSRIs and SNRIs, are commonly used to treat anxiety disorders. Benzodiazepines may be used for short-term relief of severe anxiety symptoms but are generally not recommended for long-term use due to the risk of dependence.

3. **Lifestyle Modifications:** Regular physical activity, a healthy diet, adequate sleep, and avoiding caffeine and alcohol can help reduce anxiety symptoms.

4. **Stress Management Techniques:** Practices like mindfulness, meditation, deep breathing exercises, and yoga can help manage stress and reduce anxiety.

5. **Support Groups:** Sharing experiences and strategies with others who have anxiety disorders can provide support and insights.

6. **Education:** Understanding anxiety disorders can empower individuals to take an active role in their treatment and reduce the stigma associated with mental health issues.

7. **Mind-Body Techniques:** Techniques like biofeedback and hypnotherapy can be beneficial for some individuals.

8. **Alternative Therapies:** Some people find relief with alternative therapies like acupuncture, massage therapy, or herbal supplements. However, it is important to consult a healthcare provider before trying these options.

9. **Avoiding Substance Abuse:** Steering clear of alcohol, drugs, and unnecessary medications can help in managing anxiety.

10. **Building a Supportive Network:** Cultivating strong relationships with family and friends provides emotional support and aids in coping.

It is important to note that the treatment and management of anxiety are highly individualized. What works effectively for one person may not be as effective for another. A combination of therapy, medication, lifestyle changes, and supportive interventions is often the most effective approach. Consulting with a healthcare provider or mental health professional is crucial in developing an appropriate treatment plan.

What medical disorders can directly cause anxiety?

Several medical conditions can directly contribute to or exacerbate anxiety symptoms. It is important to note that anxiety can sometimes be a symptom of an underlying medical issue. Here are some medical disorders that are known to be associated with anxiety:

1. **Endocrine Disorders:**
   - **Hyperthyroidism:** Overactive thyroid gland can lead to symptoms similar to anxiety, like nervousness, rapid heartbeat, and difficulty concentrating.
   - **Hypothyroidism:** Underactive thyroid can also cause anxiety-like symptoms along with fatigue and weight gain.
   - **Cushing's Disease:** Overproduction of cortisol can lead to symptoms of anxiety.
2. **Cardiovascular Diseases:**
   - **Heart Disease:** People with heart conditions may experience anxiety, particularly concerning their health and symptoms.
   - **Hypertension (High Blood Pressure):** While hypertension itself may not cause anxiety, the stress of managing a chronic condition can lead to anxiety.
3. **Respiratory Disorders:**
   - **Chronic Obstructive Pulmonary Disease (COPD) and Asthma:** Difficulty breathing can lead to feelings of anxiety and panic.
4. **Neurological Disorders:**
   - **Epilepsy:** Some types of seizures can be associated with anxiety.
   - **Parkinson's Disease:** Anxiety can be a symptom of Parkinson's and a side effect of medications used to treat it.

5. **Metabolic Disorders:**
   - **Diabetes:** Fluctuations in blood sugar levels can affect mood and anxiety levels.
6. **Substance Abuse and Withdrawal:**
   - **Alcohol, Drugs, and Medication:** Use and withdrawal from substances, including caffeine and prescription medications (like steroids), can cause anxiety symptoms.
7. **Gastrointestinal Conditions:**
   - **Irritable Bowel Syndrome (IBS):** Chronic GI issues can lead to or exacerbate anxiety.
8. **Chronic Pain Conditions:**
   - Ongoing pain can lead to anxiety, partly due to the stress of managing a chronic condition.
9. **Hormonal Imbalances:**
   - **Menopause:** Hormonal changes during menopause can cause symptoms of anxiety.
   - **Premenstrual Syndrome (PMS) and Premenstrual Dysphoric Disorder (PMDD):** Hormonal fluctuations can also affect mood and anxiety levels.
10. **Infections:**
    - Certain infections, particularly those affecting the brain and central nervous system, can have psychological symptoms including anxiety.
11. **Autoimmune Diseases:**
    - Conditions like lupus and rheumatoid arthritis, due to chronic pain and the stress of managing the disease, can be linked to anxiety.
12. **Cancer:**
    - Anxiety can be a reaction to a cancer diagnosis, the stress of treatment, and concerns about prognosis.

It is crucial for individuals experiencing anxiety to undergo a thorough medical evaluation to rule out or address any potential underlying medical issues. The treatment for anxiety in the context of these conditions often involves managing the underlying medical condition along with the anxiety symptoms.

What drugs can cause anxiety?

Several medications and substances can induce or exacerbate anxiety symptoms. It is important to be aware of these, especially if you have a predisposition to anxiety. Here are some common substances known to potentially cause anxiety:

1. **Stimulants:**
   - **Caffeine:** Found in coffee, tea, chocolate, and some soft drinks; high doses can increase anxiety and nervousness.
   - **Amphetamines:** Including ADHD medications (like Adderall) and recreational drugs.
   - **Cocaine:** A potent stimulant that can cause significant anxiety during use and withdrawal.
2. **Corticosteroids:**
   - Used to treat a variety of conditions, these drugs can have side effects including increased anxiety, agitation, and mood swings.
3. **Decongestants:**
   - Over-the-counter cold and allergy medications containing pseudoephedrine or phenylephrine can increase anxiety.
4. **Antidepressants:**
   - Some people may experience increased anxiety when starting certain antidepressants, particularly selective serotonin reuptake inhibitors (SSRIs). This is usually temporary.
5. **Thyroid Medications:**
   - Overmedication with thyroid hormone replacements can lead to symptoms of hyperthyroidism, including anxiety.
6. **Birth Control Pills:**
   - Hormonal fluctuations due to birth control pills can affect mood and anxiety levels in some women.
7. **Weight Loss Medications:**
   - Certain diet pills, especially those containing stimulants, can increase anxiety.
8. **Withdrawal from Drugs:**
   - Withdrawal from substances like alcohol, benzodiazepines (e.g., Xanax, Valium), and narcotics can cause significant anxiety and panic.
9. **Blood Pressure Medications:**
   - Beta-blockers and ACE inhibitors, used to manage hypertension, can sometimes cause

anxiety or exacerbate existing anxiety symptoms.

10. **Antipsychotic Medications:**
    - Some antipsychotics can have side effects that include anxiety.
11. **Alcohol:**
    - While alcohol may initially act as a sedative, its use and withdrawal can significantly increase anxiety.
12. **Nicotine and Smoking Cessation Aids:**
    - Nicotine is a stimulant and can increase anxiety. Additionally, some smoking cessation aids can also contribute to anxiety.
13. **Cannabis:**
    - While some find cannabis relaxing, others may experience increased anxiety and paranoia, especially with high THC strains.

It is important to remember that the way individuals react to drugs can vary greatly. What causes anxiety in one person may not affect another in the same way. If you suspect that a medication or substance is contributing to your anxiety, it is important to consult with a healthcare provider. They can help assess the situation and make any necessary adjustments to your treatment. Additionally, never stop a prescribed medication without consulting your healthcare provider, as this can sometimes worsen symptoms or lead to other complications.

What can be the result of anxiety?

Anxiety, especially when chronic and unmanaged, can have a wide range of effects on an individual's health, both mental and physical, as well as on their overall quality of life. Here are some of the potential outcomes and complications associated with anxiety:

Physical Health Effects

1. **Cardiovascular Problems:** Chronic anxiety can contribute to heart diseases, including heart palpitations, increased heart rate, elevated blood pressure, and increased risk of heart attacks.
2. **Weakened Immune System:** Prolonged stress and anxiety can weaken the immune system, making the body more susceptible to infections and illnesses.
3. **Gastrointestinal Issues:** Anxiety can lead to gastrointestinal problems like irritable bowel syndrome (IBS), ulcers, and chronic indigestion.
4. **Respiratory Issues:** It can exacerbate respiratory disorders such as asthma and chronic obstructive pulmonary disease (COPD).
5. **Muscle Tension:** Chronic muscle tension and pain, especially in the neck and back, can result from prolonged anxiety.
6. **Other Physical Symptoms:** Headaches, dizziness, fatigue, and other physical symptoms are commonly associated with anxiety.

Mental Health Impact

1. **Increased Risk of Depression:** There is a strong link between anxiety disorders and the development of depression.
2. **Substance Abuse:** Some individuals may turn to alcohol or drugs as a way to self-medicate their anxiety, leading to substance abuse issues.
3. **Sleep Disorders:** Difficulty falling asleep, staying asleep, or experiencing restful sleep is common in those with anxiety.
4. **Impaired Cognitive Functioning:** Anxiety can affect concentration, memory, and decision-making abilities.

Impact on Daily Life

1. **Reduced Quality of Life:** Chronic anxiety can interfere with work, school, relationships, and social activities.
2. **Avoidance Behaviors:** People with anxiety may avoid certain situations, places, or activities that they fear will trigger their anxiety.
3. **Strained Relationships:** Anxiety can put a strain on personal and professional relationships.

Long-Term Risks

1. **Chronic Health Conditions:** Long-term, unmanaged anxiety can contribute to the development of chronic health conditions like heart disease.
2. **Psychological Disorders:** Persistent anxiety can increase the risk of developing other mental health disorders.

Coping and Management

To manage anxiety and mitigate its effects, various strategies can be employed, including:

- **Professional Therapy:** Such as cognitive-behavioral therapy (CBT), which is effective in treating anxiety disorders.
- **Medications:** Including antidepressants, anti-anxiety medications, and beta-blockers.
- **Lifestyle Changes:** Regular exercise, a healthy diet, sufficient sleep, and mindfulness practices can help manage symptoms.
- **Stress Management Techniques:** Like deep breathing exercises, meditation, and yoga.
- **Support Networks:** Engaging with supportive family, friends, or joining support groups.

It is important to seek professional help if anxiety is affecting your life. Early intervention can prevent complications and improve quality of life. Remember, anxiety is a common and treatable condition, and seeking help is a sign of strength, not weakness.

How is anxiety treated?

Anxiety, a common mental health condition, can be effectively treated through a combination of therapeutic approaches, medication, lifestyle changes, and self-help strategies. Treatment is often tailored to the individual, as what works for one person might not be as effective for another. Here is an overview of the main treatment modalities for anxiety:

1. Psychological Therapies

1. **Cognitive Behavioral Therapy (CBT):**
   - This is one of the most effective therapies for anxiety. CBT focuses on identifying, understanding, and changing thinking and behavior patterns. It helps individuals challenge distorted thinking and change their reactions to anxiety-provoking situations.
2. **Exposure Therapy:**
   - Often used for specific phobias or OCD, exposure therapy involves gradual exposure to the source of anxiety in a controlled, safe environment to help reduce fear and anxiety responses.
3. **Acceptance and Commitment Therapy (ACT):**
   - ACT involves accepting anxiety symptoms rather than fighting them, while committing to behavior change aligned with personal values.
4. **Psychotherapy:**
   - Traditional talk therapy can help individuals understand the root causes of their anxiety and develop strategies to cope with them.

2. Medication

1. **Selective Serotonin Reuptake Inhibitors (SSRIs):**
   - These are commonly prescribed antidepressants that can help reduce anxiety symptoms.
2. **Serotonin-Norepinephrine Reuptake Inhibitors (SNRIs):**
   - Another class of antidepressants that can be effective in treating anxiety.
3. **Benzodiazepines:**
   - These are sedatives that can quickly reduce anxiety symptoms but are typically used for short-term relief due to risks of dependence.
4. **Beta-Blockers:**
   - Primarily used for heart conditions, beta-blockers can also help control physical symptoms of anxiety, like rapid heart rate and trembling.
5. **Buspirone:**
   - An anxiolytic that can be used for chronic anxiety treatment.

3. Lifestyle Modifications

1. **Regular Exercise:**
   - Physical activity is known to reduce anxiety symptoms and improve mood.
2. **Balanced Diet:**
   - A healthy diet can impact overall mental health positively.
3. **Adequate Sleep:**
   - Ensuring sufficient and quality sleep can help reduce anxiety.
4. **Mindfulness and Relaxation Techniques:**
   - Practices such as meditation, deep breathing exercises, and yoga can help manage stress and anxiety.
5. **Limiting Alcohol and Caffeine:**
   - Both substances can exacerbate anxiety and should be consumed in moderation.

4. Alternative Therapies

1. **Acupuncture:**
   - Some find acupuncture helpful for reducing anxiety symptoms.
2. **Herbal Supplements:**
   - Certain herbs like chamomile and valerian root are believed to have calming effects, but it is important to consult a doctor before use.
3. **Aromatherapy:**
   - Essential oils like lavender have been reported to have a calming effect.

5. Self-Help Strategies

1. **Self-Care:** Taking time for personal care and engaging in enjoyable activities.
2. **Support Groups:** Sharing experiences and coping strategies with others facing similar challenges.
3. **Stress Management:** Learning to manage stress through various techniques.

6. Technology-Assisted Interventions

1. **Online Therapy and Counseling:**
   - Digital platforms offer access to mental health professionals and online CBT programs.
2. **Mindfulness Apps:**
   - Apps can provide guided meditation and relaxation exercises.

It is important to note that treatment should be individualized, and what works for one person may not work for another. Consulting with a healthcare provider or mental health professional is crucial in developing an appropriate treatment plan. Also, never stop or change medication without consulting a healthcare professional, as this can sometimes worsen symptoms or lead to other complications.

What is the management of OCD?

Obsessive-Compulsive Disorder (OCD) is a chronic mental health disorder characterized by uncontrollable, recurring thoughts (obsessions) and behaviors (compulsions) that the individual feels compelled to repeat. Effective management of OCD typically involves a combination of therapeutic strategies, medication, self-help techniques, and lifestyle modifications.

1. Psychological Therapies

1. **Cognitive Behavioral Therapy (CBT):**
   - Especially a type of CBT known as Exposure and Response Prevention (ERP). This involves gradual exposure to the source of the obsession and learning to resist the urge to engage in compulsive behaviors.
2. **Acceptance and Commitment Therapy (ACT):**
   - Helps patients accept their thoughts without acting on them and commit to actions that align with their values.
3. **Other Forms of Psychotherapy:**
   - Such as psychodynamic therapy, which may help some individuals understand the underlying emotional basis of their OCD.

2. Medication

1. **Selective Serotonin Reuptake Inhibitors (SSRIs):**
   - These are commonly used to help reduce the symptoms of OCD by increasing the level of serotonin in the brain.
2. **Tricyclic Antidepressants (TCAs):**
   - In particular, clomipramine (Anafranil) has been effective for OCD, but it might have more side effects than SSRIs.
3. **Combination Therapy:**
   - Sometimes, a combination of medications may be necessary, depending on the individual's response to treatment.

3. Lifestyle Modifications

1. **Regular Exercise:**
   - Physical activity is known to improve mood and reduce anxiety, which can help manage OCD symptoms.
2. **Balanced Diet:**
   - A healthy diet can have a positive impact on overall well-being and mental health.
3. **Adequate Sleep:**
   - Good sleep hygiene is important for managing OCD symptoms.

4. **Mindfulness and Relaxation Techniques:**
   - Practices such as meditation, yoga, and deep breathing can help reduce stress and anxiety associated with OCD.

4. Self-Help Strategies

1. **Education:**
   - Understanding OCD and being informed about the condition can help individuals manage their symptoms more effectively.
2. **Support Groups:**
   - Sharing experiences and coping strategies with others who have OCD can provide support and reduce feelings of isolation.
3. **Stress Management:**
   - Developing effective stress management techniques can be beneficial.

5. Alternative Therapies

1. **Neurofeedback:**
   - Some evidence suggests neurofeedback may be helpful for some individuals with OCD.
2. **Herbal Supplements and Nutraceuticals:**
   - While there is limited evidence, some people find certain supplements helpful, but it is important to discuss this with a healthcare provider before starting any new treatment.

6. Advanced Treatment Options

1. **Deep Brain Stimulation (DBS):**
   - For severe cases of OCD that do not respond to conventional treatments, DBS or other forms of neuromodulation may be considered.
2. **Transcranial Magnetic Stimulation (TMS):**
   - A non-invasive procedure that uses magnetic fields to stimulate nerve cells in the brain and can be effective for some individuals with OCD.

Working with Healthcare Professionals

- **Regular Monitoring and Adjustment:** Treatment plans should be regularly reviewed and adjusted as needed by healthcare professionals.
- **Combination of Treatments:** Often, a combination of therapy, medication, and lifestyle changes yields the best results.

Remember, the management of OCD is highly individualized. What works for one person might not work for another, and it often takes time to find the most effective treatment plan. It is important for individuals with OCD to work closely with their healthcare providers to find the best approach for their specific needs.

How is panic disorder treated?

Panic disorder, characterized by recurrent and unexpected panic attacks along with persistent concern about having more attacks, can be effectively managed and treated with a combination of psychotherapy, medication, lifestyle changes, and self-help strategies. Treatment is often personalized, as what works for one person might not be as effective for another.

1. Psychotherapy

1. **Cognitive Behavioral Therapy (CBT):**
   - This is the most effective form of psychotherapy for panic disorder. CBT focuses on identifying, understanding, and changing thinking and behavior patterns. It helps individuals learn to react differently to the fears and physical sensations associated with panic attacks.
2. **Exposure Therapy:**
   - Involves gradual exposure to the sensations of panic in a safe and controlled environment, making them less frightening.

2. Medication

1. **Selective Serotonin Reuptake Inhibitors (SSRIs):**
   - These are typically the first choice in medication for panic disorder. Examples include fluoxetine (Prozac), sertraline (Zoloft), and paroxetine (Paxil).
2. **Serotonin-Norepinephrine Reuptake Inhibitors (SNRIs):**
   - Medications like venlafaxine (Effexor XR) can also be effective for panic disorder.
3. **Benzodiazepines:**
   - Fast-acting sedatives that can quickly reduce panic attack symptoms. However, they can be habit-forming and are typically used only on a short-term basis due to risks of dependence.
4. **Other Antidepressants:**
   - In some cases, other types of antidepressants may be prescribed.

3. Lifestyle Modifications

1. **Regular Exercise:**
   - Physical activity can help manage anxiety and improve mood.
2. **Balanced Diet:**
   - A healthy diet can impact overall well-being and mental health.
3. **Adequate Sleep:**
   - Good sleep hygiene can help reduce anxiety and improve emotional regulation.
4. **Mindfulness and Relaxation Techniques:**
   - Practices such as meditation, yoga, and deep breathing exercises can help manage stress and reduce anxiety symptoms.

4. Self-Help Strategies

1. **Understanding the Disorder:**
   - Being informed about panic disorder can help individuals manage their symptoms more effectively.
2. **Stress Management:**
   - Developing effective stress management techniques is crucial.
3. **Support Networks:**
   - Engaging with supportive friends and family or joining support groups can provide emotional support.
4. **Avoiding Alcohol and Caffeine:**
   - These substances can trigger or worsen panic attacks in some people.

5. Alternative Treatments

1. **Herbal Supplements and Nutraceuticals:**
   - Some individuals find relief with certain supplements, but it is important to discuss this with a healthcare provider before starting any new treatment.
2. **Acupuncture or Acupressure:**
   - These techniques may provide some individuals with relief from anxiety symptoms.

6. Advanced Treatment Options

1. **Transcranial Magnetic Stimulation (TMS):**
   - For treatment-resistant panic disorder, TMS might be an option.

It is important to note that treatment for panic disorder is highly individualized. Consulting with a healthcare provider or mental health professional is crucial for developing an appropriate treatment plan. Also, it is common for treatment strategies to be adjusted over time based on the individual's response to therapy and medication. Patience and persistence are key, as it can take some time to find the most effective approach for each individual.

What is the treatment of phobias?

The treatment of phobias, which are intense, irrational fears of specific objects, situations, or activities, typically involves psychotherapy, self-help strategies, and in some cases, medication. The goal of treatment is to reduce fear and anxiety symptoms and to help individuals manage their reactions to the object or situation they fear. Here is an overview of the common treatment approaches for phobias:

1. Psychotherapy

1. **Exposure Therapy:**
   - One of the most effective treatments for phobias. It involves gradual, controlled exposure to the feared object or situation. The exposure process often follows a hierarchy, starting from the least fearful situation and gradually moving to more challenging situations.
   - This therapy helps individuals build confidence and desensitize their responses to the feared object or situation.
2. **Cognitive Behavioral Therapy (CBT):**
   - CBT is used to identify and challenge negative thoughts associated with the phobia and to develop healthier thinking patterns.
   - It also involves learning coping skills and techniques to manage anxiety responses.

2. Medication

While medication is not typically used as the primary treatment for phobias, it can be helpful in certain situations:

1. **Beta-Blockers:**
   - Used to manage physical symptoms of anxiety, such as a rapid heartbeat, that can accompany a phobic reaction.
2. **Sedatives (Benzodiazepines):**
   - May be used for short-term relief of acute anxiety symptoms. However, they have the

potential for dependence and are generally not recommended for long-term use.

3. **Antidepressants:**
   - SSRIs (Selective Serotonin Reuptake Inhibitors) are sometimes used, particularly if the phobia co-occurs with depression or other anxiety disorders.

3. Lifestyle Modifications and Self-Help Strategies

1. **Relaxation Techniques:**
   - Practices such as deep breathing exercises, meditation, and yoga can help reduce anxiety symptoms.
2. **Mindfulness:**
   - Being present in the moment and acknowledging and accepting one's feelings and thoughts without judgment can be beneficial.
3. **Regular Exercise:**
   - Physical activity can help reduce stress and anxiety.
4. **Healthy Diet:**
   - A balanced diet can contribute to overall well-being and better mental health.

4. Support Groups and Peer Support

1. **Sharing Experiences:**
   - Talking with others who have similar phobias can provide insights and strategies for managing symptoms.

5. Education

1. **Understanding the Phobia:**
   - Learning about phobias and understanding that they are common and treatable can be reassuring and empowering.

6. Alternative Treatments

1. **Acupuncture or Herbal Supplements:**
   - Some individuals might find these alternative approaches helpful in managing anxiety, though they should always be discussed with a healthcare provider first.

7. Virtual Reality Therapy

1. **Simulated Exposure:**
   - Virtual reality technology is increasingly being used to simulate exposure to the feared object or situation in a controlled and safe environment.

It is important to note that the approach to treating phobias should be tailored to the individual's specific needs and severity of the phobia. Consulting with a mental health professional is crucial for developing an appropriate treatment plan. Additionally, patience and persistence are key, as overcoming phobias can take time and gradual exposure.

What is the treatment for Social anxiety disorder (social phobia)?

Social Anxiety Disorder, also known as social phobia, is characterized by intense anxiety or fear of being judged, negatively evaluated, or rejected in a social or performance situation. The treatment for Social Anxiety Disorder typically involves a combination of psychotherapy, medication, and self-help strategies. It is important to tailor the treatment to the individual's specific needs and severity of the disorder.

1. Psychotherapy

1. **Cognitive Behavioral Therapy (CBT):**
   - CBT is the most effective form of psychotherapy for treating Social Anxiety Disorder. It helps individuals identify and challenge negative thoughts about social situations and learn and practice social skills.
   - CBT may also include exposure therapy, where individuals gradually and systematically confront the situations they fear in a controlled way.
2. **Group Therapy:**
   - Group therapy can be particularly beneficial for social anxiety, as it provides a safe and supportive environment to practice social skills and face fears.

2. Medication

Medication can help reduce the symptoms of Social Anxiety Disorder, especially in severe cases or when psychotherapy alone. Here is has not been effective:

1. **Selective Serotonin Reuptake Inhibitors (SSRIs):**
   - SSRIs are commonly prescribed for Social Anxiety Disorder. Examples include sertraline (Zoloft), paroxetine (Paxil), and fluoxetine (Prozac).
2. **Serotonin-Norepinephrine Reuptake Inhibitors (SNRIs):**

- SNRIs like venlafaxine (Effexor XR) can also be effective.

3. **Benzodiazepines:**
   - These are sedatives that can quickly reduce anxiety symptoms. However, they can be habit-forming and are typically used only in the short term.

4. **Beta-Blockers:**
   - Used primarily to manage physical symptoms of anxiety, such as trembling and a racing heart, especially in specific situations like public speaking.

3. Lifestyle Modifications and Self-Help Strategies

1. **Stress Management Techniques:**
   - Practices such as mindfulness, meditation, and yoga can help manage overall stress and anxiety levels.

2. **Regular Exercise:**
   - Physical activity is known to improve mood and reduce symptoms of anxiety.

3. **Healthy Diet:**
   - A balanced diet can contribute to overall well-being.

4. **Adequate Sleep:**
   - Good sleep hygiene is important for managing anxiety.

4. Support Groups and Peer Support

1. **Sharing Experiences:**
   - Engaging with others who have similar challenges can provide support and coping strategies.

5. Building Social Skills

1. **Social Skills Training:**
   - This can be part of therapy and involves learning and practicing new skills in small, manageable steps.

6. Exposure to Social Situations

1. **Gradual Exposure:**
   - Gradually facing social situations that cause anxiety can help build confidence and reduce anxiety over time.

7. Alternative Treatments

1. **Herbal Supplements and Nutraceuticals:**
   - Some individuals find certain supplements helpful, but it is important to discuss this with a healthcare provider before starting any new treatment.

It is crucial for individuals with Social Anxiety Disorder to seek help from a mental health professional who can help develop an appropriate treatment plan. Treatment effectiveness can vary from person to person, and sometimes it takes time to find the most effective approach. Additi-onally, never stop or change medication without consulting a healthcare professional, as this can sometimes worsen symptoms or lead to other complications.

What is the treatment for specific phobias?

Treatment for specific phobias, which are intense, irrational fears of specific objects or situations, typically involves psychotherapy, particularly exposure therapy, and may sometimes include medication. The goal of treatment is to reduce fear and anxiety and to help individuals manage their reactions to the object or situation they fear.

1. Psychotherapy

1. **Exposure Therapy:**
   - The most effective form of treatment for specific phobias. It involves controlled, gradual exposure to the feared object or situation. The process usually follows a hierarchy, starting from the least frightening situation and gradually progressing to more challenging ones.
   - This therapy aims to help individuals build tolerance and eventually desensitize their response to the feared object or situation.

2. **Cognitive Behavioral Therapy (CBT):**
   - CBT can be used alongside exposure therapy. It helps individuals identify and challenge negative thoughts related to the phobia and develop healthier thinking patterns.
   - CBT also involves learning and practicing coping skills and relaxation techniques to manage anxiety.

2. Medication

Medication is generally not the primary treatment for specific phobias but can be helpful in certain situations, particularly for managing anxiety symptoms:

1. **Beta-Blockers:**
   - Used to control physical symptoms of anxiety, such as a rapid heartbeat, that can accompany a phobic reaction.
2. **Sedatives (Benzodiazepines):**
   - May be used for short-term relief of acute anxiety symptoms. However, due to the potential for dependence, they are generally not recommended for long-term use.

3. Self-Help Strategies

1. **Gradual Exposure:**
   - Individuals can practice exposure themselves by gradually and repeatedly exposing themselves to the phobia trigger.
2. **Relaxation Techniques:**
   - Techniques such as deep breathing exercises, meditation, and yoga can help reduce anxiety symptoms.
3. **Lifestyle Changes:**
   - Regular physical activity, a healthy diet, and adequate sleep can improve overall well-being and reduce anxiety.

4. Support Groups and Peer Support

1. **Sharing Experiences:**
   - Engaging with others who have overcome similar fears can provide encouragement and practical advice.

5. Virtual Reality Therapy

1. **Simulated Exposure:**
   - Virtual reality technology can simulate exposure to the feared object or situation in a controlled and safe environment, making it a useful tool for treatment.

6. Educational Approach

1. **Understanding the Phobia:**
   - Learning about phobias and understanding that they are common and treatable can be reassuring and empowering.

Treatment for specific phobias is usually highly effective, especially when the individual is motivated and actively participates in the treatment process. In many cases, therapy can significantly reduce or even eliminate phobic reactions. It is important for individuals to seek help from a mental health professional who can guide them in developing an appropriate and effective treatment plan.

What is the treatment for Agoraphobia?

Agoraphobia, a disorder characterized by an intense fear of being in places where escape might be difficult or help might not be available, especially in the event of having a panic attack, is treatable with a combination of psychotherapy, medication, and self-help strategies. Treatment is aimed at reducing anxiety symptoms and improving the individual's ability to function in daily life. Here is an overview of the common treatment approaches:

1. Psychotherapy

1. **Cognitive Behavioral Therapy (CBT):**
   - This is the most effective form of psychotherapy for agoraphobia. CBT focuses on identifying, understanding, and changing thinking and behavior patterns. It helps individuals learn to challenge and overcome fear and anxiety related to being in certain places or situations.
   - CBT often includes exposure therapy, where individuals are gradually and systematically exposed to the situations they fear in a controlled way.
2. **Exposure Therapy:**
   - Involves repeated exposure to the source of fear in a safe and controlled environment, which helps reduce fear and anxiety over time.

2. Medication

Medication can be an important part of treatment, especially for those with severe symptoms:

1. **Selective Serotonin Reuptake Inhibitors (SSRIs):**
   - SSRIs are commonly prescribed for agoraphobia and are generally considered first-line medication for this condition.
2. **Serotonin-Norepinephrine Reuptake Inhibitors (SNRIs):**
   - SNRIs may also be effective for treating agoraphobia.
3. **Benzodiazepines:**
   - These are sedatives that can help reduce symptoms of anxiety. However, they can be habit-forming and are generally used only for short-term relief.

3. Lifestyle Modifications and Self-Help Strategies

1. **Stress Management Techniques:**
   - Practices such as mindfulness, meditation, yoga, and deep breathing exercises can help manage stress and anxiety.
2. **Regular Exercise:**
   - Physical activity is known to improve mood and reduce symptoms of anxiety.
3. **Healthy Diet:**
   - A balanced diet can contribute to overall well-being.
4. **Adequate Sleep:**
   - Ensuring sufficient and restful sleep is important for managing anxiety.

4. Support Groups and Peer Support

1. **Engaging with Others:**
   - Sharing experiences and coping strategies with others who have similar challenges can provide support and reduce feelings of isolation.

5. Gradual Exposure to Feared Situations

1. **Systematic Desensitization:**
   - Gradually facing feared situations under controlled conditions can help build confidence and reduce anxiety over time.

6. Developing Coping Skills

1. **Learning and Practicing Coping Skills:**
   - This includes learning how to calm oneself during anxiety-provoking situations and how to gradually face and overcome fears.

It is important for individuals with agoraphobia to seek help from a mental health professional who can guide them in developing an appropriate treatment plan. Treatment effectiveness can vary from person to person, and sometimes it takes time to find the most effective approach. Additionally, never stop or change medication without consulting a healthcare professional, as this can sometimes worsen symptoms or lead to other complications.

What is the drug treatment of depression?

Drug treatment for depression primarily involves antidepressant medications. These medications work by balancing chemicals in your brain called neurotransmitters that affect mood and emotions. Here is an overview of the main types of antidepressants used in treating depression:

1. Selective Serotonin Reuptake Inhibitors (SSRIs)

- **Examples:** Fluoxetine (Prozac), Sertraline (Zoloft), Paroxetine (Paxil), Citalopram (Celexa), and Escitalopram (Lexapro).
- **How They Work:** They increase the level of serotonin in the brain and are typically considered the first-line treatment due to their relatively mild side effects.

2. Serotonin and Norepinephrine Reuptake Inhibitors (SNRIs)

- **Examples:** Venlafaxine (Effexor XR), Duloxetine (Cymbalta), and Desvenlafaxine (Presto).
- **How They Work:** These drugs increase the levels of both serotonin and norepinephrine neurotransmitters.

3. Tricyclic Antidepressants (TCAs)

- **Examples:** Amitriptyline, Nortriptyline (Pamelor), Imipramine (Tofranil), and Desipramine (Norpramin).
- **How They Work:** TCAs affect several neurotransmitters in the brain and are more potent but typically have more side effects than SSRIs and SNRIs.

4. Monoamine Oxidase Inhibitors (MAOIs)

- **Examples:** Tranylcypromine (Parnate), Phenelzine (Nardil), and Isocarboxazid (Marplan).
- **How They Work:** They work by inhibiting the activity of monoamine oxidase, an enzyme that breaks down neurotransmitters in the brain.
- **Note:** MAOIs can have serious side effects and require a strict diet due to dangerous (and potentially deadly) interactions with certain foods and medications.

5. Atypical Antidepressants

- **Examples:** Bupropion (Wellbutrin), Mirtazapine (Remeron), Trazodone, and Vilazodone (Viibryd).
- **How They Work:** These medications affect the brain's neurotransmitters differently than the typical antidepressants.

6. Other Medications

- In some cases, other medications might be used in combination with antidepressants to enhance their effectiveness. These can include mood stabilizers, antipsychotics, or anti-anxiety medications.

Considerations in Antidepressant Use

- **Finding the Right Medication:** It may take some time to find the most effective medication with the fewest side effects.
- **Side Effects:** While antidepressants can be highly effective, they can also cause side effects, which vary depending on the specific medication.
- **Duration of Treatment:** Antidepressants usually take several weeks to start working and may require long-term use.
- **Risks and Precautions:** Some antidepressants can increase the risk of suicidal thoughts and behavior, particularly in young adults. Regular monitoring by a healthcare provider is crucial.

Psychotherapy and Lifestyle Changes

- Besides medication, psychotherapy, and lifestyle changes like exercise, diet, and stress management techniques are integral parts of a comprehensive treatment plan for depression.

Conclusion

It is essential for anyone considering antidepressants to consult with a healthcare provider to determine the most appropriate treatment for their situation. The choice of medication will depend on the individual's specific symptoms, medical history, other medications they may be taking, and individual preferences.

How to manage psychotic symptoms?

Managing psychotic symptoms, which can include delusions, hallucinations, disordered thinking, and significant impairments in insight and judgment, requires a comprehensive approach that often involves medication, psychotherapy, and support strategies. Here is an overview of how psychotic symptoms are typically managed:

1. Medication

1. **Antipsychotics:**
   - These are the primary medications used to treat psychotic symptoms. They are divided into two classes: typical (first-generation) antipsychotics and atypical (second-generation) antipsychotics.
   - Typical Antipsychotics include haloperidol, chlorpromazine, and fluphenazine.
   - Atypical Antipsychotics include risperidone, olanzapine, quetiapine, aripiprazole, and clozapine.
   - Antipsychotics work by affecting the brain's neurotransmitters, particularly dopamine, to reduce psychotic symptoms.
2. **Side Effects Management:**
   - Antipsychotic medications can have side effects, ranging from weight gain and drowsiness to movement disorders. Managing these side effects is crucial and might involve adjusting the dosage or switching medications.

2. Psychotherapy

1. **Cognitive Behavioral Therapy (CBT):**
   - CBT can be helpful in managing the symptoms of psychosis. It involves helping the patient recognize and challenge distorted perceptions and beliefs.
2. **Family Therapy:**
   - Involving family members in therapy can provide better support and understanding for the person experiencing psychosis.
3. **Psychoeducation:**
   - Educating the patient and their family about psychosis and its management can be empowering and can improve treatment adherence.
4. **Supportive Psychotherapy:**
   - This can include counseling and support, crisis intervention, and helping the individual develop coping strategies.

3. Support Strategies

1. **Social Support:**
   - Encouragement and support from family, friends, and support groups can be very beneficial.
2. **Rehabilitation Programs:**
   - These programs focus on social skills training, vocational rehabilitation, and other life skills.
3. **Case Management:**
   - Helps in coordinating care, managing healthcare services, and ensuring the patient's needs are met.

4. Lifestyle Modifications

1. **Stress Reduction:**
   - Techniques such as mindfulness, relaxation exercises, and yoga can help manage stress, which can exacerbate psychotic symptoms.
2. **Healthy Living:**
   - Regular exercise, a balanced diet, and sufficient sleep are important for overall well-being.
3. **Avoiding Substance Abuse:**
   - Alcohol and drugs can worsen psychotic symptoms and interfere with medications.

5. Monitoring and Safety

1. **Regular Check-Ups:**
   - Regular follow-ups with healthcare providers are important to monitor the progress and make any necessary adjustments in treatment.
2. **Safety and Crisis Planning:**
   - Having a plan for how to respond in a crisis, including emergency contacts and procedures, is important.
3. **Compliance with Treatment:**
   - Adherence to treatment plans, including taking medications as prescribed, is crucial for managing symptoms effectively.

6. Community Resources

1. **Access to Community Resources:**
   - Utilizing community resources, such as support groups and health services, can provide additional support.

Managing psychotic symptoms is often a long-term process that requires a combination of strategies. It is important for individuals experiencing psychosis and their families to work closely with healthcare providers to develop an effective treatment plan. Regular monitoring and adjustments to the treatment plan are often necessary to ensure the best possible outcomes.

What are additional Therapies for Depression?

In addition to the primary treatments for depression, such as medication and psychotherapy, several additional therapies can be effective in managing symptoms and improving overall well-being. These therapies can be used alongside mainstream treatments to provide a more holistic approach to managing depression:

1. Lifestyle Changes and Self-Care

- **Regular Exercise:** Physical activity has been shown to have an antidepressant effect.
- **Balanced Diet:** A healthy diet, possibly including omega-3 fatty acids and B vitamins, can affect mood.
- **Adequate Sleep:** Good sleep hygiene is crucial for mental health.
- **Mindfulness and Meditation:** Practices like yoga and meditation can reduce stress and improve mood.

2. Psychoeducation

- Learning about depression can empower individuals to understand and manage their condition better.

3. Social Support

- Strengthening relationships with family and friends and participating in community or group activities can provide emotional support and reduce isolation.

4. Stress Reduction Techniques

- Techniques like deep breathing, progressive muscle relaxation, and mindfulness can help manage stress, which can exacerbate depression.

5. Light Therapy

- Especially for Seasonal Affective Disorder (SAD), exposure to bright light can help regulate mood.

6. Cognitive Behavioral Therapy (CBT)

- CBT is a standard psychotherapy for depression, focusing on identifying and changing negative thought patterns and behaviors.

7. Behavioral Activation

- Encourages engagement in activities that are rewarding and enjoyable to combat the inertia and anhedonia of depression.

8. Mindfulness-Based Cognitive Therapy (MBCT)

- Combines mindfulness practices with elements of cognitive therapy to prevent relapse in people who have had recurrent episodes of depression.

9. Art and Music Therapy

- Creative therapies like art and music therapy can offer a non-verbal outlet for emotions and stress relief.

10. Animal-Assisted Therapy

- Interaction with animals, such as pet therapy, can improve mood and reduce stress.

11. Peer Support and Support Groups

- Sharing experiences and coping strategies can be beneficial, especially in group settings.

12. Complementary and Alternative Medicine (CAM)

- This includes acupuncture, aromatherapy, and herbal supplements (like St. John's Wort and SAMe). Note: It is important to discuss these with a healthcare provider before use, as they can interact with other medications.

13. Transcranial Magnetic Stimulation (TMS)

- For treatment-resistant depression, TMS uses magnetic fields to stimulate nerve cells in the brain.

14. Electroconvulsive Therapy (ECT)

- Used for severe, treatment-resistant depression or when rapid response is needed.

15. Computerized Cognitive Behavioral Therapy (CCBT)

- Using computer-based programs to deliver CBT to individuals.

16. Vocational Rehabilitation

- For those whose work life is significantly affected by depression.

17. Environmental Modifications

- Adjusting work and home environments to reduce stressors and improve comfort and functionality.

It is important to approach the treatment of depression in a comprehensive manner that addresses both the psychological and physical aspects of the disorder. A combination of treatments tailored to the individual's specific needs is often the most effective approach. Consulting with healthcare providers is crucial to determine the best combination of treatments.

How is Treatment-Resistant Depression managed?

Treatment-Resistant Depression (TRD) refers to depression that does not respond to typical treatments like antidepressants and psychotherapy. Managing TRD can be challenging and often requires a comprehensive and sometimes innovative approach. Here is an overview of strategies used to manage treatment-resistant depression:

1. Medication Strategies

1. **Adjusting Current Medications:**
   - This can include increasing the dose, reducing it, or changing the timing of the dose.
2. **Switching Antidepressants:**
   - If one class of antidepressant does not work, switching to another class or a different medication within the same class may be effective.
3. **Combination Therapy:**
   - Using two different types of antidepressants together or combining antidepressants with other types of medications (like mood stabilizers or antipsychotics).
4. **Augmentation:**
   - Adding a non-antidepressant medication that can enhance the effects of antidepressants, such as lithium, thyroid medication, or atypical antipsychotics.

2. Psychotherapy

1. **Intensifying Psychotherapy:**
   - Increasing the frequency or duration of sessions, or trying different therapy modalities like cognitive-behavioral therapy (CBT), dialectical behavior therapy (DBT), or psychodynamic therapy.
2. **Combination of Different Therapies:**
   - Combining different types of psychotherapy can be more effective than one type alone.

3. Lifestyle Modifications and Complementary Therapies

1. **Regular Exercise:**
   - Physical activity has been shown to help alleviate symptoms of depression.
2. **Dietary Changes:**
   - A healthy diet, possibly supplemented with omega-3 fatty acids, B vitamins, and other nutrients that can influence mood.
3. **Mindfulness and Stress Reduction Techniques:**
   - Practices like meditation, yoga, and relaxation techniques.

4. **Sleep Hygiene:**
   - Improving sleep patterns and quality can significantly impact depression.

4. Advanced Treatment Options

1. **Electroconvulsive Therapy (ECT):**
   - Particularly effective for severe depression that has not responded to other treatments.
2. **Transcranial Magnetic Stimulation (TMS):**
   - A non-invasive procedure that uses magnetic fields to stimulate nerve cells in the brain.
3. **Vagus Nerve Stimulation (VNS) or Deep Brain Stimulation (DBS):**
   - Surgical options that involve stimulating specific areas of the brain.
4. **Ketamine or Esketamine Treatment:**
   - These are newer treatments that have shown promise for rapid improvement of symptoms in some patients with TRD.

5. Holistic and Alternative Approaches

1. **Acupuncture:**
   - Some people find relief from depression symptoms with acupuncture.
2. **Herbal Supplements and Nutraceuticals:**
   - Supplements like St. John's Wort, SAMe, or omega-3 fatty acids might be beneficial for some individuals, but it is important to discuss this with a healthcare provider due to potential interactions with other medications.

6. Peer Support and Community Resources

1. **Support Groups:**
   - Engaging with others facing similar challenges can provide emotional support and coping strategies.
2. **Online Resources:**
   - Websites, forums, and online therapy can be additional sources of support.

Conclusion

Managing treatment-resistant depression often involves trial and error to find the right combination of therapies. It is crucial for individuals to work closely with their healthcare providers to develop an effective treatment plan. Regular monitoring and adjustments to the treatment plan are often necessary to ensure the best possible outcomes. Patience and persistence are key, as finding the most effective approach can take time.

What is a medical Electroconvulsive Therapy (ECT)?

Electroconvulsive Therapy (ECT) is a medical treatment most commonly used for severe major depression which has not responded to other treatment methods. It can also be effective for bipolar disorder and schizophrenia. ECT is one of the fastest ways to relieve symptoms in severely depressed or suicidal patients. It is also very effective for patients who suffer from mania or other mental illnesses.

How ECT Works

1. **Procedure:** During ECT, small electric currents are passed through the brain, intentionally triggering a brief seizure. ECT seems to cause changes in brain chemistry that can quickly reverse symptoms of certain mental health conditions.
2. **Anesthesia and Muscle Relaxants:** The procedure is done under general anesthesia, and muscle relaxants are given to prevent convulsions. This means the patient is asleep and does not feel or remember the procedure afterwards.
3. **Frequency:** ECT treatments are typically given two to three times a week for a total of six to 12 treatments. The number of treatments varies based on the individual's response.

Indications for ECT

1. **Severe Depression:** Particularly when accompanied by psychosis, a high risk of suicide, or resistance to other treatments.
2. **Mania:** As part of bipolar disorder, especially when it does not respond to medication.
3. **Catatonia:** Including extreme physical immobility or excessive, abnormal movements.
4. **Schizophrenia:** Especially when accompanied by severe symptoms like hallucinations, delusions, or catatonia.

ECT's Effectiveness

- ECT is often highly effective for severe depression, with many patients experiencing significant improvements. It is considered one of the fastest ways to relieve symptoms in severely depressed or suicidal individuals.

Side Effects and Risks

- **Memory Loss:** Short-term memory loss is common after ECT. Long-term memory loss and other cognitive deficits can also occur but are less common.
- **Physical Side Effects:** Immediately after treatment, patients may experience confusion, disorientation, nausea, headache, and muscle soreness.
- **Medical Risks:** As with any procedure involving anesthesia, there are risks associated with the anesthesia itself.

Modern ECT

- Modern ECT is much safer and more humane than its portrayal in old movies and media. It is conducted with strict medical supervision, with attention to patient comfort and minimizing side effects.

Conclusion

While ECT can be very effective, particularly for severe depression, the decision to use it is typically made after careful consideration and consultation with psychiatrists and other medical professionals. It is often reserved for cases where other treatments have failed or when there is a need for a rapid response, such as in severe cases where there is a risk of suicide.

How effective is ECT?

Electroconvulsive Therapy (ECT) is considered a highly effective treatment for certain psychiatric conditions, particularly for severe depression, acute mania, and some forms of schizophrenia. The effectiveness of ECT can be assessed in various aspects:

1. Efficacy in Severe Depression:

- **Response Rate:** ECT has a high response rate for severe depression, with estimates suggesting that approximately 70-90% of patients show significant improvement. This is notably higher compared to antidepressant medications, particularly in treatment-resistant cases.
- **Speed of Response:** ECT often produces a quicker response than medication. It can be particularly life-saving in cases of severe depression with a high risk of suicide.

2. Bipolar Disorder:

- **Mania:** ECT is effective in treating acute manic episodes, particularly when patients have not responded to mood stabilizers or antipsychotic medications.
- **Depressive Episodes:** It is also beneficial in treating the depressive phase of bipolar disorder, especially when rapid stabilization is needed.

3. Schizophrenia:

- ECT can be effective for certain individuals with schizophrenia, particularly those with catatonia, extreme agitation, or severe psychotic symptoms unresponsive to antipsychotic medications.

4. Other Conditions:

- While less commonly used, ECT might be effective in certain cases of Parkinson's disease and neuroleptic malignant syndrome.

5. Long-Term Outcomes:

- **Maintenance Therapy:** To sustain the benefits of ECT, maintenance therapy, which can include continuation of ECT (albeit at a less frequent schedule), medications, or a combination of both, is often required.
- **Relapse Rates:** Relapse can occur following ECT. Studies indicate that without ongoing treatment (medication or continuation/maintenance ECT), relapse rates in the first six months post-ECT can be high.

6. Cognitive Side Effects:

- The main drawback of ECT is its cognitive side effects, including transient memory impairments. Modern techniques have reduced these risks significantly, but they still exist.

7. Quality of Life:

- Many patients report a significant improvement in quality of life and functioning after ECT, particularly when other treatments have failed.

Conclusion:

ECT is a valuable treatment option, especially for severe and treatment-resistant cases. Its effectiveness in rapidly alleviating symptoms of severe depression and other mental health disorders makes it a vital tool in psychiatric care. However, the decision to use ECT is typically made after careful consideration, weighing the potential benefits against the risks and side effects. It is most often used when other treatments have not been effective, or when there is a need for rapid treatment response.

How does electroconvulsive therapy (ECT) work?

Electroconvulsive Therapy (ECT) is a medical procedure that involves delivering controlled electrical currents to the brain to induce a brief seizure. Despite its historical controversy and somewhat dramatic portrayal in media, ECT has evolved significantly and is now a safe and effective treatment for certain psychiatric disorders. The exact mechanisms by which ECT exerts its therapeutic effects are not completely understood, but here is a general overview of how it works:

Mechanism of Action

1. **Electrical Stimulation:** In ECT, electrical currents are passed through the brain for a short duration, typically a few seconds, using electrodes placed on the scalp. This stimulation causes a brief, controlled seizure lasting for about a minute.
2. **Neurochemical Changes:** The induced seizure is believed to trigger a cascade of neurochemical events in the brain. It stimulates the release of neurotransmitters, such as serotonin, dopamine, and norepinephrine, which play a key role in mood regulation.
3. **Neuroplasticity:** ECT may enhance neuroplasticity, which is the brain's ability to reorganize and form new neural connections. This can help alleviate symptoms of mental health disorders.
4. **Brain Wave Patterns:** ECT appears to normalize the patterns of brain wave activity, especially in areas of the brain responsible for mood regulation.
5. **Neuroendocrine Regulation:** The therapy also influences the hypothalamic-pituitary-adrenal axis, which is involved in stress response and mood regulation.

Conditions Treated

1. **Severe Depression:** Particularly when accompanied by psychosis or a significant risk of suicide, or when it is unresponsive to medication and psychotherapy.
2. **Bipolar Disorder:** Effective in treating both manic and depressive episodes, especially when rapid stabilization is needed.
3. **Treatment-Resistant Schizophrenia:** Particularly beneficial for catatonic schizophrenia and schizophrenia with severe psychotic symptoms unresponsive to medication.
4. **Other Conditions:** In some cases, ECT is used for treating severe cases of Parkinson's disease, catatonia, and neuroleptic malignant syndrome.

Procedure

1. **Anesthesia and Muscle Relaxants:** ECT is performed under general anesthesia with muscle relaxants to ensure that the patient is asleep and does not feel pain or consciously experience the seizure.
2. **Electrode Placement:** Electrodes can be placed on both sides of the head (bilateral ECT) or on one side (unilateral ECT). Unilateral ECT is generally associated with fewer cognitive side effects but may be less effective than bilateral ECT.
3. **Frequency of Treatments:** ECT is typically administered two to three times a week for a total of six to twelve sessions, depending on the patient's response.

Efficacy and Safety

- ECT is one of the most effective treatments for severe depression, with a high response rate, especially in treatment-resistant cases.
- Modern ECT is considered safe when performed under controlled conditions with anesthesia. The most common side effect is short-term memory loss, which usually resolves within weeks of treatment.

Conclusion

ECT remains a vital treatment option for severe and treatment-resistant mental health conditions. Its ability to provide rapid and significant improvements in symptoms, especially where other treatments have failed, makes it an important tool in psychiatric care. However, due to its nature and potential side effects, the decision to use ECT is made carefully, considering individual patient factors and overall health.

What are indications for ECT?

Electroconvulsive Therapy (ECT) is a medical treatment that is primarily used for a range of severe mental health conditions. It is often considered when other treatments, such as medications and psychotherapy, have not been effective, or when a rapid response is needed. Here are the main indications for ECT:

1. Major Depressive Disorder

- **Severe Depression:** Especially cases that are treatment-resistant, meaning they haven't responded to medications and psychotherapy.
- **Depression with Psychotic Features:** Depression accompanied by delusions or hallucinations.

- **Depressive Episode with High Suicide Risk:** ECT can be life-saving in cases where there is a significant risk of suicide, as it often provides a quicker response than medication.
- **Catatonic Features:** In cases of severe depression where the patient experiences catatonia (an extreme lack of movement or speech).

2. Bipolar Disorder

- **Manic Episodes:** Particularly when they are severe, treatment-resistant, or pose a significant risk to the patient or others.
- **Bipolar Depression:** When depressive episodes in bipolar disorder are severe and have not responded to other treatments.

3. Schizophrenia

- **Treatment-Resistant Schizophrenia:** Especially in patients who do not respond to antipsychotic medications.
- **Catatonic Schizophrenia:** ECT can be particularly effective for schizophrenia with catatonic features.

4. Other Conditions

- **Neuroleptic Malignant Syndrome:** A life-threatening reaction to antipsychotic medications.
- **Parkinson's Disease:** In some cases, ECT can help alleviate symptoms.
- **Acute Agitation and Aggression:** In some severe cases of mental illness where agitation and aggression are extreme and pose a risk.

5. Special Situations

- **Pregnancy:** ECT can be a safer alternative to psychotropic medications for severe psychiatric conditions during pregnancy.
- **Rapid Symptom Relief Needed:** Situations where it is crucial to rapidly alleviate psychiatric symptoms due to the severity of the condition or the risk of harm.

Conclusion

ECT is usually considered a second-line treatment, typically used when other treatments have failed or when the situation is life-threatening and an immediate response is required. It is important to note that the decision to use ECT is made on a case-by-case basis, taking into account the individual's medical history, current health status, and specific symptoms. The procedure is carried out under strict medical supervision with the aim of maximizing benefits while minimizing risks.

What are the contraindications of ECT therapy?

Electroconvulsive Therapy (ECT) is generally considered safe, but like all medical procedures, it has certain contraindications. These contraindications can be absolute, meaning ECT should not be used, or relative, meaning the risks and benefits must be carefully weighed. Here are the main contraindications:

Absolute Contraindications

There are very few absolute contraindications for ECT, but they include conditions where the risk of a serious adverse event is extremely high:

1. **Recent Myocardial Infarction (Heart Attack):** Performing ECT shortly after a heart attack can be risky due to the strain on the heart.
2. **Recent Cerebral Hemorrhage or Other Severe Intracranial Processes:** ECT could potentially worsen these conditions or lead to complications.

Relative Contraindications

These conditions require careful consideration and often necessitate special precautions or Modifications to the ECT procedure:

1. **Cardiovascular Issues:** Such as severe heart disease, hypertension, or arrhythmias. While ECT can be performed, it must be done with close cardiac monitoring.
2. **Cerebrovascular Disease:** Including a history of stroke, aneurysms, or significant carotid artery stenosis.
3. **Severe Osteoporosis or Bone Fractures:** Due to the risk of fractures during the muscle contractions induced by ECT.
4. **Severe Pulmonary Conditions:** Like chronic obstructive pulmonary disease (COPD) or asthma, which might be exacerbated by the procedure.
5. **Increased Intracranial Pressure:** Caution is needed due to the risk of further increasing intracranial pressure.
6. **Glaucoma:** ECT may transiently increase intraocular pressure.
7. **Pregnancy:** While ECT is generally considered safe during pregnancy, special precautions are necessary to minimize risks to the fetus.
8. **Space-Occupying Brain Lesions:** Due to the risk of increasing intracranial pressure or causing herniation.

9. **Deep Brain Stimulation Devices or Other Neurostimulators:** The interaction between these devices and ECT needs to be carefully evaluated.

10. **History of Malignant Hyperthermia:** A rare reaction to certain types of anesthesia, which is relevant since ECT requires general anesthesia.

Precautions and Risk Assessment

- **Pre-ECT Evaluation:** It is crucial for individuals to undergo a thorough pre-ECT evaluation, including a physical examination, psychiatric assessment, and sometimes specialized tests like an electrocardiogram (EKG) or brain imaging, to identify any potential risks.
- **Anesthesiology Consultation:** Consultation with an anesthesiologist is important to assess risks related to anesthesia, especially in the presence of medical comorbidities.

Conclusion

While ECT is safe for most individuals, the decision to proceed with ECT should be made after a thorough evaluation and discussion of the potential risks and benefits, especially for those with relative contraindications. In many cases, the potential benefits of ECT in alleviating severe psychiatric symptoms outweigh the risks, but this balance must be carefully assessed for each individual.

What are the long-term effects of ECT?

Electroconvulsive therapy (ECT) is a medical treatment most commonly used for patients with severe major depression or bipolar disorder that has not responded to other treatments. It involves a brief electrical stimulation of the brain while the patient is under anesthesia.

The long-term effects of ECT can vary from person to person and depend on various factors such as the individual's overall health, the specific mental health condition being treated, and the ECT treatment protocol. Some of the potential long-term effects include:

1. **Cognitive Changes:** The most common long-term effect of ECT is changes in cognitive function. This can include memory loss, particularly of events around the time of the treatment, and difficulties with learning and retaining new information. However, these effects are typically temporary and often resolve within weeks or months after the treatment ends.

2. **Psychological Impact:** Some patients report long-term psychological changes after ECT, such as changes in personality or a feeling of being different in some way. However, these effects are not well understood and are not commonly reported.

3. **Relapse of Symptoms:** For some individuals, the benefits of ECT in terms of symptom relief for depression or bipolar disorder may diminish over time. This can lead to a relapse of symptoms, which may require further treatment.

4. **Physical Side Effects:** Long-term physical side effects from ECT are rare but can include prolonged headaches, muscle aches, or nausea.

5. **Improved Quality of Life:** On the positive side, many patients experience a significant improvement in their quality of life over the long term. ECT can be highly effective in treating severe depression and other mental health conditions, leading to improved mood, better functioning, and a reduced risk of suicide.

It is important to discuss the potential risks and benefits of ECT with a healthcare professional, who can provide personalized information based on an individual's health history and specific circumstances. ECT is generally considered safe and effective, particularly when other treatments have failed, but it is important to weigh the potential long-term effects against the potential benefits.

What are the immediate negative side effects of ECT?

Electroconvulsive therapy (ECT) can have several immediate negative side effects, which typically occur shortly after the treatment session. These side effects are usually temporary and can vary in intensity from person to person. Some of the most common immediate side effects include:

1. **Confusion:** Immediately after an ECT session, a patient may experience confusion, which can range from mild to severe. This confusion typically resolves within a few minutes to hours but can sometimes last longer.

2. **Memory Loss:** Short-term memory loss is a common side effect of ECT. Patients may have trouble recalling events that occurred right before and after the treatment. This memory loss is usually temporary, but in rare cases, it can be more persistent.

3. **Physical Side Effects:** These can include headache, muscle soreness, nausea, and vomiting. These symptoms are typically mild and can be managed with medications.

4. **Disorientation:** Patients may feel disoriented upon waking from the anesthesia, not knowing where they are or why they are there. This usually resolves as the anesthesia wears off.

5. **Heart Rate and Blood Pressure Changes:** ECT can cause transient changes in heart rate and blood pressure. These are closely monitored during the procedure to manage any significant fluctuations.

6. **Anesthetic Side Effects:** As with any procedure involving anesthesia, there can be side effects from the anesthetic itself, such as grogginess, dry mouth, or sore throat.

7. **Emotional Response:** Some patients may experience an immediate emotional response following ECT, including fear, anxiety, or distress. This is typically short-lived and can be addressed with supportive care.

It is important to note that while these side effects can be concerning, they are generally well-managed by healthcare professionals. ECT is a highly controlled and monitored procedure, and the benefits in treating severe depression, bipolar disorder, and certain other mental health conditions can outweigh these immediate side effects for many patients. Always consult with a healthcare provider for a thorough discussion of the risks and benefits of ECT in individual cases.

What is the success rate of ECT?

The success rate of Electroconvulsive Therapy (ECT) is generally considered to be quite high, especially for certain mental health conditions. However, the specific success rate can vary depending on factors such as the condition being treated, the severity of the condition, and the individual patient's response to the treatment. Here are some key points regarding the success rate of ECT:

1. **Major Depression:** ECT is most commonly used for severe major depressive disorder, particularly when it is treatment-resistant. In these cases, ECT has a high success rate, often cited as being effective in about 70% to 90% of cases.

2. **Treatment-Resistant Conditions:** ECT is particularly effective for treatment-resistant depression and other mental health conditions that have not responded to medications or other therapies. It often works where other treatments have failed.

3. **Bipolar Disorder:** ECT is also effective in treating bipolar disorder, especially during severe manic or mixed episodes, as well as in depressive phases that do not respond to other treatments.

4. **Schizophrenia and Other Conditions:** While less commonly used for schizophrenia, ECT can be effective, particularly in treatment-resistant cases or when rapid symptom relief is needed.

5. **Speed of Response:** One of the advantages of ECT is the rapid improvement of symptoms in many cases, which is particularly important in life-threatening situations like severe suicidal ideation.

6. **Long-Term Efficacy:** The long-term success of ECT depends on various factors, including follow-up care, maintenance treatments if needed, and the use of medication or psychotherapy to manage symptoms after the initial ECT course.

7. **Relapse Rates:** It is important to note that while ECT can be very effective initially, there is a risk of relapse. Studies suggest that without follow-up treatment, relapse rates can be high, but maintenance ECT and/or medication can significantly reduce this risk.

In conclusion, ECT is a highly effective treatment for certain psychiatric conditions, especially when other treatments have not been effective. However, individual responses can vary, and it is important for patients to discuss the potential benefits and risks with their healthcare provider.

What is Pediatric Depression?

Pediatric depression refers to depression that occurs in children and adolescents. It is a serious mental health issue that can significantly impact a child's life, affecting their social interactions, school performance, and overall development. Understanding pediatric depression involves recognizing its unique manifestations, causes, and treatment approaches in younger populations.

Characteristics of Pediatric Depression

1. **Symptoms:** While some symptoms of depression in children and adolescents are similar to those in adults, they can also present differently. Common symptoms include:
   - Persistent sadness or low mood.
   - Irritability or anger, often more pronounced than in adults.
   - Loss of interest in previously enjoyable activities.

- Changes in appetite and sleep patterns.
- Fatigue or low energy.
- Feelings of worthlessness or guilt.
- Difficulty concentrating.
- Somatic complaints, like headaches or stomachaches without a clear medical cause.
- In severe cases, thoughts of death or suicide.

2. **Age-Related Differences:** Younger children might have trouble articulating their feelings and may demonstrate their distress through behavior changes, such as increased irritability, clinginess, or changes in play. Adolescents may exhibit more classic symptoms of depression or engage in risky behaviors.

Causes

The causes of pediatric depression are multifactorial, including:

- **Genetic Factors:** A family history of depression or other mental health disorders can increase risk.
- **Environmental Factors:** Stressful life events, trauma, bullying, or family issues.
- **Biological Factors:** Changes in brain chemistry or hormonal fluctuations, especially during adolescence.
- **Psychological Factors:** Low self-esteem, chronic anxiety, or coping issues.

Treatment

1. **Psychotherapy:** Cognitive-behavioral therapy (CBT) and other forms of psychotherapy are often effective in treating pediatric depression.
2. **Medication:** Antidepressants may be used, particularly in moderate to severe cases, but with careful monitoring due to concerns about their effects on developing brains.
3. **Family Therapy and Support:** Involving the family in treatment can be beneficial.
4. **Lifestyle Changes:** Regular exercise, healthy diet, and sufficient sleep can help manage symptoms.

Challenges and Considerations

- **Diagnosis:** Diagnosing depression in children can be challenging as symptoms often overlap with other developmental issues or mental health disorders.
- **Stigma:** There is still a stigma surrounding mental health issues in children, which can delay seeking treatment.
- **Developmental Impact:** Untreated depression can have significant impacts on a child's emotional, social, and cognitive development.

Early identification and appropriate treatment of pediatric depression are crucial for the wellbeing and long-term prognosis of the child. If depression is suspected in a child or adolescent, it is important to seek evaluation and treatment from a healthcare professional specializing in pediatric mental health.

What are the dangers in treating pediatrics patients for depression?

Treating pediatric patients for depression involves several challenges and potential dangers that healthcare professionals must carefully consider. These risks arise from the unique developmental, psychological, and biological characteristics of children and adolescents. Here are some key concerns:

1. **Medication Side Effects and Risks:**
   - Antidepressants, particularly selective serotonin reuptake inhibitors (SSRIs), are commonly used to treat depression in adults, but their effects on children and adolescents can be different. There is a risk of increased suicidal thoughts or behaviors, especially during the first few weeks of treatment or when the dose is changed.
   - **Developmental Impact:** The long-term impact of antidepressants on the developing brain is not fully understood, raising concerns about growth, cognitive development, and emotional regulation.
   - **Physical Side Effects:** These can include weight gain, gastrointestinal issues, sleep disturbances, and other physical symptoms.
2. **Psychosocial Impacts:**
   - **Stigma:** Children and adolescents treated for depression might face stigma from peers, which can exacerbate feelings of isolation or difference.
   - **Self-Image:** Being labeled with a mental health diagnosis can impact a young person's self-esteem and self-image during critical developmental years.

3. **Therapeutic Challenges:**
   - **Communication:** Younger children, in particular, may have difficulty expressing their feelings or understanding their condition, making it harder to diagnose and treat effectively.
   - **Engagement in Therapy:** Engaging children and adolescents in therapy can be challenging, especially if they are resistant or lack insight into their condition.
4. **Misdiagnosis and Overmedication:**
   - **Complex Diagnosis:** Symptoms of depression in children can overlap with other developmental disorders or mental health issues, leading to misdiagnosis.
   - **Overmedication:** There is a concern about the tendency to medicate behavioral and emotional problems in children without sufficient exploration of other therapeutic options.
5. **Family and Environmental Factors:**
   - **Family Dynamics:** Treatment must often involve family dynamics, which can be complex and sensitive.
   - **Environmental Influences:** External factors like bullying, social media pressure, and family issues can significantly impact treatment effectiveness.
6. **Comorbid Conditions:**
   - Many children and adolescents with depression also have other mental health conditions like anxiety disorders, ADHD, or substance abuse problems, which can complicate treatment.
7. **Long-Term Outcomes:**
   - The long-term effects of early-onset depression and its treatment are not entirely understood, raising concerns about future mental health, social functioning, and quality of life.

Given these challenges, it is crucial for treatment to be individualized, closely monitored, and often multi-faceted, incorporating psychotherapy, family involvement, lifestyle changes, and, when necessary, medication. Collaboration between healthcare providers, parents, educators, and the young patients themselves is key to effectively managing pediatric depression. Regular follow-up and adjustment of treatment plans are essential to address the changing needs of children and adolescents as they grow and develop.

What are the guidelines for treating pediatric depression?

Treating pediatric depression requires a careful, evidence-based approach that takes into account the unique psychological, developmental, and physiological characteristics of children and adolescents. Clinical guidelines for treating pediatric depression often include the following key elements:

1. **Comprehensive Assessment:**
   - **Clinical Evaluation:** This includes a thorough psychiatric evaluation to diagnose depression, differentiate it from other mental health disorders, and assess its severity.
   - **Medical Examination:** To rule out any medical conditions that may be contributing to depressive symptoms.
   - **Psychosocial Evaluation:** Assessing the child's environment, including family, school, and peer relationships.
2. **Psychoeducation:**
   - Educating the patient and their family about depression, its symptoms, causes, and treatment options.
   - Addressing any misconceptions and stigma associated with mental health disorders.
3. **Psychotherapy:**
   - **Cognitive-Behavioral Therapy (CBT):** Often the first-line treatment, especially for mild to moderate depression. CBT focuses on changing negative thought patterns and behaviors.
   - **Interpersonal Therapy (IPT):** Addresses interpersonal issues and aims to improve communication skills and increase social support.
   - **Family Therapy:** Can be beneficial, especially if family conflicts or dynamics are contributing to the child's depression.
4. **Pharmacotherapy:**
   - Considered for moderate to severe depression, or when psychotherapy alone is insufficient.
   - Selective Serotonin Reuptake Inhibitors (SSRIs) are commonly prescribed, but it is essential to start with low doses and monitor closely for side effects, particularly for any signs of increased suicidal thoughts or behaviors.

- Regular follow-ups are crucial to monitor the effectiveness and any side effects of medication.

5. **Monitoring and Follow-up:**
   - Regular and close monitoring of symptoms, side effects, and overall well-being.
   - Adjustment of treatment plans as needed based on the child's response to treatment.
6. **Management of Suicidal Risk:**
   - Assessing risk factors for suicide and developing a safety plan.
   - Involvement of family members in monitoring and supporting the child.
7. **Collaboration and Coordination of Care:**
   - Involvement of a multidisciplinary team including pediatricians, psychiatrists, psychologists, school personnel, and social workers.
   - Ensuring communication and coordination among all parties involved in the child's care.
8. **Treatment of Comorbid Conditions:**
   - Addressing any co-occurring mental health disorders such as anxiety, ADHD, or substance use disorders.
9. **School Involvement:**
   - Working with school officials to provide academic support and accommodations as needed.
10. **Prevention and Early Intervention:**
    - Identifying at-risk children and adolescents for early intervention.
    - Implementing preventive measures like resilience-building and stress management techniques.

It is important to note that these guidelines can vary by region and are subject to change as new research emerges. Treatment should always be tailored to the individual needs of the child or adolescent and carried out by qualified health professionals. Families should engage in open dialogue with healthcare providers to ensure a clear understanding of the treatment plan and to advocate for the best interests of their child.

How do you treat resistant depression in pediatric population?

Treating resistant depression in the pediatric population, where standard treatments like psychotherapy and first-line antidepressants have not been effective, requires a more comprehensive and often multi-modal approach. Here are the key strategies commonly employed:

1. **Re-evaluation of Diagnosis:** It is crucial to reassess the diagnosis to ensure that it is accurate. Misdiagnosis can lead to ineffective treatment. Comorbid conditions, such as anxiety disorders, ADHD, or learning disabilities, should also be identified and treated.
2. **Optimization of Current Treatment:**
   - **Medication Adjustment:** This may involve increasing the dose within safe limits, if not already at the maximum recommended level.
   - **Enhancing Psychotherapy:** Intensifying the frequency or duration of sessions, or trying different therapeutic approaches like Cognitive Behavioral Therapy (CBT), Dialectical Behavior Therapy (DBT), or Family Therapy.
3. **Medication Review and Changes:**
   - **Switching Antidepressants:** If the current medication is not effective, switching to a different antidepressant, often from a different class, may be beneficial.
   - **Augmentation Strategies:** Adding another medication to the current antidepressant, such as a mood stabilizer, antipsychotic, or another type of antidepressant, can sometimes enhance efficacy.
4. **Specialized Therapies:**
   - **Electroconvulsive Therapy (ECT):** In cases of severe, life-threatening depression or when other treatments have failed, ECT may be considered, although it is used cautiously and less frequently in children and adolescents.
   - **Transcranial Magnetic Stimulation (TMS):** For adolescents, TMS has shown some promise as a treatment for resistant depression.
5. **Comprehensive Psychosocial Interventions:**
   - Addressing environmental factors such as family dynamics, school issues, and peer relationships.
   - Strengthening social support systems and enhancing coping skills.

6. **Lifestyle Modifications:**
   - Encouraging regular physical activity, healthy eating, and good sleep hygiene.
   - Mindfulness practices, stress management techniques, and other complementary therapies.
7. **Close Monitoring and Follow-up:**
   - Regularly monitoring for side effects, suicidal thoughts, and changes in symptoms.
   - Adjusting the treatment plan as needed based on the patient's response.
8. **Collaborative Care:**
   - Involving a multidisciplinary team including pediatricians, child psychiatrists, psychologists, and possibly other specialists.
   - Engaging the family and school in the treatment process.
9. **Clinical Trials or Experimental Therapies:**
   - In some cases, participation in clinical trials for new treatments or experimental therapies might be an option, particularly when standard treatments have failed.
10. **Support and Education for Families:**
    - Providing resources and education to families to help them understand and support their child's condition and treatment.

It is important to approach treatment with patience and persistence, as finding the right combination of therapies can take time. Each child or adolescent is unique, and what works for one individual might not work for another. The safety and wellbeing of the child should always be the primary concern, and decisions should be made collaboratively with the child, family, and healthcare providers.

Is there a relationship between antidepressants and suicidality in youths?

Yes, there is a recognized relationship between the use of antidepressants, particularly selective serotonin reuptake inhibitors (SSRIs), and an increased risk of suicidality (suicidal thoughts and behaviors) in children, adolescents, and young adults. This relationship has been the subject of extensive research and has led to specific regulatory actions and clinical guidelines.

1. **FDA Black Box Warning:** In 2004, the U.S. Food and Drug Administration (FDA) issued a "black box warning" for antidepressants, indicating that these medications may increase the risk of suicidal thinking and behavior in children and adolescents. This warning was later extended to include young adults up to age 24.
2. **Research Findings:** Studies have shown that while SSRIs and other antidepressants can be effective in treating depression in young people, they can also increase the risk of suicidal thoughts and behaviors, especially during the first few weeks of treatment or when the dose is changed.
3. **Mechanism:** The exact mechanism behind this increased risk is not fully understood. It is hypothesized that antidepressants may lead to increased energy and motivation before mood improves, which might enable suicidal behavior in individuals already having suicidal thoughts.
4. **Risk-Benefit Analysis:** When prescribing antidepressants to youths, healthcare providers conduct a careful risk-benefit analysis. While there is a risk of increased suicidality, untreated depression itself is a major risk factor for suicide. Therefore, the potential benefits of antidepressants in alleviating severe depression must be weighed against their risks.
5. **Close Monitoring:** It is crucial for healthcare providers to closely monitor young patients for any increase in suicidal thoughts or behaviors, especially during the initial period of treatment or when doses are adjusted. Families and caregivers are also advised to monitor for changes in behavior and to report any concerns to the healthcare provider immediately.
6. **Individualized Treatment:** Decisions regarding the use of antidepressants in young people should be highly individualized, taking into consideration the severity of depression, previous treatment responses, and the presence of other mental health conditions.
7. **Alternative Treatments:** In some cases, other treatments such as psychotherapy (e.g., cognitive-behavioral therapy) might be recommended as the first-line treatment, with medication considered only if these approaches are insufficient.
8. **Informed Consent:** It is important for healthcare providers to discuss the risks and benefits of

antidepressants with both the patient and their guardians, ensuring that they are making an informed decision about treatment.

Overall, the relationship between antidepressants and suicidality in youths underscores the importance of careful assessment, close monitoring, and a comprehensive treatment approach when managing pediatric depression.

So, what are the recommendations when treating pediatric depression?

Treating pediatric depression effectively requires a careful, multifaceted approach. The recommendations often include a combination of psychotherapy, pharmacotherapy, and comprehensive support. Here are the key recommendations:

1. **Initial Evaluation and Diagnosis:**
   - Conduct a thorough psychiatric evaluation to confirm the diagnosis of depression.
   - Rule out other medical conditions or mental health disorders that might mimic or contribute to depressive symptoms.
   - Assess the severity of depression and any risk factors, including suicidality.
2. **Psychoeducation:**
   - Educate the patient and their family about depression, its symptoms, causes, and treatment options.
   - Address any misconceptions and stigma about mental health.
3. **Psychotherapy:**
   - **First-line Treatment for Mild to Moderate Depression:** Cognitive Behavioral Therapy (CBT), Interpersonal Therapy (IPT), or other evidence-based psycho-therapies.
   - Family therapy may be beneficial, especially if family dynamics are contributing to the child's depression.
4. **Pharmacotherapy:**
   - For moderate to severe depression or when psychotherapy alone is insufficient, consider antidepressant medication.
   - SSRIs (Selective Serotonin Reuptake Inhibitors) are commonly the first choice.
   - Close monitoring for any side effects, particularly for increased risk of suicidal thoughts or behaviors, especially in the initial weeks of treatment or during dose changes.
5. **Monitoring and Follow-Up:**
   - Regular follow-up appointments to monitor the effectiveness of treatment and adjust as necessary.
   - Monitor for side effects of medications and changes in symptoms.
6. **Management of Suicidal Risk:**
   - Conduct regular assessments for suicidal thoughts or behaviors.
   - Develop a safety plan and involve family members in monitoring and supporting the child.
7. **Collaborative Care:**
   - Involve a multidisciplinary team, including pediatricians, psychiatrists, psychologists, school counselors, and social workers.
   - Ensure communication among all parties involved in the child's care.
8. **Supportive Interventions:**
   - Encourage healthy lifestyle habits, including regular physical activity, a balanced diet, and adequate sleep.
   - Support the child in building a strong social support network.
9. **Treatment of Comorbid Conditions:**
   - Address any co-occurring mental health disorders such as anxiety or ADHD.
10. **School Involvement:**
    - Collaborate with school personnel to support the child's educational needs.
11. **Patient and Family Engagement:**
    - Actively involve the child and their family in treatment decisions.
    - Provide support and resources to families to help them understand and manage the child's depression.
12. **Consideration of Cultural and Individual Factors:**
    - Tailor the treatment to the cultural background and individual circumstances of the child and family.

It is important to note that these recommendations can vary based on individual cases and evolving clinical guidelines. Treatment should always be tailored to the specific needs of the child or adolescent and carried out by qualified health professionals. Regular reassessment and adjustment of the treatment plan are essential to ensure the best outcomes.

What tests should be done before treating pediatric depression with TCAs?

Before treating pediatric depression with tricyclic antidepressants (TCAs), several important tests and evaluations should be conducted to ensure the safety and appropriateness of this treatment. TCAs are not typically the first-line treatment for pediatric depression due to their side effect profile and potential risks, but they may be considered in certain cases where other treatments have failed or are not suitable. Here are the key steps and tests that are generally recommended:

1. **Comprehensive Psychiatric Evaluation:**
   - A thorough assessment to confirm the diagnosis of depression and to rule out other mental health disorders.
   - Evaluation of the severity of symptoms and assessment of any suicidal ideation or behavior.
2. **Medical History and Physical Examination:**
   - A complete medical history to identify any co-existing medical conditions, previous r esponses to medications, and potential contraindications.
   - A physical examination to assess overall health and to identify any physical issues that might affect treatment.
3. **Baseline Electrocardiogram (ECG):**
   - An ECG is important before initiating TCA treatment due to the risk of cardiac side effects, such as changes in heart rhythm and conduction.
   - TCAs can prolong the QT interval, so it is crucial to ensure the patient does not have any pre-existing cardiac conditions or a predisposition to arrhythmias.
4. **Laboratory Tests:**
   - Blood tests, including a complete blood count (CBC), liver function tests, and renal function tests, to establish baseline health and to identify any potential issues that might affect medication metabolism or increase the risk of side effects.
   - Thyroid function tests, as thyroid disorders can sometimes mimic or exacerbate depressive symptoms.
5. **Medication Review:**
   - Review of all current medications (including over-the-counter drugs and herbal supplements) to check for potential drug interactions.
6. **Risk Assessment for Side Effects:**
   - Evaluating the risk of common side effects of TCAs, such as anticholinergic effects (dry mouth, constipation, urinary retention), orthostatic hypotension, weight gain, and sedation.
   - Assessing the risk of more serious side effects, including cardiac effects and the potential for overdose.
7. **Family History:**
   - Inquiring about family history, especially regarding heart disease, sudden cardiac death, or mental health disorders, as this may influence treatment decisions.
8. **Informed Consent:**
   - Discussing the potential risks and benefits of TCA treatment with both the patient and their parents or guardians.
   - Ensuring that they understand the importance of medication adherence and regular follow-up.
9. **Baseline Symptom Measurement:**
   - Establishing a baseline for depression severity to help monitor treatment response and side effects.

Given the potential risks associated with TCAs, they are usually considered only after other treatment options, such as SSRIs (Selective Serotonin Reuptake Inhibitors), have been tried and have not been effective or have caused intolerable side effects. The decision to use TCAs in pediatric depression should always be made with caution, and under the close supervision of a qualified healthcare professional. Regular monitoring and follow-up are essential to ensure patient safety and to assess treatment efficacy.

How should depression during Pregnancy be treated?

Treating depression during pregnancy is crucial for the health of both the mother and the developing fetus.

However, it poses unique challenges due to the potential risks of various treatments to the fetus. Here are general guidelines for treating depression during pregnancy:

1. **Thorough Evaluation:**
   - A comprehensive assessment by a healthcare provider to diagnose depression and evaluate its severity.
   - Consideration of the woman's psychiatric history, including previous episodes of depression and treatment responses.
2. **Psychotherapy:**
   - Often the first-line treatment, particularly for mild to moderate depression.
   - Cognitive-Behavioral Therapy (CBT) and Interpersonal Therapy (IPT) are effective and do not have the risks associated with medications.
   - Counseling can provide support and strategies to manage symptoms.
3. **Medication:**
   - For moderate to severe depression, or when psychotherapy alone is insufficient, medication may be necessary.
   - The decision to use antidepressant medication during pregnancy is complex. It requires a careful risk-benefit analysis, considering the risks of untreated depression against the potential risks of medication to the fetus.
   - Selective Serotonin Reuptake Inhibitors (SSRIs) are commonly used, but some SSRIs have been associated with specific birth defects, albeit the risk is generally low.
   - The choice of medication should be individualized based on the woman's prior response to antidepressants, the safety profile of the medication, and consultation with a psychiatrist.
4. **Lifestyle Modifications:**
   - Regular physical activity, balanced nutrition, adequate sleep, and stress reduction techniques can be beneficial.
   - Support from family, friends, and support groups is important.
5. **Close Monitoring:**
   - Regular follow-up appointments to monitor the mother's mood and the pregnancy.
   - Monitoring for any medication side effects.
6. **Collaborative Care:**
   - Care should involve a team approach, including obstetricians, psychiatrists, and primary care providers.
   - Communication between healthcare providers is essential for coordinated care.
7. **Risk of Postpartum Depression:**
   - Women with depression during pregnancy are at higher risk for postpartum depression, so planning for support and treatment after delivery is important.
8. **Alternative Treatments:**
   - Some women may choose to explore alter native treatments like acupuncture, light therapy, or omega-3 fatty acids. However, the efficacy and safety of these treatments during pregnancy should be discussed with a healthcare provider.
9. **Informed Decision Making:**
   - Providing comprehensive information to the expectant mother, enabling her to make informed decisions about her treatment.
10. **Emergency Situations:**
    - In cases of severe depression, more acute interventions may be necessary, including hospitalization or electroconvulsive therapy (ECT), especially if there is a risk of harm to the mother or fetus.

It is important to individualize treatment plans based on the specific needs and circumstances of the pregnant woman. The goal is to optimize the mother's mental health while minimizing risks to the developing fetus. Collaboration and open communication between the woman and her healthcare providers are key to achieving the best outcomes.

What are the risks to infants whose mothers were on antidepressants?

Exposure to antidepressants during pregnancy can pose risks to the developing fetus and the new-born infant. These risks depend on various factors, including the type of antidepressant, the dose, the timing during pregnancy, and individual differences in maternal and fetal metabolism. Here are some of the potential risks:

1. **Congenital Malformations:**
   - Some studies have suggested a small increase in the risk of certain birth defects, particularly heart defects, with the use of specific antidepressants (especially certain SSRIs) during pregnancy. However, the overall risk remains low.
2. **Neonatal Adaptation Syndrome:**
   - Infants exposed to antidepressants, particularly SSRIs and SNRIs (serotonin-norepinephrine reuptake inhibitors), late in the third trimester may experience neonatal adaptation syndrome. Symptoms can include respiratory distress, feeding difficulties, irritability, and jitteriness. These symptoms are generally mild and resolve within a few days to weeks after birth.
3. **Persistent Pulmonary Hypertension of the New-born (PPHN):**
   - A rare but serious condition, PPHN is more common in infants whose mothers took SSRIs during the second half of the pregnancy. However, the absolute risk is still low.
4. **Preterm Birth:**
   - Some studies have found an association between the use of antidepressants during pregnancy and a slightly increased risk of preterm birth.
5. **Low Birth Weight:**
   - There may be a slightly increased risk of giving birth to a baby with low birth weight.
6. **Developmental Delays:**
   - Research on the long-term developmental outcomes of children exposed to antidepressants in utero is ongoing. Some studies suggest potential impacts on motor development or increased risk of psychiatric disorders, but findings are not conclusive.
7. **Withdrawal Symptoms:**
   - In some cases, new-borns may exhibit withdrawal-like symptoms such as tremors, sleep disturbances, and high-pitched crying if the mother used antidepressants during pregnancy.

It is important to note that the risks associated with the use of antidepressants during pregnancy must be balanced against the risks of untreated maternal depression, which can also adversely affect both maternal and fetal well- being. Untreated depression in pregnancy can lead to poor nutrition, smoking, drinking, suicidal behavior, and reduced adherence to prenatal care, all of which can negatively impact fetal development and pregnancy outcomes.

Therefore, the decision to use antidepressants during pregnancy should be made collaboratively by the woman and her healthcare providers, taking into account the severity of her depression, her response to other treatments, and the specific risks associated with the medication. Close monitoring of both the mother and the infant is essential.

What is postpartum depression?

Postpartum depression (PPD) is a serious mental health condition that affects some women after childbirth. It involves more than just the "baby blues," which are relatively mild and usually resolve within two weeks after delivery. PPD can develop anywhere from a few weeks to a year after childbirth, and it is characterized by longer-lasting and more severe symptoms that can significantly impact a mother's ability to function and care for her baby. Key aspects of postpartum depression include:

Symptoms

Symptoms of postpartum depression can vary but often include:

- Persistent feelings of sadness, hopelessness, or emptiness.
- Loss of interest or pleasure in most activities, including those previously enjoyed.
- Changes in appetite or weight.
- Sleep disturbances, either insomnia or sleeping too much.
- Fatigue or loss of energy.
- Feelings of worthlessness or excessive guilt.
- Difficulty thinking, concentrating, or making decisions.
- Irritability or excessive crying.
- Anxiety and panic attacks.
- Thoughts of harming oneself or the baby.
- A lack of interest in the baby, not feeling bonded to the baby, or feeling overly anxious about the baby's health and well-being.

Causes

The exact cause of postpartum depression is not known,

but it is likely due to a combination of physical, emotional, and lifestyle factors, including:

- Hormonal changes after childbirth.
- Physical exhaustion and sleep deprivation.
- Stress from the new responsibility of caring for a new-born.
- Emotional factors such as self-image, family dynamics, or a history of depression or anxiety.
- Lack of support from partner, family, or friends.

Risk Factors

Certain factors may increase the risk of developing postpartum depression, such as:

- A history of depression, either during pregnancy or at other times.
- A family history of depression or other mental health disorders.
- A lack of support from family or friends.
- Anxiety or negative feelings about the pregnancy.
- Complications in pregnancy, birth, or breastfeeding.
- Stressful life events during pregnancy or shortly after giving birth.

Treatment

Effective treatments for postpartum depression include:

- **Psychotherapy:** Talking therapies, such as cognitive-behavioral therapy (CBT) or interpersonal therapy (IPT), can be very effective.
- **Medication:** Antidepressants may be prescribed, and the choice of medication may take into account whether the mother is breastfeeding.
- **Support Groups:** Joining a support group can provide validation and encouragement from others who have had similar experiences.
- **Self-Care:** Practices such as getting adequate rest, nutrition, physical activity, and time for oneself can be beneficial.

Importance of Treatment

It is important for women experiencing symptoms of postpartum depression to seek treatment as early as possible. Untreated postpartum depression can affect the mother's health and her ability to connect with and care for her baby, and it can have long-term effects on the child's development.

Postpartum depression is a common and serious condition, but with the right treatment and support, most women can make a full recovery. It is crucial for new mothers and their families to recognize the signs of postpartum depression and seek help promptly.

How to go about antidepressants and Breastfeeding?

Balancing the use of antidepressants while breastfeeding is an important consideration for new mothers dealing with depression or anxiety. The goal is to treat the mother's mental health condition effectively while minimizing any potential risks to the nursing infant. Here are key points to consider when addressing antidepressants and breastfeeding:

1. **Consult Healthcare Providers:**
   - It is crucial to discuss medication options with healthcare providers who are knowledgeable about both mental health and breastfeeding. This may include a psychiatrist, an obstetrician/gynecologist, a pediatrician, and a lactation consultant.
2. **Choosing the Right Antidepressant:**
   - Certain antidepressants are considered safer for use during breastfeeding due to lower levels of excretion into breast milk and fewer reported effects on the infant.
   - SSRIs (Selective Serotonin Reuptake Inhibitors), particularly sertraline (Zoloft) and paroxetine (Paxil), are often preferred due to their relatively favorable safety profile in breastfeeding mothers and their infants.
   - Bupropion (Wellbutrin) and tricyclic antidepressants (TCAs) like nortriptyline and amitriptyline are also considered relatively safe options.
3. **Monitoring the Infant:**
   - The baby should be monitored for any side effects, such as unusual irritability, changes in feeding habits, or sleep disturbances. If any concerns arise, they should be addressed immediately with the pediatrician.
4. **Timing of Medication:**
   - Taking the medication right after breastfeeding or before the baby's longest sleep period can reduce the infant's exposure to the medication.
5. **Dosage and Treatment Plan:**
   - Using the lowest effective dose can help

- minimize the amount of medication passed to the infant through breast milk.
- The treatment plan should be regularly reviewed and adjusted as necessary, taking into account the mother's mental health needs and the wellbeing of the infant.

6. **Benefits vs. Risks:**
   - The decision to use antidepressants while breastfeeding involves weighing the benefits of treating the mother's depression against any potential risks to the infant.
   - Untreated maternal depression has its own risks, both for the mother and the baby, including impacts on bonding and care.
7. **Alternative Treatments:**
   - If medication is a concern, other treatment options like psychotherapy can be effective for managing depression and anxiety and are safe for breastfeeding mothers.
8. **Informed Decision Making:**
   - Mothers should be provided with comprehensive information to make an informed decision about the use of antidepressants while breastfeeding.
9. **Support and Education:**
   - Emotional and practical support, along with education about managing depression during the postpartum period, can be beneficial.
10. **Coordination of Care:**
    - Coordinated care between the mother's and baby's healthcare providers ensures that both the mother's mental health and the baby's wellbeing are being closely monitored.

Remember, the decision to use antidepressants while breastfeeding should be made on an individual basis, considering the specific circumstances and needs of the mother and her baby. With careful management and proper support, many women successfully continue breastfeeding while taking antidepressants.

Are special precautions necessary while using antidepressants in the Elderly?

Yes, special precautions are necessary when using antidepressants in elderly patients. Older adults often have different responses to medications compared to younger individuals, due to factors like altered drug metabolism, increased likelihood of comorbidities, and higher sensitivity to side effects. Here are key considerations and precautions:

1. **Start Low, Go Slow:**
   - Begin with a lower dose than you would in younger adults. Elderly patients often metabolize drugs more slowly and are more sensitive to their effects.
   - Gradually increase the dose if needed, closely monitoring for effectiveness and side effects.
2. **Monitor for Side Effects:**
   - Elderly patients are more susceptible to side effects such as dizziness, falls, confusion, hyponatremia (low sodium levels), and cardiac effects.
   - Particular attention should be paid to risks like orthostatic hypotension, which can increase fall risk.
3. **Be Cautious with Certain Antidepressants**:
   - Tricyclic antidepressants (TCAs) are generally avoided in older adults due to their anticholinergic effects and potential to cause cardiac arrhythmias.
   - SSRIs are often preferred due to their more favorable side effect profile, but they are not without risks, including gastrointestinal bleeding, especially if the patient is also taking NSAIDs or anticoagulants.
4. **Evaluate Drug Interactions:**
   - The elderly often take multiple medications, increasing the risk of drug-drug interactions. Review all medications (including over-the-counter drugs and supplements) to avoid interactions.
5. **Consider Underlying Health Conditions:**
   - Tailor the choice of antidepressant to the patient's medical history. For example, certain antidepressants should be avoided in patients with heart disease, glaucoma, or prostate hypertrophy.
6. **Watch for Worsening or Emergence of Conditions:**
   - Be vigilant for the worsening of coexisting conditions like diabetes, heart disease, or kidney disease.
   - Monitor cognitive function, as some antidepressants can cause or worsen cognitive impairment.

7. **Assess Renal and Hepatic Function:**
   - Kidney and liver functions tend to decline with age, affecting drug metabolism and clearance. Regular monitoring is important.
8. **Suicide Risk:**
   - Monitor closely for signs of suicidal ideation, as depression in the elderly can sometimes be linked to a higher risk of suicide.
9. **Regular Follow-up and Monitoring:**
   - Frequent follow-ups are necessary to monitor the efficacy and side effects of the medication.
   - Adjust the treatment plan as needed based on the patient's response and tolerance.
10. **Non-Pharmacological Approaches:**
    - Consider integrating psychotherapy, exercise, and social engagement, which can be particularly beneficial for the elderly.
11. **Duration of Treatment:**
    - Be mindful of the duration of treatment. Elderly patients might need a longer course of treatment to prevent relapse.
12. **Gradual Discontinuation:**
    - If discontinuing an antidepressant, taper it off slowly to avoid withdrawal symptoms.

When treating depression in the elderly, it is important to maintain a holistic view of the patient's health, considering both psychological and physiological aspects. Collaboration with other healthcare professionals involved in the patient's care can also enhance treatment outcomes.

When to hospitalize in depression?

Hospitalization for depression is considered under certain circumstances when the severity of the condition poses a significant risk to the patient or others, or when outpatient treatment is insufficient. Here are key situations when hospitalization may be necessary:

1. **Suicidal Ideation or Attempts:**
   - If a patient is actively suicidal, expresses a plan or intent to harm themselves, or has recently attempted suicide, hospitalization is often required for safety and intensive treatment.
2. **Homicidal Ideation:**
   - If the patient expresses thoughts of harming others, immediate hospitalization is necessary to ensure the safety of others.
3. **Severe Depression with Psychotic Features:**
   - If the patient experiences severe depression accompanied by psychotic symptoms (such as hallucinations or delusions), hospitalization may be needed for comprehensive treatment and safety.
4. **Inability to Care for Self:**
   - If depression has rendered the patient unable to care for themselves, including not eating, bathing, or managing basic daily activities, and there is no support system in place at home.
5. **Significant Risk of Deterioration:**
   - If there is a high risk that the patient's condition will rapidly worsen without close monitoring and immediate intervention.
6. **Failure of Outpatient Treatment:**
   - If outpatient treatment, including therapy and medication, has been ineffective, and the patient's condition is not improving or is worsening.
7. **Need for Electroconvulsive Therapy (ECT):**
   - In cases where ECT is considered as a treatment option, especially for severe or treatment-resistant depression, hospitalization may be necessary for the duration of the treatment course.
8. **Severe Co-morbid Psychiatric or Medical Conditions:**
   - If there are co-occurring psychiatric or medical conditions that complicate the treatment of depression and require an integrated approach that can be best provided in a hospital setting.
9. **Detoxification from Substance Abuse:**
   - If the patient is struggling with substance abuse in addition to depression, and requires detoxification and dual diagnosis treatment.
10. **Lack of Supportive Environment:**
    - If the patient lacks a supportive home environment or is in a situation where the home

environment may exacerbate their depression (e.g., exposure to abuse, neglect, or significant stressors).

11. **Severe Impairment in Judgment or Functioning:**
    - If depression significantly impairs the patient's judgment, insight, or ability to function, and there are concerns about their ability to make safe decisions.

The decision to hospitalize a patient for depression is made based on a careful assessment of the risks and benefits, the severity of symptoms, and the individual's specific circumstances. It is often a collaborative decision involving mental health professionals, the patient, and their family or caregivers. Hospitalization provides a safe environment for intensive treatment and stabilization, often allowing for a quicker adjustment of medications, close monitoring of side effects, and provision of therapy and other supportive measures.

What is fatal insomnia, (FI)?

Fatal Insomnia (FI) is a rare and fatal degenerative brain disorder. It is divided into two types: Familial Fatal Insomnia (FFI) and Sporadic Fatal Insomnia (SFI). FFI is a hereditary condition caused by a mutation in the PRNP gene, which also causes Creutzfeldt-Jakob disease and other prion diseases. SFI, on the other hand, occurs spontaneously without a known genetic cause.

Characteristics of Fatal Insomnia:

1. **Insomnia:** As the name suggests, a prominent feature is a severe disruption of sleep patterns. This includes difficulty falling asleep and staying asleep, leading to progressive and severe insomnia.
2. **Neurological and Physical Symptoms:** The disorder typically involves a range of other symptoms, such as:
    - Motor dysfunction, including coordination problems and stiffness.
    - Cognitive impairments, like memory loss and confusion.
    - Autonomic nervous system disturbances, which can include hyperhidrosis (excessive sweating), fever, hypertension, and tachycardia (rapid heart rate).
    - Psychiatric manifestations, including paranoia, hallucinations, and panic attacks.
3. **Progressive Course:** FI is a progressive condition that worsens over time, often rapidly. It usually begins with mild symptoms and gradually advances to more severe neurological and physical symptoms.
4. **Fatal Outcome:** Unfortunately, there is no cure or effective treatment to halt the progression of FI. It is invariably fatal, with the duration from onset of symptoms to death typically ranging from a few months to a few years.

Diagnosis:

- **Genetic Testing:** For FFI, genetic testing can confirm the presence of the PRNP gene mutation.
- **Medical History and Symptom Assessment:** A thorough review of symptoms and medical history is essential.
- **Neurological Exams and Imaging:** Brain imaging and neurological exams can help rule out other causes of the symptoms.
- **Sleep Studies:** Polysomnography can assess sleep disturbances.

Research and Treatment:

- **Experimental Treatments:** Due to its rarity, treatment options are limited and generally focus on symptomatic relief.
- **Ongoing Research:** Research is ongoing to better understand prion diseases and to develop potential treatments.

Fatal Insomnia is a complex and rare condition that represents a significant challenge in neurology and sleep medicine. The study of such rare disorders often provides insights into more common neurodegenerative diseases and advances our understanding of brain function and disease.

What Complications can arise during treatment for Depression with SSRIs?

Treatment with selective serotonin reuptake inhibitors (SSRIs), a class of drugs commonly used to treat depression, can lead to various complications and side effects. While SSRIs are generally safe and effective for many people, they can cause issues in some individuals, particularly if not closely monitored. Here are some potential complications and side effects associated with SSRIs:

1. **Gastrointestinal Issues:** Common side effects include nausea, diarrhea, and constipation. These are often mild and may resolve over time.

2. **Sexual Dysfunction:** SSRIs can cause problems such as reduced sexual desire, difficulty achieving orgasm, or erectile dysfunction.
3. **Weight Gain:** Long-term use of some SSRIs can lead to weight gain.
4. **Sleep Disturbances:** Some individuals may experience insomnia or, conversely, excessive sleepiness.
5. **Increased Anxiety or Agitation:** Especially early in the treatment, SSRIs can increase feelings of restlessness, anxiety, or agitation.
6. **Emotional Blunting:** Some people on SSRIs report feeling emotionally "numb" or less able to experience strong emotions.
7. **Serotonin Syndrome:** A rare but potentially life-threatening condition can occur, particularly if SSRIs are taken in combination with other medications that increase serotonin levels, such as other antidepressants, certain pain or migraine medications, and some herbal supplements. Symptoms include agitation, confusion, rapid heart rate, high blood pressure, dilated pupils, muscle rigidity, and in severe cases, seizures.
8. **Bleeding Risks:** SSRIs can affect platelet aggregation, leading to an increased risk of bleeding, especially if taken with other medications that affect bleeding, like anticoagulants or NSAIDs.
9. **Hyponatremia:** Especially in older adults, SSRIs can lead to a drop in sodium levels in the blood, which can cause symptoms ranging from headache and confusion to seizures.
10. **Withdrawal Symptoms:** Abruptly stopping SSRIs can lead to withdrawal symptoms, such as dizziness, tingling sensations, fatigue, vivid dreams, and irritability or agitation.
11. **Suicidal Thoughts and Behaviors:** Particularly in children, adolescents, and young adults, SSRIs can increase the risk of suicidal thoughts and behaviors, especially during the initial period of treatment.
12. **Bone Density Reduction:** Long-term use of SSRIs has been associated with a reduction in bone mineral density, increasing the risk of fractures.
13. **Interactions with Other Medications:** SSRIs can interact with a wide range of medications, leading to increased side effects or decreased effectiveness of one or more of the medications.

When prescribing SSRIs, healthcare providers typically start with the lowest possible effective dose and monitor patients closely, particularly at the beginning of treatment and during dose changes. It is important for patients to communicate openly with their healthcare providers about any side effects or concerns they have while taking SSRIs. Adjustments to the treatment plan, including changes in medication, dosage, or addition of other therapies, can often manage side effects effectively.

What Complications can arise during treatment for Depression with Tricyclic antidepressants?

Tricyclic antidepressants (TCAs) are an older class of antidepressant medications used for treating depression. While effective, they are often associated with more side effects and potential complications compared to newer classes of antidepressants like selective serotonin reuptake inhibitors (SSRIs). Some of the key complications and side effects associated with TCAs include:

1. **Anticholinergic Effects:** TCAs often cause side effects related to their anticholinergic activity, such as dry mouth, blurred vision, constipation, urinary retention, and confusion. These effects can be particularly troublesome for elderly patients.
2. **Cardiovascular Issues:** TCAs can affect heart rhythm and function, leading to complications like tachycardia (fast heart rate), arrhythmias, and orthostatic hypotension (a drop in blood pressure upon standing), which can increase the risk of falls, especially in the elderly.
3. **Weight Gain:** Long-term use of TCAs is associated with weight gain in some patients.
4. **Sedation:** Many TCAs have a sedative effect, which can cause drowsiness and impair the ability to drive or operate machinery. This can also be beneficial for patients with insomnia related to depression.
5. **Lower Seizure Threshold:** TCAs can lower the seizure threshold, increasing the risk of seizures, particularly in individuals with a history of epilepsy or other conditions that predispose to seizures.
6. **Suicidal Thoughts and Behaviors:** As with other antidepressants, TCAs can increase the risk of suicidal thoughts and behaviors, especially in children, adolescents, and young adults.

7. **Overdose Risk:** TCAs can be toxic in overdose, much more so than SSRIs. Overdose can lead to life-threatening conditions, such as cardiac arrhythmias, severe hypotension, seizures, and coma.
8. **Sexual Dysfunction:** Sexual side effects, such as reduced libido, difficulty achieving orgasm, or erectile dysfunction, can occur with TCA use.
9. **Withdrawal Symptoms:** Discontinuing TCAs abruptly can lead to withdrawal symptoms like nausea, headache, and malaise. Therefore, they should be tapered off gradually under medical supervision.
10. **Interactions with Other Medications:** TCAs can interact with various other medications, leading to increased side effects or reduced efficacy. This includes interactions with certain psychiatric medications, heart medications, and substances like alcohol.
11. **Serotonin Syndrome:** Although less common than with SSRIs, combining TCAs with other medications that increase serotonin levels can lead to serotonin syndrome, a potentially life-threatening condition.
12. **Hyponatremia:** TCAs can cause a drop in sodium levels in the blood, particularly in older adults, which can lead to symptoms ranging from confusion and lethargy to seizures.

Because of these potential side effects and complications, TCAs are generally not the first-line treatment for depression, especially in older adults or those with certain medical conditions. However, they can be effective for some patients, particularly those who have not responded to other antidepressants. When prescribing TCAs, healthcare providers closely monitor patients, particularly at the beginning of treatment and during dose adjustments, and tailor the treatment plan based on individual patient needs and responses.

What is mania?

Mania is a state of abnormally elevated or irritable mood, arousal, and energy levels. It is most commonly seen in bipolar disorder, a mental health condition characterized by extreme mood swings that include emotional highs (mania or hypomania) and lows (depression). Mania is a defining feature of Bipolar I disorder, and its presence can significantly impact an individual's life and functioning. Here are key characteristics of mania:

Symptoms of Mania

1. **Elevated Mood:** Excessive happiness, euphoria, extreme optimism, or an inflated sense of self-esteem or grandiosity.
2. **Increased Irritability:** In some cases, mania can manifest as irritability or aggressive behavior rather than an elevated mood.
3. **Decreased Need for Sleep:** Feeling rested after only a few hours of sleep or inability to sleep.
4. **Racing Thoughts and Rapid Speech:** Jumping quickly from one idea to another or speaking so rapidly that it is hard for others to follow.
5. **Distractibility:** Inability to concentrate or being easily distracted by irrelevant stimuli.
6. **Increased Activity or Energy:** High levels of energy, restlessness, or an increase in goal-directed activities. This can include taking on multiple new projects or having an excessive involvement in pleasurable but risky activities.
7. **Impulsivity or Risky Behavior:** Engaging in reckless behavior, such as excessive spending, making rash decisions, or risky sexual behavior.

Duration and Severity

- To be classified as a manic episode, these symptoms must last for at least one week (or any duration if hospitalization is necessary) and represent a noticeable change from the person's usual behavior.
- The symptoms should be severe enough to cause significant distress or impairment in social, occupational, or other important areas of functioning, or to necessitate hospitalization to prevent harm to oneself or others.
- In some cases, manic episodes can include psychotic features such as delusions or hallucinations.

Hypomania vs. Mania

- Hypomania is a milder form of mania, characterized by similar but less severe symptoms. Hypomanic episodes do not lead to the significant functional impairment that manic episodes do and do not include psychotic features. Hypomania is a feature of Bipolar II disorder.

Treatment

- Treatment of mania often involves a combination of mood stabilizers (like lithium or valproate), antipsychotic medications, and psychotherapy.
- In severe cases, especially when there are psychotic features or a risk of harm to oneself or others, hospitalization may be necessary to ensure safety and stabilize the mood.

Recognizing and treating mania is critical, as it can lead to risky behaviors and have serious repercussions on a person's relationships, job, and overall well-being. If you or someone you know is experiencing symptoms of mania, it is important to seek professional help from a healthcare provider.

What does Mania feel like?

Experiencing mania can vary from person to person, but it generally involves a period of extremely high energy, euphoria, or irritability, along with other significant changes in behavior and mood. Here is how individuals often describe what mania feels like:

1. **Elevated Mood:** People may feel an overwhelming sense of euphoria or extreme happiness. This can feel like being on top of the world, often without a clear reason.
2. **Increased Energy and Restlessness:** There is often a dramatic increase in energy levels. People may feel hyperactive, restless, and find it hard to stay still. They might be constantly moving or feel an urge to engage in many activities at once.
3. **Reduced Need for Sleep:** Many people experience a significantly reduced need for sleep. They might feel fully rested after only a few hours of sleep or go without sleep for long periods.
4. **Racing Thoughts:** Thoughts may race uncontrollably, often jumping rapidly from one idea to another. This can make it difficult to concentrate or focus on a single task.
5. **Rapid Speech:** People often talk more than usual, speak very quickly, and may jump around to different topics. This rapid speech can be hard for others to follow.
6. **Grandiosity or Inflated Self-Esteem:** There can be an inflated sense of self-importance or abilities. People might feel like they have special powers, talents, or are destined for greatness.
7. **Impulsivity and Risk-Taking Behaviors:** Mania often leads to impulsive decisions without considering the consequences. This can include reckless driving, spending sprees, risky sexual behavior, or unwise business investments.
8. **Irritability or Agitation:** In some cases, mania can manifest as irritability or agitation, especially if someone's ideas or plans are challenged or if they feel constrained.
9. **Detachment from Reality:** In severe cases, mania can include psychotic symptoms, such as delusions (strongly held beliefs in things that are not true) or hallucinations (seeing or hearing things that aren't there).
10. **Feelings of Invincibility:** A sense of invulnerability or ignoring personal limitations, which can lead to overcommitting or engaging in dangerous activities.

While the experience of mania can feel exhilarating and productive to some, it often leads to significant problems in life, relationships, and work. It is important to recognize that these feelings and behaviors are symptoms of a disorder and not just heightened states of creativity or productivity. Mania is often followed by a depressive episode, which can be severe.

If you or someone you know is experiencing symptoms of mania, it is important to seek help from a healthcare professional. Effective treatments are available, and early intervention can help manage the symptoms and prevent complications.

What are the physical signs of mania?

The physical signs of mania, a phase of bipolar disorder, can vary but typically include several key indicators. These might include:

1. **Increased Energy and Activity Levels:** Individuals experiencing mania often show remarkably high energy levels. They might appear unusually active, restless, or agitated.
2. **Reduced Need for Sleep:** One of the most common signs of mania is a decreased need for sleep. People in a manic phase can go with very little or no sleep for days without feeling tired.
3. **Rapid Speech:** During manic episodes, individuals often speak rapidly, sometimes so fast that it is hard for others to follow. They might also abruptly change topics or feel a pressure to keep talking.
4. **Physical Agitation or Restlessness:** This can manifest as an inability to sit still, constant

movement, fidgeting, or engaging in multiple activities at once.

5. **Impulsiveness and Risky Behaviors:** Engaging in behaviors that are unusual for the individual, like reckless driving, spending sprees, or impulsive decision-making.
6. **Heightened Physical Reactions:** This could include increased libido, drug or alcohol abuse, or engaging in physically demanding activities without apparent fatigue.
7. **Changes in Appetite:** This could either be an increase or decrease in appetite, sometimes resulting in significant weight loss or gain.
8. **Dress and Grooming Changes:** Some people in a manic phase may dress more flamboyantly or neglect their personal grooming.

It is important to note that these signs can vary widely among individuals and should be assessed by a healthcare professional for an accurate diagnosis. Mania can have a significant impact on a person's life and relationships, and appropriate treatment is crucial for managing the symptoms.

What can cause mania?

Mania is most commonly associated with bipolar disorder, but there are several factors and conditions that can trigger or contribute to manic episodes. These include:

1. **Bipolar Disorder:** Mania is a key characteristic of bipolar disorder, particularly Bipolar I disorder. In this condition, individuals experience episodes of extreme mood elevation (mania) along with periods of depression.
2. **Medications and Substances:** Certain medications, particularly antidepressants, can trigger mania in some individuals, especially if they have bipolar disorder. Likewise, the use of stimulant drugs, such as cocaine or amphetamines, can induce manic-like symptoms.
3. **Brain Chemistry and Structure:** Imbalances in neurotransmitters (brain chemicals) and structural brain changes are believed to contribute to the development of manic episodes.
4. **Genetic Factors:** There is a strong genetic component to bipolar disorder. Individuals with a family history of bipolar disorder are at a higher risk of developing the condition and experiencing mania.
5. **Sleep Deprivation:** Lack of sleep can trigger manic episodes in some people, particularly those with bipolar disorder.
6. **Stress:** Significant life stressors, such as the death of a loved one, major life changes, or high levels of stress, can precipitate a manic episode.
7. **Seasonal Changes:** For some individuals, seasonal changes can influence mood and behavior. For instance, manic episodes are more common during the spring and summer months.
8. **Medical Conditions:** Certain neurological or medical conditions can present with manic symptoms. These include multiple sclerosis, stroke, traumatic brain injury, and hyperthyroidism.
9. **Substance Withdrawal:** Withdrawal from alcohol or drugs, especially sedatives, can lead to symptoms of mania.

It is important to note that the manifestation of mania can vary significantly from person to person, and the exact cause of manic episodes can be complex and multifactorial. If mania or bipolar disorder is suspected, it is crucial to seek professional medical evaluation and treatment. Proper management often involves a combination of medication, psychotherapy, lifestyle changes, and support.

What are signs of mixed mania in bipolar disorder?

Mixed mania, also known as a mixed episode or mixed features, in bipolar disorder is characterized by the simultaneous occurrence of manic and depressive symptoms. This can be a particularly complex and distressing state for individuals, as they experience conflicting symptoms. Key signs of mixed mania include:

1. **Agitation or Irritability:** This is a common sign where an individual may feel extremely restless and irritable. This agitation can be more intense than what is typically seen in either mania or depression alone.
2. **Rapid Mood Swings:** Experiencing rapid and intense shifts in mood, often without any apparent reason. This can include feeling euphoric one moment and profoundly sad or hopeless the next.
3. **High Energy with Low Mood:** Individuals may have the high energy and restlessness typical of mania but feel depressed, hopeless, or empty at the same time.

4. **Racing Thoughts with Sadness:** Experiencing racing thoughts or pressured speech (common in mania) while having predominantly depressive content in thoughts.

5. **Increased Risk-Taking with Depressive Thoughts:** Engaging in risky, impulsive behaviors (a characteristic of mania) while feeling despair or having thoughts of self-harm.

6. **Difficulty Concentrating:** This can be a result of the combined overactivity (mania) and low motivation or indecisiveness (depression).

7. **Sleep Disturbances:** Trouble sleeping is common, which may include insomnia or restless sleep. This symptom overlaps both manic and depressive states.

8. **Changes in Appetite:** This could manifest as either increased or decreased appetite, reflecting the mixed influence of both manic and depressive symptoms.

9. **Feelings of Worthlessness or Guilt:** Despite having high energy or agitation, individuals might experience intense feelings of guilt or worthlessness, which are more typical of depressive states.

10. **Suicidal Thoughts:** The risk of suicide can be high in mixed episodes, due to the combination of depressive symptoms with the energy and impulsivity of mania.

Mixed episodes can be particularly challenging to treat, as they encompass symptoms of both poles of bipolar disorder. It is crucial for individuals experiencing these symptoms to seek professional help. Treatment usually involves a combination of mood stabilizers, psychotherapy, and sometimes antipsychotic medication, tailored to manage the complexity and severity of the symptoms.

What medications trigger mania?

Certain medications and substances have the potential to trigger manic episodes, particularly in individuals with bipolar disorder or those predisposed to it. It is important to note that while these medications can trigger mania, they may be safe and effective for many individuals when used appropriately. The following are some types of medications known to potentially trigger mania:

1. **Antidepressants:** The most common trigger for medication-induced mania is the use of antidepressants, especially in individuals with undiagnosed bipolar disorder. This includes selective serotonin reuptake inhibitors (SSRIs), tricyclic antidepressants, and monoamine oxidase inhibitors (MAOIs).

2. **Corticosteroids:** Medications like prednisone, often used for inflammatory conditions, can induce manic symptoms in some individuals.

3. **Stimulants:** Medications used to treat attention-deficit/hyperactivity disorder (ADHD), such as amphetamine and dextroamphetamine (Adderall), methylphenidate (Ritalin), and others, can trigger mania or hypomania.

4. **Dopamine Agonists:** Used in the treatment of Parkinson's disease and sometimes restless legs syndrome, these medications can induce manic-like symptoms.

5. **Illicit Drugs and Stimulants:** Substances such as cocaine, ecstasy (MDMA), and methamphetamine can induce manic episodes.

6. **Thyroid Medications:** Over-replacement of thyroid hormones, leading to hyperthyroidism, can trigger mania in susceptible individuals.

7. **Non-prescription Drugs and Supplements:** Certain over-the-counter medications and supplements, especially those with stimulant properties, can potentially trigger mania.

8. **Caffeine and Alcohol:** In some sensitive individuals, excessive caffeine or alcohol consumption can contribute to the onset of manic symptoms.

9. **Antiviral Drugs:** Certain medications used to treat HIV/AIDS and hepatitis C have been associated with triggering mania in some cases.

It is important for individuals with bipolar disorder or those at risk for it to inform their healthcare providers about their condition before starting any new medication. Additionally, any changes in mood or behavior should be promptly discussed with a healthcare provider. The management of bipolar disorder often requires a careful balance of medications to stabilize mood without triggering manic or depressive episodes.

How to treat bipolar disorder in pregnancy?

Treating bipolar disorder during pregnancy requires careful consideration and management, as both the disorder and the medications used to treat it can pose risks to the mother and the developing fetus. Here are some general guidelines for treating bipolar disorder in pregnancy:

1. **Consultation with Healthcare Providers:** It is essential for pregnant women with bipolar disorder to work closely with their psychiatrist, obstetrician, and possibly a perinatal psychiatrist. This collaboration ensures the risks and benefits of treatment are carefully weighed.
2. **Medication Management:** Some medications used for bipolar disorder can be teratogenic (harmful to the developing fetus) or carry other risks during pregnancy. However, discontinuing medication can also be risky due to the potential for relapse. Decisions about medication should be individualized:
   - Lithium, while effective, carries a risk of congenital abnormalities, particularly when used in the first trimester. However, the absolute risk is relatively low. Lithium levels must be closely monitored during pregnancy.
   - Anticonvulsants like valproate and carbamazepine are generally avoided due to high teratogenic risks.
   - Atypical antipsychotics may be used, but there is limited data on their safety in pregnancy. They might be considered when the benefits outweigh the risks.
   - With any medication, the lowest effective dose should be used.
3. **Psychotherapy:** Psychotherapy, particularly cognitive behavioral therapy (CBT) and interpersonal therapy, can be beneficial during pregnancy, providing support without the risks associated with medications.
4. **Monitoring and Support:** Close monitoring of the mother's mental health throughout pregnancy and the postpartum period is crucial. This includes regular appointments with mental health professionals.
5. **Lifestyle Modifications:** Stress management techniques, regular exercise, adequate sleep, and a healthy diet can help manage symptoms of bipolar disorder during pregnancy.
6. **Planning for the Postpartum Period:** Women with bipolar disorder are at a high risk for postpartum mood episodes. Plans for close monitoring and support after delivery should be in place.
7. **Breastfeeding Considerations:** Decisions about breastfeeding need to consider the medication being used and its effects on the new-born. Some medications for bipolar disorder can be excreted in breast milk.
8. **Fetal Monitoring:** Depending on the medications used, additional fetal monitoring might be recommended to ensure the baby's health.

It is important to note that treatment decisions should be highly individualized, taking into account the severity of the bipolar disorder, the woman's history with the illness, her response to previous treatments, and the specific risks associated with treatment options. The goal is to maintain the best possible mental health for the mother while minimizing risks to the developing fetus.

What are the symptoms of hypomania?

Hypomania is a milder form of mania, often seen in bipolar II disorder. While it shares some characteristics with mania, the symptoms are less severe and do not typically cause significant disruption in daily life or require hospitalization. However, they can still be impactful and noticeable. Common symptoms of hypomania include:

1. **Elevated or Irritable Mood:** Feeling unusually "high," euphoric, or irritable for an extended period.
2. **Increased Energy and Activity Levels:** A noticeable increase in energy and activity, including social, work, or personal projects.
3. **Decreased Need for Sleep:** Feeling rested after only a few hours of sleep.
4. **More Talkative than Usual:** Talking more or feeling a pressure to keep talking.
5. **Racing Thoughts:** Experiencing a rapid flow of ideas or the feeling that thoughts are jumping from topic to topic.
6. **Distractibility:** Easily distracted by unimportant or irrelevant external stimuli.
7. **Increased Self-Esteem or Grandiosity:** Inflated self-esteem or grandiosity, often unrealistic.
8. **Engaging in Risky Behaviors:** More likely to engage in behavior that could have serious consequences, such as reckless driving, spending sprees, or impulsive business decisions.
9. **Enhanced Creativity and Productivity:** Feeling more creative or productive, often manifesting in taking on multiple projects at once.
10. **Heightened Sociability:** Increased sociability, such as a sudden surge in socializing or making lots of new friends.

Unlike mania, hypomania does not involve psychosis (such as hallucinations or delusions) and its impact on functioning is not as severe. However, it can still lead to significant distress or impaired functioning, and it often precedes or follows depressive episodes in bipolar II disorder. Therefore, recognizing and treating hypomania is crucial in the overall management of bipolar disorder. Treatment typically involves mood stabilizers, psychotherapy, and lifestyle changes to help manage symptoms and prevent progression to more severe episodes.

What is the difference between mania and hypomania?

Mania and hypomania are both states characterized by elevated mood and increased energy, but they differ significantly in their intensity, duration, and impact on a person's functioning. These differences are crucial for the diagnosis and treatment of bipolar disorders. Here is a comparison:

1. **Intensity of Symptoms:**
   - **Mania:** More severe symptoms. The mood elevation can be extreme, often accompanied by high levels of energy, euphoria, or irritability.
   - **Hypomania:** Less severe. The mood elevation is noticeable but not as extreme. People often feel more energetic and more productive.
2. **Duration:**
   - **Mania:** To be classified as mania, symptoms must last for at least one week or require hospitalization.
   - **Hypomania:** Symptoms need to last at least four days in a row and are clearly different from the person's non-depressed mood.
3. **Impact on Functioning:**
   - **Mania:** Can significantly impair a person's ability to function in daily life. It may lead to psychotic symptoms (delusions, hallucinations) and often requires hospitalization.
   - **Hypomania:** Does not cause significant impairment in social or occupational functioning. People often continue their routine activities, and it may not be immediately obvious to others that something is wrong.
4. **Psychotic Features:**
   - **Mania:** May include psychotic features like hallucinations or delusions.
   - **Hypomania:** Does not include psychosis.
5. **Association with Bipolar Disorder:**
   - **Mania:** A hallmark of Bipolar I Disorder.
   - **Hypomania:** Typically associated with Bipolar II Disorder, where it alternates with episodes of depression.
6. **Behavioral Changes:**
   - **Mania:** Behaviors are often more extreme, including reckless or dangerous activities, poor judgment, and impulsivity.
   - **Hypomania:** Behaviors, while elevated, are less extreme. Increased creativity and productivity are common.
7. **Consequences:**
   - **Mania:** The consequences can be severe, including legal problems, financial issues, and relationship breakdowns.
   - **Hypomania:** The consequences are usually less severe but can still impact relationships and life decisions.

It is important to note that both mania and hypomania are serious conditions that require professional medical evaluation and treatment. Recognition and management of these episodes are crucial in the overall care of bipolar disorder.

What drugs are used for Mania?

The treatment of mania typically involves the use of medications known as mood stabilizers and antipsychotics. These drugs help control the symptoms of mania, such as high energy levels, reduced need for sleep, and rapid speech. The choice of medication depends on the individual's specific symptoms, previous treatment response, and potential side effects. Commonly used medications for mania include:

1. **Mood Stabilizers:**
   - **Lithium:** One of the most widely used and studied medications for the treatment of mania. Lithium can be very effective in controlling mania and preventing the recurrence of both manic and depressive episodes.
   - **Valproate (**Valproic Acid or Divalproex Sodium): Often used for rapid-cycling bipolar disorder and mixed episodes. It is also frequently chosen for individuals who don't respond well to lithium.
   - **Carbamazepine:** Another option for treating mania, particularly in people who don't respond to lithium or valproate.

- **Lamotrigine:** Mainly used for the maintenance treatment of bipolar disorder, especially in preventing depressive episodes. It is less effective for acute mania.

2. **Antipsychotics:**
   - **Atypical Antipsychotics** (such as olanzapine, risperidone, quetiapine, aripiprazole, ziprasidone, and lurasidone): These are often used, either alone or in combination with mood stabilizers, to treat manic episodes. They can be particularly useful when psychotic symptoms (like delusions or hallucinations) are present.
   - **Typical Antipsychotics:** Less commonly used today due to their side effect profile but can be effective in certain cases.
3. **Benzodiazepines:**
   - Medications like lorazepam or clonazepam can be used for short-term management of acute manic symptoms, particularly agitation or insomnia. They are usually used in combination with mood stabilizers or antipsychotics.
4. **Calcium Channel Blockers:**
   - Although not typically a first-line treatment, some calcium channel blockers (such as verapamil) have shown effectiveness in treating mania, particularly in individuals who cannot tolerate the side effects of standard treatments.

It is important to note that the treatment of mania often requires careful monitoring by a healthcare professional, as the effectiveness and side effects of these medications can vary greatly among individuals. In addition, medication treatment is often more effective when combined with psychotherapy, lifestyle changes, and regular monitoring of mood symptoms.

How many episodes of bipolar I can be diagnosed?

The diagnosis of bipolar I disorder does not depend on the number of episodes a person has had. Rather, it is based on the presence of at least one manic episode. This manic episode may be preceded by or followed by hypomanic or major depressive episodes, but these are not required for the diagnosis.

In bipolar I disorder, the manic episode is a distinct period of abnormally and persistently elevated, expansive, or irritable mood, and abnormally and persistently increased activity or energy lasting at least one week, and present most of the day, nearly every day.

It is important to note that the diagnosis and treatment of bipolar I disorder and any other mental health conditions should be carried out by a qualified healthcare professional. They will consider the individual's specific symptoms, their duration, and the impact on the person's life. The number and pattern of episodes can vary greatly between individuals.

What is bipolar II?

Bipolar II disorder is a type of mood disorder characterized by a pattern of depressive episodes and hypomanic episodes, but without the full-blown manic episodes that are typical of Bipolar I disorder.

Here are the key features of Bipolar II disorder:

1. **Hypomanic Episodes:** These are periods of elevated, expansive, or irritable mood and increased activity or energy that are clearly different from the individual's usual non-depressed mood. Hypomanic episodes in Bipolar II disorder are less severe than manic episodes in Bipolar I disorder. They last at least four consecutive days and are observable by others, but are not severe enough to cause major impairment in social or occupational functioning or to necessitate hospitalization.
2. **Major Depressive Episodes:** These episodes involve symptoms such as a depressed mood or loss of interest or pleasure in almost all activities, along with other symptoms like significant weight loss or gain, insomnia or hypersomnia, psychomotor agitation or retardation, fatigue, feelings of worthlessness or excessive guilt, diminished ability to think or concentrate, and recurrent thoughts of death or suicide. For a diagnosis of Bipolar II disorder, the individual must have experienced at least one such episode.
3. **No History of Manic Episodes:** Unlike Bipolar I disorder, individuals with Bipolar II disorder have never experienced a full manic episode.

It is important to differentiate Bipolar II disorder from major depressive disorder, especially since the hypomanic episodes can sometimes be overlooked or mistaken for a "normal" mood state, especially if they are not causing obvious distress or impairment. The diagnosis and treatment of bipolar disorders should be managed by qualified healthcare professionals.

What is alcohol withdrawal?

Alcohol withdrawal refers to a range of symptoms that can occur when an individual who has been drinking heavily for weeks, months, or years suddenly stops or significantly reduces their alcohol consumption. These symptoms are the result of the central nervous system adjusting to the absence of alcohol. Severity of withdrawal symptoms can vary widely, depending on the length and intensity of alcohol use, and they can range from mild to severe.

Key aspects of alcohol withdrawal include:

1. **Timing:** Symptoms typically begin within hours of the last drink and can last for several days.
2. **Symptoms:** These can range from mild to severe and can include:
   - Anxiety
   - Sweating
   - Tremors (shakiness, particularly in the hands)
   - Insomnia
   - Nausea or vomiting
   - Headache
   - Agitation
   - Increased heart rate and blood pressure
3. **Severe Symptoms: In some cases, severe withdrawal symptoms occur, such as:**
   - Hallucinations (seeing or hearing things that are not there).
   - Seizures.
   - Delirium tremens (DTs), a serious condition that may include confusion, rapid heartbeat, fever, and in severe cases, can be life-threatening.
4. **Progression:** Symptoms typically begin to appear when blood alcohol level decreases significantly or reaches zero, and they peak in intensity at 24 to 48 hours after the last drink.
5. **Treatment:** Treatment of alcohol withdrawal may involve:
   - Medical monitoring to ensure safety.
   - Medications to reduce withdrawal symptoms (such as benzodiazepines).
   - Fluids and treatment of other medical conditions that may be present.
   - Long-term treatment for alcohol dependence or abuse, including therapy and support groups.

It is crucial to note that alcohol withdrawal can be dangerous, and in some cases, life-threatening. Medical supervision is highly recommended for individuals experiencing significant withdrawal symptoms, especially if they have a history of severe alcohol use or previous withdrawal complications.

What is the cause of alcohol withdrawal?

The cause of alcohol withdrawal is primarily related to how prolonged alcohol use affects the brain's functioning and neurochemistry. Here is a more detailed explanation:

1. **Neurochemical Adaptation:** Alcohol is a central nervous system depressant. With regular and heavy use, the brain starts to adapt to its depressant effects. This adaptation is partly achieved by altering the balance of neurotransmitters – chemicals that transmit signals in the brain.
2. **GABA and Glutamate:** Alcohol enhances the effect of GABA (gamma-aminobutyric acid), a neurotransmitter that produces feelings of relaxation and calm. Simultaneously, it inhibits the effects of glutamate, a neurotransmitter associated with excitability. Over time, the brain adjusts to these effects by reducing its GABA activity and increasing glutamate activity.
3. **Withdrawal of Alcohol:** When alcohol is suddenly removed (or significantly reduced), the brain remains in a hyper-excited state due to the increased glutamate activity and decreased GABA activity. This heightened state of nervous system activity leads to the symptoms of withdrawal.
4. **Physical Dependence:** With continuous exposure to alcohol, the body becomes dependent on it to maintain neurological balance. When alcohol is no longer present, this balance is disrupted, causing physical withdrawal symptoms.
5. **Tolerance:** Over time, individuals who drink heavily often develop a tolerance to alcohol, meaning they need to consume more to achieve the same effects. This increased consumption exacerbates the neurochemical imbalance and, in turn, can lead to more severe withdrawal symptoms when alcohol use is reduced or stopped.
6. **Genetic and Environmental Factors:** Genetic predispositions and environmental factors, such as stress or trauma, can also play a role in the development and severity of alcohol withdrawal.

It is important to understand that alcohol withdrawal can be a serious medical condition, especially for those who have been drinking heavily for a long period. Medical supervision is often necessary during the withdrawal process to manage the symptoms safely.

What are the symptoms of alcohol withdrawal?

The symptoms of alcohol withdrawal can vary in severity, ranging from mild to potentially life-threatening. They usually start within a few hours to a few days after the last drink and can last for several days. The most common symptoms include:

1. **Psychological Symptoms:**
   - Anxiety or nervousness
   - Depression
   - Irritability
   - Mood swings
   - Confusion
   - Nightmares
   - Difficulty thinking clearly
2. **Physical Symptoms:**
   - Headache
   - Sweating, especially the palms of the hands or the face
   - Nausea and vomiting
   - Loss of appetite
   - Insomnia or disturbed sleep
   - Fatigue
   - Rapid heart rate (tachycardia)
   - Paleness
   - Eyes, nose, or palms appearing redder than usual
   - Shaky hands or tremors
   - Clammy skin
3. **Severe Symptoms:**
   - Hallucinations (seeing or hearing things that aren't there)
   - Seizures
   - High fever
   - Severe confusion
   - Agitation
   - Delirium tremens (DTs), a severe form of withdrawal that can include vivid hallucinations and delusions, severe confusion, fever, and seizures. DTs are a medical emergency.

The severity and combination of symptoms can vary based on several factors, such as the duration and intensity of alcohol use, the presence of co-occurring medical or psychiatric conditions, previous withdrawal experiences, and individual physiological factors.

It is important for individuals undergoing alcohol withdrawal, especially if they experience severe symptoms, to seek medical attention. Alcohol withdrawal can be dangerous and, in some cases, life-threatening, requiring professional medical supervision and treatment.

How is alcohol withdrawal diagnosed?

Diagnosing alcohol withdrawal typically involves a combination of medical evaluation, patient history, and sometimes the use of specific assessment tools. Here is a general overview of the process:

1. **Medical Evaluation and History:**
   - **Symptom Assessment:** The healthcare provider will ask about the symptoms the individual is experiencing. This includes their type, severity, and onset.
   - **Drinking History:** Detailed information about the individual's alcohol use is crucial. This includes the amount and frequency of alcohol consumption, the last time alcohol was consumed, and any previous experiences with withdrawal.
   - **Medical History:** Information about any past medical issues, especially those related to liver or neurological conditions, and any current or past mental health issues.
2. **Physical Examination:**
   - The doctor will perform a physical exam to check for physical signs of alcohol withdrawal, such as tremors, sweating, an irregular heartbeat, and dehydration.
   - They may also check for any co-occurring medical conditions that could be influenced by alcohol use or withdrawal.
3. **Laboratory Tests:**
   - Blood tests might be conducted to assess overall health, liver function, and to check for other substances in the system.
   - Blood Alcohol Concentration (BAC) may also be measured.

4. **Use of Assessment Tools:**
   - Tools like the Clinical Institute Withdrawal Assessment for Alcohol (CIWA-Ar) scale can be used. This scale assesses the severity of withdrawal symptoms and helps in guiding treatment decisions.
5. **Psychiatric Evaluation:**
   - If there are signs of co-occurring mental health disorders, a psychiatric evaluation may be necessary.
6. **Monitoring for Severe Withdrawal Symptoms:**
   - In some cases, especially if the individual is at risk for severe withdrawal symptoms like seizures or delirium tremens (DTs), they may be observed or admitted for monitoring.

It is important to note that diagnosing alcohol withdrawal is a clinical process and needs to be performed by a healthcare professional. They will take into account the individual's specific situation, including their physical and mental health history, to make a diagnosis and recommend the appropriate treatment. The goal is to ensure a safe withdrawal process and to address any long-term issues related to alcohol use.

How alcohol withdrawal is treated?

Treatment for alcohol withdrawal is tailored to the individual's specific symptoms and their severity. It often involves a combination of medical management, support, and long-term treatment strategies for alcohol dependence. Here is an overview:

1. **Medical Supervision:**
   - For moderate to severe withdrawal symptoms, treatment typically occurs in a hospital or a specialized detoxification facility. This allows for close monitoring and management of symptoms.
   - Mild withdrawal symptoms may be managed at home, but this should only be done under the guidance of a healthcare provider.
2. **Medication:**
   - **Benzodiazepines:** These are commonly used to reduce withdrawal symptoms, particularly anxiety, seizures, and to prevent complications like delirium tremens (DTs). Examples include diazepam (Valium), lorazepam (Ativan), and chlordiazepoxide (Librium).
   - **Anticonvulsants:** Sometimes used for seizure prevention.
   - **Beta-blockers and alpha-2 agonists:** These can help reduce autonomic symptoms like rapid heart rate and high blood pressure.
   - **Nutritional Support:** Supplements, especially thiamine (vitamin B1), are often given to prevent or treat Wernicke-Korsakoff syndrome, a neurological disorder that can result from long-term heavy drinking.
3. **Fluids and Nutrition:**
   - Rehydration and restoration of nutritional balance are important, as dehydration and malnutrition are common in individuals with chronic alcohol use.
4. **Monitoring and Support:**
   - Regular monitoring of vital signs and symptoms to adjust treatment as needed.
   - Psychological and emotional support is also important.
5. **Long-term Treatment for Alcohol Dependence:**
   - Detoxification is only the first step in treating alcohol dependence. Long-term treatment typically includes counseling, support groups (like Alcoholics Anonymous), and sometimes medications to help maintain sobriety.
   - Therapy can include cognitive-behavioral therapy, motivational enhancement therapy, and family therapy.
6. **Treatment of Co-occurring Disorders:**
   - If there are co-occurring mental health disorders, these should also be treated, as they can play a role in alcohol use and relapse.

The approach to treating alcohol withdrawal is to ensure safety, manage symptoms, prevent complications, and then provide a pathway to long-term recovery from alcohol dependence. It is crucial to seek professional medical advice for alcohol withdrawal treatment, as the process can be complex and, in some cases, life-threatening.

How long will the effects last for alcohol withdrawal?

The duration of alcohol withdrawal symptoms can vary significantly from person to person, depending on various factors like the severity of alcohol dependence, the individual's overall health, and their history of alcohol use and withdrawal. Generally, the timeline can be described as follows:

1. **Early Withdrawal:**
   - Symptoms can begin as early as 6 hours after the last drink.
   - Early symptoms often include anxiety, shaking, nausea, insomnia, and gastrointestinal disturbances.
2. **Peak Intensity:**
   - Symptoms typically reach their peak intensity between 24 to 72 hours after the last drink.
   - This is often when symptoms are most uncomfortable and potentially dangerous. Severe symptoms like seizures or hallucinations (especially tactile or visual hallucinations) can occur during this time.
3. **Delirium Tremens (DTs):**
   - Delirium tremens is a severe form of alcohol withdrawal that typically develops 2 to 3 days after the last drink but can occur up to 7-10 days later.
   - DTs can include confusion, rapid heartbeat, fever, and seizures. It is considered a medical emergency.
4. **Late Withdrawal:**
   - Some symptoms, particularly psychological ones like mood swings, sleep disturbances, and cravings, can persist for weeks or even months. This is sometimes referred to as protracted or prolonged withdrawal.
   - The severity of these prolonged symptoms usually diminishes over time.
5. **Factors Influencing Duration:**
   - The length of time one has been drinking, the amount of alcohol typically consumed, previous withdrawal experiences, overall health, and the presence of co-occurring mental health or medical conditions all influence the duration and severity of withdrawal symptoms.

It is important to note that while the acute phase of withdrawal is temporary, recovering from alcohol dependence is a longer process that often requires ongoing treatment and support. If you or someone you know is going through alcohol withdrawal, it is crucial to seek medical assistance, as withdrawal can be dangerous and professional guidance can significantly aid in managing the process safely and effectively.

How can I take care of alcohol withdrawal myself?

Taking care of yourself during alcohol withdrawal is crucial, as it can be a challenging process both physically and emotionally. If you are going through alcohol withdrawal, here are some steps you can take to ensure a safer and more comfortable experience:

1. **Seek Medical Advice:**
   - Consult a healthcare provider before attempting to quit, especially if you have been drinking heavily or have a history of severe withdrawal symptoms. They can assess your situation and recommend the safest approach to withdrawal.
2. **Stay Hydrated:**
   - Drink plenty of fluids to stay hydrated. Withdrawal often leads to sweating and vomiting, which can cause dehydration.
3. **Eat a Balanced Diet:**
   - Your body needs nutrients to recover. Try to eat balanced meals, even if you don't feel like eating. Nutritional supplements may be necessary.
4. **Rest and Relax:**
   - Get plenty of sleep and rest. Your body is going through a stressful process, and rest is essential for recovery.
5. **Avoid Triggers:**
   - Stay away from environments or situations where you might be tempted to drink. This includes avoiding contact with people who encourage drinking.
6. **Seek Support:**
   - Reach out to supportive friends and family. Consider joining a support group like Alcoholics Anonymous (AA) where you can find encouragement from others who have gone through similar experiences.
7. **Manage Stress:**
   - Practice stress management techniques like deep breathing exercises, meditation, yoga, or light physical activity, as per your doctor's advice.

8. **Monitor Your Symptoms:**
   - Keep track of your withdrawal symptoms. If they worsen or you experience severe symptoms like seizures, hallucinations, or extreme confusion, seek medical attention immediately.
9. **Plan for Long-term Recovery:**
   - Think about your long-term treatment plan for alcohol use disorder. This might include therapy, counseling, medication, and ongoing support groups.
10. **Avoid Substituting Addictions:**
    - Be cautious not to replace alcohol with other addictive substances or unhealthy habits.

Remember, alcohol withdrawal can be dangerous, and the safest approach is under medical supervision, particularly if you expect to experience moderate to severe withdrawal symptoms. The process of recovery from alcohol dependence is ongoing and often requires long-term strategies and support.

While you are being treated for alcohol withdrawal:

Being treated for alcohol withdrawal, especially in a medically supervised setting, involves specific considerations and steps to ensure safety and effectiveness. Here is what typically happens and what you should be aware of during the treatment process:

1. **Medical Supervision:**
   - You'll be closely monitored by healthcare professionals. They will track your vital signs, withdrawal symptoms, and overall health to adjust treatment as needed.
2. **Medication Management:**
   - Medications may be prescribed to manage withdrawal symptoms. Commonly used medications include benzodiazepines to reduce anxiety and risk of seizures, and others for specific symptoms like nausea or headaches.
   - Follow the prescribed medication regimen strictly and communicate any side effects to your healthcare provider.
3. **Hydration and Nutrition:**
   - You might receive fluids and nutrients through an IV if you are dehydrated or unable to eat.
   - If you are able to eat, focus on a balanced diet to help replenish nutrients.
4. **Rest and Sleep:**
   - Adequate rest is crucial. Withdrawal can disrupt your sleep patterns, so you might be given a quiet environment and possibly medication to help you sleep.
5. **Emotional Support:**
   - Withdrawal can be emotionally taxing. You might have access to counseling or therapy during this time.
   - Support groups or meetings might be part of the treatment program.
6. **Monitoring for Complications:**
   - The medical team will be vigilant for any signs of severe withdrawal symptoms like delirium tremens (DTs), seizures, or hallucinations.
7. **Education and Planning:**
   - You might receive education about alcohol dependence and withdrawal.
   - The treatment team will also start discussing long-term recovery plans, including therapy, support groups, and strategies to prevent relapse.
8. **Environment:**
   - The treatment environment is typically calm and safe, designed to reduce stress and triggers.
9. **Involvement of Family and Friends:**
   - Depending on the situation, family members or close friends might be involved in the process, offering support and learning how they can help in your recovery journey.
10. **Preparation for Discharge and Aftercare:**
    - As you progress through withdrawal, the focus will gradually shift to aftercare planning. This includes arranging for ongoing treatment, whether it is outpatient therapy, support groups, or other forms of care.

It is important to follow the guidance of the healthcare professionals during this process and to be open about how you are feeling, both physically and emotionally. The goal of the treatment is not only to safely manage the immediate withdrawal symptoms but also to set a foundation for long-term recovery from alcohol dependence.

What can be done to help prevent alcohol withdrawal?

Preventing alcohol withdrawal primarily involves managing and moderating alcohol consumption or abstaining from alcohol altogether. This can be challenging, especially for individuals who have developed a dependence on alcohol. Here are some strategies and considerations for preventing alcohol withdrawal:

1. **Moderate Drinking:**
   - Follow guidelines for moderate drinking (which vary by country and organization). Typically, this means up to one drink per day for women and up to two drinks per day for men.
2. **Abstinence:**
   - If you have a history of alcohol dependence or difficulty controlling your drinking, abstaining from alcohol is the safest approach.
3. **Seek Professional Help:**
   - If you are struggling to control your drinking, consult a healthcare provider or a mental health professional specializing in substance abuse. They can provide guidance and treatment options.
4. **Gradual Reduction:**
   - For those who drink heavily, it is often safer to reduce alcohol consumption gradually under medical supervision rather than stopping abruptly. This can help minimize withdrawal symptoms.
5. **Treatment Programs:**
   - Consider enrolling in a treatment program for alcohol dependence. These programs can offer medical, psychological, and peer support.
6. **Support Groups:**
   - Joining a support group like Alcoholics Anonymous (AA) can provide encouragement and understanding from others who have faced similar challenges.
7. **Lifestyle Changes:**
   - Engage in healthy activities that promote overall wellbeing and help reduce stress, such as exercise, hobbies, or socializing in non-alcohol-centered environments.
8. **Therapy and Counseling:**
   - Counseling or therapy, especially cognitive-behavioral therapy, can be effective in addressing the underlying issues related to alcohol use and developing coping strategies.
9. **Medication:**
   - In some cases, medications can be prescribed to help reduce the desire to drink or manage underlying conditions that contribute to alcohol use.
10. **Awareness of Risk Factors:**
    - Be aware of personal risk factors, such as a family history of alcoholism or co-occurring mental health disorders, and take proactive steps to address them.
11. **Educate Yourself:**
    - Understanding the risks associated with heavy drinking and the benefits of reducing alcohol intake can be motivating.
12. **Support from Family and Friends:**
    - Encourage support from loved ones, as their understanding and encouragement can be crucial.

Prevention of alcohol withdrawal is about managing alcohol consumption in a healthy and responsible way. If dependence has already developed, it is important to seek professional help to manage the condition safely and effectively.

What is amnesia?

Amnesia refers to a loss of memories, such as facts, information, and experiences. Unlike a temporary lapse in memory, amnesia can be a symptom of a more serious condition, typically involving parts of the brain that control memory processing. There are several types of amnesia, each with distinct causes and characteristics:

1. **Anterograde Amnesia:**
   - This is the inability to form new memories following the onset of an amnesia-causing event. People with anterograde amnesia can recall their past but have difficulty creating new memories.
2. **Retrograde Amnesia:**
   - This involves the loss of memories that were formed before the onset of amnesia. The person may forget events that occurred,

personal information, and even their own identity, but they can typically form new memories.

3. **Transient Global Amnesia:**
   - A temporary, sudden loss of memory that is not caused by a neurological condition like epilepsy or stroke. It is rare and tends to resolve within hours.
4. **Dissociative Amnesia:**
   - This is often linked to trauma or stress and involves forgetting specific information, usually about a traumatic or stressful event. Dissociative amnesia can be selective or generalized.
5. **Infantile/Childhood Amnesia:**
   - This is the normal inability of adults to remember the first few years of their childhood.
6. **Drug-Induced Amnesia:**
   - Certain medications and substances can impair memory formation.

Causes of Amnesia: Amnesia can result from several causes, including:

- Brain Injury: Such as from a blow to the head.
- Stroke
- Alcohol Abuse: Particularly chronic alcoholism, which can lead to Wernicke-Korsakoff syndrome.
- Certain Diseases or Infections: Like Alzheimer's disease, other dementias, HIV/AIDS, tuberculosis, and syphilis that affect the brain.
- Seizures
- Psychological Trauma: Especially in dissociative amnesia.
- Lack of Oxygen to the Brain: Such as from a heart attack, respiratory distress, or carbon monoxide poisoning.

Treatment: Treatment for amnesia focuses on the underlying cause. In some cases, especially when the amnesia is caused by psychological trauma, psychotherapy can be beneficial. Occupational or cognitive therapy helps some people to learn new ways of remembering information. For amnesia caused by physical damage to the brain, treatment usually involves supportive strategies to enhance the person's remaining memory and cognitive function.

What happens in the brain in amnesia?

In amnesia, various disruptions occur in the brain's processes that are responsible for creating, storing, and retrieving memories. The specific nature of these disruptions depends on the type of amnesia and its cause. Here is an overview of what happens in the brain in cases of amnesia:

1. **Damage to Memory-Related Brain Regions:**
   - The hippocampus, located in the temporal lobe, is crucial for forming new memories. Damage to the hippocampus often results in anterograde amnesia, where a person cannot form new memories.
   - The amygdala, also in the temporal lobe, is involved in processing emotions, which affects the strength and retention of memories, especially emotionally charged ones.
   - The prefrontal cortex is involved in retrieving and organizing memories, and damage here can lead to problems with memory retrieval.
2. **Neurotransmitter Disruption:**
   - Certain neurotransmitters, like acetylcholine, are essential for memory and learning. Disruption in their levels or functioning can impact memory formation and retrieval.
   - Alcohol and some drugs can interfere with neurotransmitter function, leading to memory impairments.
3. **Neural Pathway Interruptions:**
   - Memory involves complex networks of neurons across different brain regions. Damage or interruption in these pathways can impair the storage and retrieval of memories.
4. **Wernicke-Korsakoff Syndrome:**
   - This condition, often associated with chronic alcoholism, results from a deficiency in thiamine (vitamin B1) and leads to severe anterograde and retrograde amnesia. It damages the mammillary bodies and other regions related to memory.
5. **Psychological Factors:**
   - In dissociative amnesia, extreme stress or trauma can cause the brain to block out memories related to the event, a mechanism thought to be a psychological defense against emotional pain.
6. **Global Cerebral Ischemia:**
   - Lack of oxygen to the brain, as seen in cardiac arrest or respiratory failure, can lead

to widespread brain damage, including areas critical for memory.

7. **Neurodegenerative Diseases:**
   - Conditions like Alzheimer's disease lead to the degeneration and death of neurons, including those in memory-related areas.
8. **Seizures:**
   - Seizures, particularly those originating in the temporal lobe, can disrupt memory formation and retrieval.

In summary, amnesia typically involves damage to or dysfunction of the parts of the brain responsible for memory processing. This can be due to physical damage, nutritional deficiencies, neurotransmitter disruptions, neurodegenerative diseases, or psychological factors. The specific nature and location of the brain damage or dysfunction determine the type of amnesia and the pattern of memory loss.

What is the working classification of amnesia?

The working classification of amnesia typically divides the condition into various types based on the nature of memory loss, its causes, and its characteristics. Here is an overview of the common classifications:

1. **By Duration:**
   - **Transient:** Short-term memory loss, as seen in transient global amnesia.
   - **Chronic:** Long-term memory loss, often due to brain injury or neurodegenerative disease.
2. **By Affected Memory Type:**
   - **Anterograde Amnesia:** Difficulty forming new memories after the onset of amnesia.
   - **Retrograde Amnesia:** Difficulty recalling memories formed before the onset of amnesia.
3. **By Etiology (Cause):**
   - **Traumatic Amnesia:** Caused by head injury.
   - **Wernicke-Korsakoff Syndrome:** Due to chronic alcohol abuse and thiamine deficiency.
   - **Global Cerebral Ischemia:** Resulting from reduced blood flow or oxygen to the brain.
   - **Post-Operative Amnesia:** Following surgery, particularly brain surgery.
   - **Dissociative Amnesia:** Psychological, often stemming from trauma or stress.
   - **Neurodegenerative Amnesia:** As part of conditions like Alzheimer's disease.
   - **Drug-Induced Amnesia:** Due to the effects of certain medications or substances.
4. **By Severity:**
   - **Mild:** Short-term, less severe impairment.
   - **Severe:** Profound memory loss affecting daily functioning.
5. **By Source of Memory:**
   - **Declarative Memory Loss:** Difficulty recalling facts and information.
   - **Non-Declarative Memory Loss:** Affecting skills and tasks one can perform without conscious recall.
6. **Special Categories:**
   - **Infantile/Childhood Amnesia:** Inability to remember early childhood.
   - **Source Amnesia:** Remembering information but not the source.
   - **Lacunar Amnesia:** Losing memory for a specific, isolated event.

Each type of amnesia can have different implications for treatment and prognosis. Diagnosing the specific type of amnesia is crucial for healthcare professionals to manage the condition effectively. This classification helps in understanding the underlying causes and directing appropriate therapeutic interventions.

What are the causes of amnesia?

Amnesia can be caused by a variety of factors, which affect the brain's ability to store, retain, and recall memories. The main causes include:

1. **Brain Injury:**
   - Traumatic brain injury (TBI) resulting from accidents, falls, sports injuries, or violence can lead to amnesia. The severity of memory loss often correlates with the severity of the injury.
2. **Stroke:**
   - A stroke can interrupt blood supply to parts of the brain, damaging areas crucial for memory processing and storage.
3. **Alcohol Abuse:**
   - Chronic alcoholism can lead to Wernicke-Korsakoff syndrome, a condition caused by

thiamine (vitamin B1) deficiency, leading to severe memory impairment.

4. **Seizures:**
   - Certain types of seizures, particularly those originating in the temporal lobe, can cause memory loss.
5. **Encephalitis:**
   - Inflammation of the brain, often due to infection (such as herpes simplex virus) or autoimmune diseases, can affect memory areas.
6. **Surgery:**
   - Brain surgery, especially in areas that control memory, can result in amnesia.
7. **Neurodegenerative Diseases:**
   - Diseases like Alzheimer's and other forms of dementia can progressively impair memory and other cognitive functions.
8. **Medications:**
   - Certain medications, particularly sedatives and some treatments for anxiety or insomnia, can impact memory formation.
9. **Lack of Oxygen (Hypoxia):**
   - Oxygen deprivation to the brain, due to events like a heart attack, respiratory distress, or carbon monoxide poisoning, can cause memory loss.
10. **Psychological Trauma:**
    - Dissociative amnesia can occur after severe stress or trauma. It is a psychological response that helps a person cope by making them unable to remember the traumatic event.
11. **Electroconvulsive Therapy (ECT):**
    - ECT, used for severe depression, can lead to short-term retrograde amnesia as a side effect.

Understanding the cause of amnesia is essential for effective treatment. In some cases, treating the underlying cause can lead to partial or full recovery of lost memories. In other cases, especially where there is permanent damage to the brain, the focus may be on managing the condition and developing compensatory strategies to deal with the memory loss.

How do you diagnose amnesia?

Diagnosing amnesia involves a combination of medical history evaluation, physical and neurological examinations, cognitive tests, and imaging studies. Here is a typical diagnostic process:

1. **Medical and Personal History:**
   - A detailed interview to gather information about the individual's medical history, recent and past events, alcohol and drug use, and family history of neurological or psychiatric conditions.
   - Understanding the circumstances in which memory loss was first noticed is crucial.
2. **Physical Examination:**
   - General physical examination to check overall health.
   - Neurological examination to assess reflexes, sensory function, balance, and other aspects of brain and nervous system health.
3. **Cognitive Tests:**
   - Neuropsychological tests to evaluate memory, problem-solving skills, attention span, counting skills, and other cognitive abilities.
   - Specific tests to differentiate between types of amnesia and to assess the severity of memory impairment.
4. **Laboratory Tests:**
   - Blood tests to check for nutritional deficiencies, thyroid function, liver function, kidney function, and signs of infections that might affect memory.
   - Toxicology screening for drugs and alcohol.
5. **Brain Imaging Studies:**
   - Magnetic Resonance Imaging (MRI) or Computed Tomography (CT) scans to detect brain damage, abnormalities, or changes in brain structure.
   - Functional imaging techniques like fMRI or PET scans may be used in some cases to assess brain activity patterns.
6. **Psychiatric Evaluation:**
   - To determine if depression, stress, or another psychological condition is contributing to or causing the memory problems.

7. **Review of Medications:**
   - Evaluating whether any current medications could be contributing to memory loss.
8. **Observation:**
   - In some cases, hospitalization for observation and detailed evaluation might be necessary, especially if symptoms suggest a rapid-onset condition like transient global amnesia or if there are safety concerns.

The diagnosis of amnesia aims to identify not just the symptoms but also the underlying causes, which can guide the appropriate treatment and management strategy. It is important for this process to be thorough to ensure accurate diagnosis and to differentiate amnesia from other conditions like dementia or temporary memory lapses.

How do you manage amnesia?

Managing amnesia involves a combination of treatments and strategies tailored to the individual's specific type and cause of memory loss, as well as their overall health and lifestyle. Here are some common approaches to managing amnesia:

1. **Treating Underlying Causes:**
   - If the amnesia is due to an underlying medical condition (like a brain injury, stroke, alcohol abuse, or infection), addressing that condition is the first step. This might involve medications, surgery, or other medical interventions.
2. **Cognitive Rehabilitation:**
   - Memory training and cognitive therapy can help some individuals. This may involve exercises to improve memory, strategies to compensate for the memory problem, and techniques to manage tasks.
3. **Occupational Therapy:**
   - Occupational therapists can assist individuals in learning new ways to carry out daily activities. They can provide tools and strategies to cope with memory loss and maintain independence.
4. **Psychological Support:**
   - Counseling or therapy can be beneficial, especially if the amnesia is related to psychological trauma (as in dissociative amnesia).
   - Support for depression, anxiety, or other mental health issues that may accompany amnesia.
5. **Medications:**
   - While there are no specific drugs to cure amnesia, medications may be prescribed to address underlying causes or associated symptoms (like depression or sleep disturbances).
6. **Lifestyle Modifications:**
   - Establishing a routine and maintaining a structured environment can help.
   - Using memory aids like notebooks, electronic devices, calendars, and timers.
   - Keeping a consistent schedule and organizing home and work environments to make them more predictable and easier to navigate.
7. **Family and Caregiver Support:**
   - Educating family members and caregivers about amnesia and ways to support the affected individual.
   - Encouraging social interaction and activities that can engage the person in a safe, comfortable environment.
8. **Safety Measures:**
   - Implementing strategies to ensure the person's safety, especially if they are prone to forgetting important tasks like turning off appliances or taking medication.
9. **Nutrition and Physical Exercise:**
   - A healthy diet and regular physical exercise can improve overall brain health and cognitive function.
10. **Monitoring and Follow-Up:**
    - Regular follow-up with healthcare providers to monitor progress and adjust treatment strategies as needed.

The management of amnesia is often multidisciplinary, involving neurologists, psychiatrists, psychologists, occupational therapists, and other healthcare professionals. The goal is to maximize the individual's functioning and quality of life while addressing any underlying issues contributing to memory loss.

What is Transient Global Amnesia (TGA)?

Transient Global Amnesia (TGA) is a temporary, sudden loss of memory that is uncharacteristic of the individual's normal behavior. It is a distinct form of amnesia due to its acute onset and relatively short duration. Key characteristics and facts about TGA include:

1. **Sudden Memory Loss:**
   - TGA is marked by an abrupt onset of anterograde amnesia, meaning the person cannot form new memories. There is often some degree of retrograde amnesia as well, meaning difficulty recalling past events.
2. **Duration:**
   - The amnesic episode typically lasts from a few hours up to 24 hours. After this period, memory gradually returns to normal, and the person regains full memory function, although they may never remember what happened during the episode.
3. **Symptoms:**
   - During an episode, the person will seem confused and repeatedly ask questions about recent events because they cannot remember the answers. Despite this memory impairment, they maintain their identity awareness and usually do not have trouble recognizing people or places.
   - Other cognitive skills, such as attention, language, and recognition, remain intact.
4. **Causes:**
   - The exact cause of TGA is unknown. Potential triggers include physical or emotional stress, strenuous activity, exposure to cold water, sexual intercourse, or minor head trauma.
   - It is not associated with any long-term neurological damage, nor is it typically considered a sign of a more serious condition like a stroke or epilepsy.
5. **Risk Factors:**
   - TGA most frequently occurs in middle-aged or older adults, usually over the age of 50.
   - There might be a vascular component or a link to migraine in some cases.
6. **Diagnosis:**
   - TGA is diagnosed based on its clinical features. Doctors rule out other causes of temporary memory loss, such as epilepsy or stroke, through a neurological examination and sometimes brain imaging or other tests.
7. **Treatment:**
   - There is no specific treatment for TGA. The focus is on patient safety and comfort during the episode.
   - Once the episode resolves, further treatment typically is not necessary, though follow-up may be recommended to rule out underlying conditions.
8. **Recurrence:**
   - While TGA can recur, most cases are one-time events.

Transient Global Amnesia is a unique and still somewhat mysterious neurological phenomenon. It is generally benign, with individuals returning to their normal state without lasting effects. However, the experience can be distressing both for the person experiencing it and for their loved ones.

What are the causes of TGA?

Transient Global Amnesia (TGA) is a mysterious and poorly understood condition, and its exact cause remains unknown. However, several theories and potential triggers have been identified based on observations and studies. It is important to note that these are not definitive causes but rather factors that may precipitate an episode of TGA:

1. **Vascular Factors:**
   - Some researchers believe that TGA might be related to temporary disruptions in blood flow to certain parts of the brain, particularly areas involved in memory and learning. However, clear evidence of ischemic events (like those in a stroke) is typically lacking in TGA cases.
2. **Migraine:**
   - There is a noted association between migraine and TGA. Some individuals who experience TGA have a history of migraines, suggesting a possible link.
3. **Physical Triggers:**
   - Episodes of TGA can sometimes be triggered by physical exertion, sexual intercourse, cold water immersion (like swimming in cold water), or minor head trauma.
4. **Emotional Stress:**
   - Psychological stress or emotional events are known triggers for TGA. This includes situations like family conflicts, emotional distress, or bereavement.

5. **Neurological Factors:**
    - There might be a temporary disruption in the hippocampus, a part of the brain crucial for forming new memories. This disruption could be due to various factors, including metabolic, epileptic, or migrainous phenomena.
6. **Venous Flow Abnormalities:**
    - Some studies have suggested that abnormalities in the venous blood flow from the brain might play a role in TGA, particularly in the context of Valsalva-like activities (activities that increase pressure in the chest and abdomen, like coughing, straining, or lifting heavy weights).
7. **Epileptic Phenomena:**
    - While not a common cause, there is some evidence to suggest that TGA might have an epileptic component in rare cases.

Despite these potential triggers, many cases of TGA occur spontaneously without an identifiable cause. The condition is still a subject of ongoing research. Importantly, TGA episodes are generally benign, with the affected individuals typically recovering fully without any lasting effects on their memory or other cognitive functions. However, due to the similarities in presentation with more serious conditions like stroke or epilepsy, medical evaluation is important to rule out other causes.

What are the Symptoms and Signs of TGA?

Transient Global Amnesia (TGA) is characterized by a sudden, temporary episode of memory loss that cannot be attributed to a more common neurological condition, like epilepsy or stroke. The primary symptoms and signs of TGA include:

1. **Sudden Memory Loss:**
    - The most striking feature is a sudden and severe impairment in forming new memories (anterograde amnesia). Individuals cannot remember recent events and cannot retain new information for more than a few minutes.
2. **Preserved Personal Identity:**
    - Despite memory loss, individuals maintain their self-awareness. They know who they are and can usually recognize family and friends.
3. **Repetitive Questioning:**
    - Due to the inability to form new memories, people with TGA often ask the same questions repeatedly because they immediately forget the answers.
4. **Lack of Other Neurological Symptoms:**
    - Unlike conditions like stroke, TGA does not typically involve other neurological deficits, such as weakness, numbness, visual disturbances, or impaired speech.
5. **Temporal Orientation:**
    - People experiencing TGA are often aware of the time and place, although they might be slightly confused due to their memory impairment.
6. **Retrograde Amnesia:**
    - Some individuals may also experience a loss of more remote memories (retrograde amnesia), forgetting events that occurred hours, days, or even years prior to the episode.
7. **Duration:**
    - TGA episodes are short-lived, typically lasting no more than 24 hours. The average duration is about 4 to 6 hours.
8. **Behavior:**
    - Individuals usually appear normal to others during an episode, aside from being somewhat puzzled or perplexed due to their memory loss.
9. **Gradual Recovery:**
    - Memory gradually returns to normal following an episode, but there is often permanent amnesia for the period of the TGA episode.
10. **No Lasting Effects:**
    - After an episode, there are generally no lasting cognitive or neurological impairments.
11. **Possible Triggers:**
    - In some cases, TGA may be preceded by a triggering event such as physical exertion, emotional stress, pain, sexual intercourse, or immersion in cold or hot water.

It is important for individuals experiencing these symptoms to receive immediate medical attention to rule out more serious conditions. While TGA is generally benign, its symptoms can resemble those of stroke, epilepsy, or other neurological disorders that require urgent treatment.

What is Asperger syndrome and its management?

Asperger syndrome is a developmental disorder that is part of the autism spectrum. It is characterized by difficulties in social interaction and nonverbal communication, along with restricted and repetitive patterns of behavior and interests. It is important to note that Asperger syndrome is no longer an official diagnosis in many countries. In 2013, it was integrated into the broader category of Autism Spectrum Disorder (ASD) in the Diagnostic and Statistical Manual of Mental Disorders 5th edition (DSM-5). However, the term is still used in some contexts.

Characteristics of Asperger Syndrome:

1. **Social Challenges:** Difficulty with social interactions, including understanding and responding to social cues and maintaining conversations.
2. **Communication Difficulties:** Problems with nonverbal communication such as facial expressions, body language, and understanding tone of voice.
3. **Restricted Interests:** Intense focus on specific topics or hobbies, often to the exclusion of other activities.
4. **Desire for Routine:** Preference for predictable, structured environments and difficulty with change.
5. **Motor Coordination:** Challenges with motor coordination and physical clumsiness are common.
6. **Normal to High Intelligence:** People with Asperger's often have average to above-average intelligence.

Management of Asperger Syndrome: While there is no cure for Asperger syndrome, various interventions and strategies can help manage symptoms and improve functioning:

1. **Behavioral Therapy:** Helps in building social skills, managing emotions, and reducing obsessive interests and repetitive routines.
2. **Cognitive Behavioral Therapy (CBT):** Can assist in addressing anxiety, depression, and other mental health issues that often accompany Asperger syndrome.
3. **Social Skills Training:** Focuses on improving interpersonal skills and understanding social cues.
4. **Occupational Therapy:** Helps in developing coordination and motor skills, and in learning how to process sensory information.
5. **Speech-Language Therapy:** Assists in improving communication skills, both verbal and nonverbal.
6. **Educational Support:** Tailored learning programs to meet individual educational needs.
7. **Parent Education and Training:** Teaches families about Asperger syndrome and coping strategies.
8. **Medications:** While there are no medications specifically for Asperger syndrome, some medications can help with symptoms such as anxiety, depression, or hyperactivity.

Support and Acceptance: Creating a supportive and understanding environment is crucial. Acceptance and encouragement from family, friends, teachers, and employers can significantly impact the well-being and success of an individual with Asperger syndrome.

Lifelong Condition: Asperger syndrome is a lifelong condition, and management focuses on acquiring skills necessary for daily living and building a fulfilling life. Many individuals with Asperger's lead successful, independent lives, often excelling in areas related to their interests.

What is the cause of Asperger syndrome?

The exact cause of Asperger syndrome, like other Autism Spectrum Disorders (ASD), is not fully understood, but it is believed to result from a complex interplay of genetic and environmental factors. Research in this area points to several key factors:

1. **Genetic Factors:**
   - A strong genetic basis is suggested, as Asperger syndrome tends to run in families. Specific genes associated with the syndrome have not been definitively identified, but multiple genes are thought to be involved.
   - Genetic studies have shown that various genetic changes or mutations can increase the risk of developing Asperger syndrome. These may not cause the condition directly but could increase susceptibility.
2. **Brain Structure and Function:**
   - Differences in certain areas of the brain's structure and function have been observed in people with Asperger syndrome. These differences

may affect the development and functioning of brain circuits that control thought and behavior.

- Neuroimaging studies have shown variations in brain development, particularly in regions responsible for social cognition and communication.

3. **Prenatal Factors:**
   - Some evidence suggests that prenatal environmental factors, such as exposure to certain drugs, chemicals, or illnesses during pregnancy, might increase the risk of a child developing Asperger syndrome. However, these findings are not conclusive and require further research.
4. **Birth Complications:**
   - There is some association between Asperger syndrome and complications during birth, particularly those involving oxygen deprivation to the baby's brain. However, this link is not clearly understood and is the subject of ongoing study.
5. **Older Parental Age:**
   - Some studies have suggested that children born to older parents may have a higher risk of developing ASD, including Asperger syndrome, although this association is not fully understood.
6. **Environmental Triggers:**
   - While much focus has been on genetic factors, environmental influences may also play a role, though specific environmental triggers have not been conclusively identified.

It is important to note that Asperger syndrome is not caused by a person's upbringing, social circumstances, or environmental factors like vaccines, which have been conclusively debunked as a cause of autism spectrum disorders.

The understanding of the causes of Asperger syndrome is still evolving. It is likely that a combination of multiple factors leads to the development of the condition, and these factors may vary from person to person.

What are the symptoms Asperger syndrome?

Asperger syndrome, a condition on the autism spectrum, is characterized by challenges in social interaction, nonverbal communication, and repetitive behaviors. It is important to remember that the presentation can vary significantly from person to person. Common symptoms include:

1. **Social Interaction Difficulties:**
   - Challenges in understanding and responding to social cues.
   - Difficulty in developing and maintaining friendships.
   - Preference for solitary activities.
   - Difficulty interpreting body language, facial expressions, and tone of voice.
2. **Restricted and Repetitive Behaviors:**
   - Strong preference for routines and schedules; distress at changes in routine.
   - Repetitive behaviors or rituals.
   - Specific and intense interests in particular subjects or activities.
   - Unusual preoccupations or rituals.
3. **Communication Challenges:**
   - Difficulty with two-way conversation; might talk at length about a favorite subject without noticing lack of interest in others.
   - Literal interpretation of language; difficulty understanding sarcasm, humor, or abstract concepts.
   - Monotone or flat speech patterns, or alternatively, a very formal way of speaking.
4. **Coordination and Physical Skills:**
   - Clumsiness, awkward movements, or atypical body language.
   - Uncoordinated motor movements.
5. **Sensory Sensitivity:**
   - Over-sensitivity or under-sensitivity to sounds, lights, textures, or other sensory stimuli.
6. **Emotional Difficulties:**
   - Difficulty in recognizing or expressing emotions.
   - Inappropriate or out-of-context emotional responses.
7. **Cognitive Abilities:**
   - Often average to above-average intelligence.
   - May excel in areas requiring detail and precision, such as mathematics, science, or art.

8. **Unique Strengths and Abilities:**
   - Intense focus and concentration on areas of interest.
   - Exceptional memory in specific areas.
   - Strong adherence to rules and honesty.
9. **Challenges with Change:**
   - Struggling with transitions or changes in routine.

These symptoms typically become apparent in early childhood, but the degree to which they affect daily functioning can vary widely. Some individuals with Asperger syndrome might require minimal support, while others might need significant assistance in daily life. It is also common for people with Asperger syndrome to have co-occurring conditions such as anxiety disorders, depression, or attention-deficit/hyperactivity disorder (ADHD).

Diagnosis and understanding of Asperger syndrome have evolved, and it is now generally considered part of the broader category of Autism Spectrum Disorder (ASD). Each person with Asperger's has a unique experience, and the presentation of symptoms can change over time, especially with support and intervention.

How is Asperger syndrome diagnosed?

Diagnosing Asperger syndrome, now typically classified under the broader category of Autism Spectrum Disorder (ASD) in many diagnostic manuals, involves a multidisciplinary assessment approach. There is no single medical test to diagnose Asperger's. Instead, the process usually includes the following steps:

1. **Developmental Screening:**
   - This is often the first step, particularly in children. A healthcare provider may use a questionnaire or checklist to gather information about a child's development and behavior.
2. **Comprehensive Diagnostic Evaluation:**
   - This more in-depth evaluation can include a variety of components:
     - **Observation:** Behavioral observation, often in different settings (e.g., at home and in a clinical environment).
     - **Interviews:** Discussions with parents or caregivers about the child's development, behavior, social interactions, and communication skills.
     - **Medical History:** Review of the individual's developmental milestones, family medical history, and any potential prenatal or birth complications.
     - **Neuropsychological and/or Psychiatric:** Assessment: Cognitive and language testing to evaluate the individual's IQ, problem-solving skills, attention span, and language abilities.
     - **Physical Examination:** To rule out other medical conditions that might mimic or contribute to the symptoms.
3. **Multidisciplinary Team:**
   - A team of specialists may be involved in the diagnosis, including pediatricians, neurologists, psychiatrists, psychologists, speech and language therapists, and occupational therapists.
4. **Diagnostic Criteria:**
   - The diagnostic criteria for ASD, as outlined in diagnostic manuals like the DSM-5 (Diagnostic and Statistical Manual of Mental Disorders, Fifth Edition), are used. Criteria include persistent deficits in social communication and social interaction across multiple contexts, as well as restricted, repetitive patterns of behavior, interests, or activities.
5. **Parent and Teacher Reports:**
   - Reports from parents, teachers, and other adults who interact with the child are crucial. They provide insight into the child's social interactions, communication skills, and behavior in different settings.
6. **Ruling Out Other Conditions:**
   - It is important to distinguish Asperger syndrome from other conditions like social communication disorder, ADHD, anxiety disorders, or other developmental disorders.
7. **Observation Over Time:**
   - In some cases, professionals might monitor the child over a period to see how their symptoms develop or change.

The process of diagnosing Asperger syndrome can be complex and requires a thorough evaluation by professionals experienced in developmental disorders. It is also an evolving process, as an individual's abilities and challenges can change over time. Early diagnosis and intervention can significantly improve outcomes, helping individuals with Asperger's to develop social, communication, and self-care skills.

How is Asperger syndrome treated?

Asperger syndrome, now typically diagnosed as part of the broader category of Autism Spectrum Disorder (ASD), does not have a cure, but various interventions and therapies can help manage symptoms and develop essential skills. Treatment is tailored to the individual's needs and often involves a combination of the following approaches:

1. **Behavioral Therapies:**
   - **Applied Behavior Analysis (ABA)** is commonly used to encourage positive behaviors and reduce negative behaviors.
   - **Cognitive Behavioral Therapy (CBT)** can help manage co-occurring conditions like anxiety and depression and can teach coping strategies for social situations.
2. **Educational Interventions:**
   - Special education services and educational interventions can be tailored to a child's specific strengths and weaknesses. These often include social skills training and structured learning environments.
3. **Social Skills Training:**
   - This focuses on developing the ability to interact more effectively with others and can include group therapy sessions or social skills groups.
4. **Speech-Language Therapy:**
   - This can help improve communication skills, including understanding and using language in social contexts.
5. **Occupational Therapy:**
   - Helps in developing everyday skills like dressing, eating, and working. It can also address sensory integration issues.
6. **Medication:**
   - While there are no medications specifically for Asperger syndrome, medications may be prescribed to address specific symptoms or co-occurring conditions, such as ADHD, anxiety, or depression.
7. **Parent Training and Family Therapy:**
   - Educating families about Asperger syndrome and providing strategies for home-based interventions is crucial. Family therapy can also help family members understand and support their loved one with Asperger's.
8. **Peer Support and Mentoring:**
   - Interacting with peers who have similar challenges can provide valuable social experiences and role models.
9. **Life Skills Coaching:**
   - For adolescents and adults, coaching in life skills, including job coaching or training in independent living skills, can be beneficial.
10. **Regular Exercise and Healthy Diet:**
    - Physical activity and a balanced diet can improve overall well-being and manage symptoms.
11. **Transition Planning:**
    - For adolescents, planning for the transition to adulthood, higher education, and employment is important.

The goal of these interventions is not to "cure" Asperger syndrome but to help the individual manage the challenges associated with it and utilize their unique strengths. Early intervention can be particularly beneficial. As people with Asperger's often have average to above-average intelligence, many are capable of leading fulfilling lives with the appropriate support and accommodations.

How long will the effects of Asperger syndrome last?

Asperger syndrome, which is now typically recognized as part of the Autism Spectrum Disorder (ASD) following the updates in diagnostic criteria, is a lifelong condition. The effects of Asperger syndrome are not temporary and usually persist throughout an individual's life. However, the manifestation of these effects can change over time, especially with intervention and support. Here are some key points to understand about the duration and progression of Asperger syndrome:

1. **Persistent Nature:**
   - The core characteristics of Asperger syndrome, such as difficulties with social communication and repetitive patterns of behavior, are generally consistent and enduring.
2. **Variable Impact:**
   - While the condition is lifelong, the impact it has on daily functioning can vary greatly from person to person and can change over time. Some individuals may learn to manage their symptoms effectively and lead relatively independent lives.

3. **Developmental Changes:**
   - Symptoms and challenges may shift as an individual grows and develops. For example, children might struggle more with behavioral issues, while adults might face more challenges with social interactions and employment.
4. **Effect of Interventions:**
   - Early and consistent interventions can significantly improve skills and coping mechanisms. With therapy and support, individuals with Asperger syndrome can develop effective communication and social skills and manage repetitive behaviors.
5. **Co-occurring Conditions:**
   - Some associated conditions or challenges, such as anxiety or depression, can be managed with appropriate treatment, which can improve overall functioning and quality of life.
6. **Adaptation and Coping:**
   - Many adults with Asperger syndrome learn to adapt to their challenges and may develop coping strategies to deal with social and communication difficulties.
7. **Social and Occupational Opportunities:**
   - Access to supportive education and employment opportunities can greatly influence the long-term outcome for individuals with Asperger syndrome.
8. **Lifelong Support:**
   - Continuous support, whether through therapy, community services, or family support, remains important throughout life.

It is important to recognize that each individual with Asperger syndrome is unique, and their abilities and challenges can be quite diverse. With the right support and accommodations, many people with Asperger syndrome can lead fulfilling and productive lives.

What are behavioral emergencies (BE)?

Behavioral emergencies (BE), also known as psychiatric or mental health emergencies, refer to situations where a person's behavior poses a direct threat to their own safety or the safety of others. This can include a wide range of situations, from severe mental health crises to reactions to stressful events. The key aspect of a behavioral emergency is that it requires immediate attention and intervention to prevent harm.

Behavioral emergencies can be caused by various underlying factors, including mental health disorders, substance abuse, psychological stress, or a combination of these and other factors. Common scenarios include:

1. **Suicidal Ideation or Attempts:**
   - Expressing a desire to harm or kill oneself, making plans for suicide, or attempting suicide.
2. **Homicidal or Violent Behavior:**
   - Threats of violence or harm towards others, or engaging in physically aggressive acts.
3. **Severe Psychosis:**
   - Experiencing a break from reality, which may involve hallucinations, delusions, or severe disorganization in thought and behavior.
4. **Severe Anxiety or Panic Attacks:**
   - Intense, overwhelming anxiety or panic that incapacitates the individual or leads to dangerous behavior.
5. **Extreme Agitation or Aggression:**
   - Highly agitated or aggressive behavior that poses a risk to oneself or others.
6. **Substance-Induced Behaviors:**
   - Behaviors caused by intoxication or withdrawal from drugs or alcohol that threaten the individual's or others' safety.
7. **Severe Mood Disturbances:**
   - Extreme episodes of mania or depression that significantly impair judgment and behavior.
8. **Self-Harming Behavior:**
   - Engaging in self-injury or self-mutilation without the intent of suicide.

The management of behavioral emergencies typically involves ensuring the immediate safety of the individual and others, providing psychiatric assessment, and implementing appropriate interventions. This might include de-escalation techniques, hospitalization, medication, counseling, or other forms of therapy, depending on the nature and severity of the emergency. In many cases, law enforcement or emergency medical services may need to be involved to help manage the situation safely.

It is important for individuals experiencing a behavioral emergency or their loved ones to seek immediate help from mental health professionals, emergency services, or crisis hotlines. Early intervention can be crucial in preventing harm and addressing the underlying causes effectively.

What are the causes of behavioral emergencies?

Behavioral emergencies arise from a complex interplay of various factors. These emergencies are situations where an individual's behavior poses an immediate risk to their own safety or the safety of others. The causes can be multifaceted and may include:

1. **Mental Health Disorders:**
   - Conditions like schizophrenia, bipolar disorder, major depression, or severe anxiety disorders can lead to behavioral emergencies, especially if they are not effectively managed.
2. **Substance Abuse and Intoxication:**
   - The use of drugs or alcohol can significantly impair judgment and self-control, leading to dangerous behaviors. Substance withdrawal can also trigger severe psychological or physical reactions.
3. **Psychological Stress:**
   - Intense stress from life events such as a traumatic experience, loss of a loved one, relationship problems, financial stress, or other significant stressors can overwhelm an individual's coping mechanisms, leading to a crisis.
4. **Neurological Disorders:**
   - Conditions like dementia, brain injuries, or seizures can lead to changes in behavior that may escalate into emergencies.
5. **Medication Side Effects:**
   - Certain medications, particularly psychiatric drugs, can have side effects that include increased agitation, suicidal thoughts, or other behavioral changes.
6. **Environmental Factors:**
   - Situational stressors, such as being in a confined space, extreme temperatures, or chaotic environments, can exacerbate underlying conditions or stress.
7. **History of Trauma or Abuse:**
   - Individuals with a history of physical, sexual, or emotional abuse or trauma are at a higher risk for behavioral crises, especially when faced with triggering events.
8. **Lack of Social Support:**
   - Isolation or lack of a supportive social network can contribute to the escalation of a crisis, especially in individuals with pre-existing mental health conditions.
9. **Poor Coping Skills:**
   - Inadequate coping mechanisms to deal with stress or emotional problems can lead to extreme reactions.
10. **Psychosocial Crises:**
    - Developmental crises, identity crises, and other psychosocial factors can sometimes culminate in acute behavioral emergencies.

It is important to recognize that a behavioral emergency is often the result of multiple interacting factors, and the specific causes can vary greatly from person to person. Identifying and understanding these causes is crucial for effectively managing and preventing future crises. This typically involves a comprehensive approach that addresses both immediate safety concerns and longer-term treatment and support.

How are behavioral emergencies evaluated?

Evaluating behavioral emergencies is a critical and sensitive process, often requiring immediate and coordinated efforts from mental health professionals, emergency medical personnel, and sometimes law enforcement. The evaluation aims to assess the risk to the individual and others, identify the underlying causes, and determine the most appropriate course of action. Here is an overview of how behavioral emergencies are typically evaluated:

1. **Initial Assessment of Safety:**
   - The first priority is to ensure the safety of the individual, responders, and others nearby. This might involve de-escalation techniques, securing the environment, or, in some cases, restraint to prevent harm.
2. **Rapid Medical Evaluation:**
   - A medical assessment is crucial to rule out medical causes of the behavior, such as a drug overdose, head injury, metabolic disturbances, or other medical conditions.
3. **Mental Status Examination:**
   - Mental health professionals conduct a mental status examination to assess the individual's current state of mind. This includes evaluating their appearance, behavior, speech,

mood, thought processes, thought content (including any delusions or hallucinations), and cognition.

4. **Gathering Information:**
   - Collecting information about the individual's medical history, psychiatric history, recent behaviors, and any current stressors or triggers. This can involve talking to family members, friends, or others who know the person well.
5. **Risk Assessment:**
   - Assessing the risk of harm to self or others is a critical part of the evaluation. This includes identifying any suicidal or homicidal thoughts, plans, and the means to carry out those plans.
6. **Substance Use Assessment:**
   - Evaluating the use of alcohol or drugs, as substance abuse can often contribute to or exacerbate behavioral emergencies.
7. **Consideration of Psychosocial Factors:**
   - Understanding the individual's social context, including family dynamics, living situation, employment status, and support networks, is important.
8. **Legal Considerations:**
   - In some cases, legal considerations such as involuntary hospitalization or psychiatric holds may need to be evaluated, especially if the person is deemed a danger to themselves or others.
9. **Development of a Management Plan:**
   - Based on the evaluation, a management plan is developed. This can include hospitalization, psychiatric treatment, counseling, medication, and follow-up care.
10. **Documentation:**
    - Accurate documentation of the assessment, decisions made, and the rationale for these decisions is important for ongoing treatment and legal reasons.

The evaluation process is dynamic and might evolve as more information becomes available or as the person's condition changes. The primary goals are to stabilize the immediate situation, prevent harm, and arrange for appropriate ongoing care and support.

How must BE patients be approached?

Approaching patients in a behavioral emergency (BE) requires a careful, empathetic, and safety-focused strategy. These situations are often volatile and can pose a risk to the patient, healthcare providers, and others nearby. Here are key guidelines for approaching patients in a BE:

1. **Ensure Safety:**
   - Assess the safety of the environment for both the patient and others. Remove potential hazards and ensure there is a clear exit path.
   - If there is a threat of violence, it may be necessary to have security personnel or law enforcement on standby.
2. **Stay Calm and Non-threatening:**
   - Approach the patient in a calm, non-threatening manner. Your own demeanor can have a significant impact on the situation.
   - Speak in a clear, gentle, and reassuring voice.
3. **Respect Personal Space:**
   - Give the patient enough physical space to avoid feeling trapped or crowded. Invading personal space can escalate agitation.
4. **Non-confrontational Stance:**
   - Avoid direct eye contact and do not stand directly in front of the patient, as these can be perceived as confrontational. Instead, use a side-on stance.
5. **Active Listening:**
   - Listen to the patient's concerns and feelings without judgment. Acknowledge their emotions and fears.
   - Avoid arguing or trying to reason with delusional thoughts, but do gently convey reality.
6. **Clear and Simple Communication:**
   - Use simple, clear, and concise language. Avoid medical jargon or complex explanations.
   - Be honest and consistent in your communication.
7. **Assess and Respond to Immediate Needs:**
   - Determine if there are immediate needs like pain, hunger, or withdrawal symptoms that need to be addressed.

8. **De-escalation Techniques:**
   - Employ de-escalation techniques such as empathizing, setting clear limits, and offering choices and reassurance.
9. **Seek to Understand the Underlying Cause:**
   - Try to determine the underlying cause of the behavioral emergency, whether it is a mental health crisis, substance use, medical issue, or a response to a stressor.
10. **Involve Mental Health Professionals:**
    - Involve mental health professionals as soon as possible for assessment and management.
11. **Document the Encounter:**
    - Document your observations and interventions. This information can be crucial for subsequent care and treatment.
12. **Plan for Emergencies:**
    - Be prepared for the situation to escalate and have a plan for how to respond, including knowing how to call for additional help.
13. **Self-Care:**
    - After the encounter, healthcare providers should also debrief and take care of their own mental health, as these situations can be stressful.

Remember, the primary goals in approaching BE patients are to ensure safety, stabilize the situation, and arrange for appropriate care and treatment. Each situation is unique and requires a tailored approach based on the patient's specific behavior and needs.

How must the patients of behavioral emergency be restrained?

In a behavioral emergency, the restraint of a patient should always be a last resort, and it is important to follow both ethical guidelines and legal regulations. The methods used can vary depending on the specific situation, the patient's condition, and the environment. Here are some general principles:

1. **Least Restrictive Measures:** Start with the least restrictive measures possible. This could include verbal de-escalation techniques or offering medications to help calm the patient.
2. **Safety First:** Ensure the safety of both the patient and healthcare providers. This involves removing any potential hazards and ensuring that the patient cannot harm themselves or others.
3. **Physical Restraints:** If physical restraints are absolutely necessary, they should be applied in a way that does not cause injury or unnecessary discomfort. Common restraints include soft limb restraints or a safety bed with controlled access.
4. **Medical Supervision:** Patients under physical restraint should be under continuous medical supervision to monitor their physical and mental condition.
5. **Legal Compliance:** Ensure that all actions comply with local laws and healthcare regulations regarding patient rights and restraint use.
6. **Documentation:** Thoroughly document the reason for the restraint, the type of restraint used, the duration of the restraint, and the patient's response.
7. **Training:** Healthcare providers involved in restraining patients should be adequately trained in safe and effective restraint techniques.
8. **Debriefing:** After the incident, it is important to debrief and review the situation to learn from it and improve future responses.

It is crucial to remember that the goal is always to protect the patient and those around them, and to use the least restrictive means necessary to resolve the situation. Restraint should never be used as a punishment or for the convenience of the staff.

What can be the complications of restraints?

The use of restraints, while sometimes necessary in behavioral emergencies, can lead to a range of complications. These complications can be physical, psychological, and legal in nature. Here are some of the key concerns:

1. **Physical Injuries:** Improper application of restraints can lead to physical injuries such as bruises, cuts, pressure sores, or even more severe injuries like fractures or nerve damage. Restrained patients might also suffer from reduced circulation, particularly if restraints are too tight or left in place for too long.
2. **Respiratory Complications:** Restraints can interfere with normal breathing, especially if a patient is placed in a prone position or if chest restraints are too tight.

3. **Decreased Cardiovascular Circulation:** Prolonged immobility due to restraints can lead to poor blood circulation, increasing the risk of deep vein thrombosis (DVT) and pulmonary embolism.

4. **Psychological Impact:** The experience of being restrained can be traumatic, leading to psychological distress, anxiety, feelings of helplessness, or post-traumatic stress disorder (PTSD), especially in patients with a history of trauma or mental illness.

5. **Agitation and Behavioral Problems:** Some patients may become more agitated, aggressive, or uncooperative after being restrained, potentially worsening the behavioral emergency.

6. **Risk of Asphyxiation:** In rare cases, improper restraint techniques or positions (like prone positioning) can lead to accidental asphyxiation.

7. **Decreased Functional Status:** Long-term use of restraints can lead to a decline in physical function due to muscle weakness and reduced mobility.

8. **Legal and Ethical Issues:** The use of restraints can raise legal and ethical concerns, particularly if it is done without proper justification, documentation, or adherence to legal standards. This can result in lawsuits or regulatory action against healthcare providers or facilities.

9. **Skin Integrity Issues:** Prolonged restraint can lead to skin breakdown, particularly in elderly or frail patients.

10. **Incontinence and Hygiene Issues:** Restraints can make it difficult for patients to attend to basic needs like using the bathroom, leading to incontinence and associated hygiene problems.

Due to these potential complications, it is important that restraints are used only when absolutely necessary, with the least restrictive method being preferred. Continuous monitoring and regular reassessment are essential to mitigate risks. Healthcare providers must be trained in the proper use of restraints and in identifying and managing potential complications.

What is the treatment of Behavioral Emergency (BE)?

The treatment of a behavioral emergency (BE) typically involves a multi-faceted approach, focusing on immediate stabilization, ensuring safety, and addressing the underlying causes. The specific treatment may vary depending on the nature of the emergency, the underlying cause, the patient's history, and the available resources. Here are some general steps and considerations:

1. **Assessment and Stabilization:** The first step is to assess the patient's physical and mental status. This includes evaluating their level of consciousness, vital signs, potential for violence, and immediate medical needs. The environment should be made safe for both the patient and healthcare providers.

2. **Verbal De-escalation:** Attempt to calm the patient using verbal de-escalation techniques. This involves speaking calmly, offering support, listening to the patient's concerns, and trying to understand their perspective. The goal is to reduce agitation without resorting to physical intervention.

3. **Medication:** If verbal de-escalation is not effective and the patient poses a danger to themselves or others, medication may be necessary. This could include antipsychotics, mood stabilizers, or sedatives, depending on the patient's symptoms and medical history.

4. **Physical Restraints:** As a last resort, if the patient is a danger to themselves or others and all other measures have failed, physical restraints may be necessary. This should be done in compliance with legal and ethical guidelines, ensuring the safety and dignity of the patient.

5. **Psychiatric Evaluation:** A comprehensive psychiatric evaluation is crucial to determine the underlying cause of the behavioral emergency. This can include a review of the patient's mental health history, current medications, substance use, and any recent stressors or triggers.

6. **Treatment of Underlying Conditions:** Address any identified underlying psychiatric or medical conditions with appropriate treatment. This could involve medication management, psychotherapy, substance abuse treatment, or other specialized interventions.

7. **Follow-up and Support:** Provide appropriate follow-up care and support. This may include referrals to mental health professionals, outpatient therapy, support groups, or social services.

8. **Crisis Intervention Team (CIT):** In some cases, especially in community settings, a CIT trained

in dealing with mental health crises can be involved in the response.

9. **Legal Considerations:** Ensure all interventions are in line with legal requirements, including obtaining consent where possible and respecting the patient's rights.

10. **Family and Caregiver Involvement:** When appropriate, involve family members or caregivers in the treatment plan, providing them with education and support.

It is important to remember that the treatment of a behavioral emergency is not just about managing the immediate crisis, but also about addressing the broader mental health needs of the individual. Collaboration among healthcare providers, mental health specialists, and the patient's support system is key to effective treatment and prevention of future crises.

What is Breath-holding spells (BHS)?

Breath-holding spells (BHS) are a common condition seen in young children, typically occurring between the ages of 6 months and 6 years. During a breath-holding spell, a child involuntarily stops breathing for a short period, which can lead to changes in their appearance or even brief loss of consciousness. It is important to note that these spells are involuntary – the child is not holding their breath on purpose.

There are two main types of breath-holding spells:

1. **Cyanotic Breath-Holding Spells:** These are the most common type and are often triggered by anger, frustration, pain, or injury. The child cries or gasps and then stops breathing, leading to cyanosis (a bluish tint to the skin, especially around the lips), due to lack of oxygen. The child may lose consciousness and have a brief period of "floppiness".

2. **Pallid Breath-Holding Spells:** These are less common and are typically triggered by a sudden, unexpected event such as a shock or a minor injury. The child does not cry before stopping breathing; instead, they often become pale (hence the name "pallid") due to a decrease in heart rate and blood pressure, leading to a fainting episode.

Both types of spells are usually brief, lasting from a few seconds to a couple of minutes. After the spell, normal breathing resumes, and the child regains consciousness. While breath-holding spells can be terrifying for parents to witness, they are generally harmless and most children outgrow them by the time they start school.

The exact cause of breath-holding spells is not completely understood, but they are thought to be related to the immature development of the autonomic nervous system, which controls involuntary functions like heart rate and breathing. There is also a genetic component, as these spells can run in families.

In terms of management:

- **Medical Evaluation:** It is important for a child experiencing breath-holding spells to be evaluated by a healthcare provider to rule out other medical conditions and to provide guidance on how to handle the spells.
- **Reassurance:** Parents and caregivers should be reassured that these spells are generally benign and self-limiting.
- **Safety Measures:** During a spell, the child should be laid on their side or back to ensure they don't hurt themselves. Do not shake the child or splash water on their face.
- **Avoiding Triggers:** If possible, avoiding known triggers can help.
- **Iron Supplements:** Some studies suggest that iron supplements can reduce the frequency of spells, especially in children with iron deficiency.
- **Education and Support:** Educating family members, caregivers, and teachers about the condition and how to respond to a spell is essential.

In most cases, breath-holding spells decrease in frequency with age and eventually stop. However, if there are concerns about the frequency, severity, or nature of the spells, or if they continue beyond the typical age range, further medical evaluation may be necessary.

What are the types of BHS?

Breath-holding spells (BHS) in children can be categorized into two primary types, each characterized by different triggers and physical responses. These types are:

1. **Cyanotic Breath-Holding Spells:**
   - **Trigger:** Usually occur in response to frustration, anger, or a painful experience.
   - **Description:** The child often cries or screams before abruptly holding their breath. In these spells, the child's body reduces breathing or stops breathing altogether, leading to cyanosis (a bluish tint to the skin, especially noticeable around the lips and face), due to a lack of oxygen.

- **Outcome:** The child may lose consciousness and, in some cases, may also exhibit brief, jerky movements which can be mistaken for a seizure. These movements are actually a reflex action due to the lack of oxygen. The child typically recovers spontaneously and resumes normal breathing.

2. **Pallid Breath-Holding Spells:**

   - **Trigger:** Often triggered by a sudden, unexpected fright, pain, or shock. Unlike cyanotic spells, they are not typically preceded by crying.
   - **Description:** The child's heart rate and blood pressure drop, leading to pallor (paleness) rather than cyanosis. This reaction is thought to be a reflex caused by the vagus nerve, which affects heart rate and blood pressure.
   - **Outcome:** The child may lose consciousness and become limp. They usually recover quickly once they start breathing again.

Both types of breath-holding spells are an involuntary response, meaning the child does not intentionally hold their breath. While these episodes can be frightening to witness, they are typically harmless and most children outgrow them by school age. However, it is always advisable for children experiencing breath-holding spells to be evaluated by a healthcare professional to rule out other possible causes and to provide guidance and reassurance to the parents or caregivers.

In rare cases, a child might have a mix of both cyanotic and pallid spells, or the type could change over time. The management and approach to each type of spell are generally similar, focusing on ensuring the child's safety during spells, reducing triggers where possible, and providing reassurance and support to the family.

What is the pathophysiology of breath-holding spells?

The pathophysiology of breath-holding spells (BHS) in children is not completely understood, but these episodes are believed to involve the autonomic nervous system, which controls involuntary body functions. The autonomic nervous system comprises the sympathetic nervous system (responsible for "fight or flight" responses) and the parasympathetic nervous system (responsible for "rest and digest" activities). Here is a closer look at the pathophysiology behind the two main types of breath-holding spells:

1. **Cyanotic Breath-Holding Spells:**

   - **Emotional Trigger:** These spells are often triggered by an emotional upset or a painful event.
   - **Hyperventilation and Breath Holding:** The initial response is usually crying or hyperventilation, followed by a forced expiration or holding the breath in.
   - **Vagal Influence:** The act of crying or screaming followed by breath-holding leads to a decrease in oxygen (hypoxia) and an increase in carbon dioxide (hypercapnia) in the blood.
   - **Physiological Response:** The reduced oxygen levels trigger a reflex in the body that may cause the child to lose consciousness. The autonomic nervous system's response to hypoxia and hypercapnia can cause a decrease in heart rate (bradycardia) and, consequently, a decrease in the brain's blood supply, leading to fainting or a seizure-like episode.

2. **Pallid Breath-Holding Spells:**

   - **Physical Trigger:** These are usually triggered by a sudden fright, pain, or shock.
   - **Vagal Activation:** The trigger leads to an intense activation of the vagus nerve, which is a key part of the parasympathetic nervous system.
   - **Bradycardia and Hypotension:** The vagal activation results in a rapid drop in heart rate (bradycardia) and blood pressure (hypotension). This decrease in cardiac output leads to reduced cerebral perfusion.
   - **Loss of Consciousness:** The reduced blood flow to the brain causes the child to become pale (pallid) and lose consciousness.

In both types, the brain's response to the altered blood gases (in cyanotic spells) or the decreased cerebral perfusion (in pallid spells) is what leads to the loss of consciousness. The brain essentially initiates a protective shutdown to reset the body's systems. When the child faints and becomes horizontal, blood flow to the brain is restored, and the child regains consciousness.

Breath-holding spells are a dramatic but usually benign expression of the immature autonomic nervous system in young children. Most children outgrow these spells by the time they start school, as their nervous system matures. Understanding the pathophysiology behind BHS can help caregivers and medical professionals better manage and reassure those who care for children experiencing these episodes.

What are brief psychotic disorders and how to manage them?

Brief Psychotic Disorder is a mental health condition characterized by sudden, temporary episodes of psychotic behavior, such as hallucinations, delusions, disorganized speech, or grossly disorganized or catatonic behavior. These episodes are brief, lasting at least a day but less than a month, and are followed by a full return to the individual's previous level of functioning. The onset can be rapid, often occurring within two weeks of a significant stressor, although a stressor is not always identifiable.

Causes and Risk Factors

The exact cause of brief psychotic disorder is unknown, but it may be associated with a combination of genetic, psychological, and environmental factors. Potential triggers include:

- Severe stress or traumatic events
- A history of psychological trauma or abuse
- A family history of psychotic disorders
- Drug use, particularly hallucinogens and stimulants

Symptoms

The symptoms of brief psychotic disorder can be severe and include:

- Hallucinations (seeing or hearing things that aren't there)
- Delusions (firmly held beliefs not supported by objective reality)
- Disorganized speech (incoherence)
- Grossly disorganized or catatonic behavior
- Emotional turmoil or overwhelming confusion

Management and Treatment

The management of brief psychotic disorder typically involves a combination of medication, psychotherapy, and support. The specific treatment plan should be tailored to the individual's needs and may include the following components:

1. **Medication:** Antipsychotic medications are commonly used to reduce or eliminate the symptoms of psychosis. In some cases, other medications like mood stabilizers or anti-depressants may be used.
2. **Psychotherapy:** Various forms of psychotherapy can be beneficial. Cognitive-behavioral therapy (CBT) can help the individual understand and change problematic thoughts and behaviors. Supportive therapy can provide emotional support and stress management.
3. **Hospitalization:** In cases where there is a risk of harm to the individual or others, or if the symptoms are severe, hospitalization may be necessary to ensure safety and stabilize the condition.
4. **Family Education and Support:** Educating the family about the disorder and involving them in the treatment process can be crucial. Support groups for family members can also be helpful.
5. **Addressing Underlying Issues:** If the psychotic episode was triggered by stress, trauma, or substance abuse, addressing these underlying issues is crucial. This might include trauma-focused therapy, stress management techniques, or substance abuse treatment.
6. **Monitoring and Follow-Up:** Regular follow-up and monitoring by healthcare professionals are important to assess treatment effectiveness and make necessary adjustments.
7. **Crisis Planning:** Developing a plan for how to handle potential future episodes can be beneficial.

Prognosis

The prognosis for brief psychotic disorder is generally good, as individuals typically recover fully with treatment. However, some individuals may go on to develop other psychiatric conditions, such as schizophrenia or bipolar disorder. Early intervention and comprehensive treatment can significantly improve outcomes.

Prevention

While it is difficult to prevent brief psychotic disorder, maintaining good mental health, managing stress, seeking early treatment for trauma or substance abuse, and having strong social support can help reduce the risk or mitigate the severity of episodes.

It is important to note that brief psychotic disorder is a serious mental health condition that requires professional treatment. If someone is suspected of having a psychotic episode, prompt medical attention is essential.

What is Catatonia and its management?

Catatonia is a complex neuropsychiatric syndrome characterized by a range of motor, behavioral, and emotional abnormalities. It is often associated with mood disorders (like bipolar disorder and depression), psychotic disorders (like schizophrenia), and other medical conditions.

Characteristics of Catatonia

Catatonia can manifest in various ways, including:

1. **Motor Symptoms:**
   - Stupor (reduced reactivity to stimuli and a tendency to remain immobile)
   - Catalepsy (maintenance of rigid body posture for extended periods)
   - Waxy flexibility (limbs remain in positions they are placed in by someone else)
   - Mutism (little to no verbal response)
   - Negativism (resistance to instructions or movement)
   - Posturing (holding unusual postures)
   - Mannerisms (odd or exaggerated movements)
   - Stereotypy (repetitive, abnormally frequent, non-goal-directed movements)
   - Agitation (not influenced by external stimuli)
2. **Other Symptoms:**
   - Grimacing
   - Echolalia (mimicking another's speech)
   - Echopraxia (mimicking another's movements)

Causes of Catatonia

Catatonia is not a disease itself but a clinical syndrome that can occur in the context of various psychiatric and medical conditions. Causes include:

- Schizophrenia and other psychotic disorders
- Bipolar disorder
- Major depressive disorder
- Neurodevelopmental disorders
- Neurological conditions (e.g., encephalitis, brain injury)
- Substance use (withdrawal or intoxication)
- Metabolic imbalances

Management of Catatonia

The management of catatonia involves several steps:

1. **Medical Evaluation:** An initial medical evaluation is crucial to identify underlying causes, including medical and neurological conditions, and to rule out other conditions that may present with similar symptoms.
2. **Treatment of Underlying Disorder:** Managing the underlying psychiatric or medical condition is a critical part of treating catatonia.
3. **Benzodiazepines:** Benzodiazepines, such as lorazepam, are often the first-line treatment. They can be remarkably effective, with rapid improvement in symptoms.
4. **Electroconvulsive Therapy (ECT):** ECT is considered for severe cases or when there is a lack of response to medications. It is particularly effective for catatonic symptoms associated with mood disorders.
5. **Supportive Care:** Ensuring the patient's safety and addressing basic needs, such as nutrition, hydration, and hygiene, are important, especially in cases of severe catatonia where the patient might be immobile.
6. **Monitoring for Complications:** Severe catatonia can lead to complications like malnutrition, dehydration, pressure sores, and blood clots due to immobility. Continuous monitoring and preventive care are essential.
7. **Physical Therapy:** This may be necessary to prevent complications of prolonged immobility.
8. **Psychotherapy and Rehabilitation:** Once acute symptoms are managed, ongoing therapy and rehabilitation may be helpful, especially if the catatonia is associated with a psychiatric disorder.

Prognosis

The prognosis of catatonia varies depending on the underlying cause, the severity of symptoms, and the response to treatment. With prompt and appropriate treatment, many patients experience significant improvement or full resolution of catatonic symptoms.

Conclusion

Catatonia is a serious clinical condition that requires prompt medical attention. Early recognition and treatment are crucial for a good outcome. Due to its diverse causes, a comprehensive approach to evaluation and management is essential.

What is cognitive therapy?

Cognitive therapy, also known as cognitive behavioral therapy (CBT), is a type of psychotherapy that focuses on changing unhelpful or destructive thought patterns, with the aim of influencing emotions and behaviors. It is based on the concept that thoughts, feelings, and behaviors are interconnected, and that altering one can change the others. Cognitive therapy is a well-established treatment approach for various mental health disorders and psychological problems.

Key Principles of Cognitive Therapy

1. **Identification of Negative Thoughts:** Cognitive therapy involves identifying negative or distorted thought patterns that contribute to emotional distress or harmful behaviors.
2. **Challenging Cognitive Distortions:** Once these thoughts are identified, the therapy works on challenging and reframing them into more realistic and positive ways of thinking.
3. **Behavioral Changes:** Cognitive therapy also involves making changes in behaviors that are contributing to psychological problems. This is based on the idea that changing one's behavior can lead to changes in thoughts and feelings.
4. **Problem Solving:** It teaches problem-solving skills to cope with difficult situations.
5. **Goal Setting:** CBT is often goal-oriented, with the therapist and client working together to set achievable goals.
6. **Skills Training:** It often involves teaching clients skills for handling stress, managing time, improving communication, or dealing with specific problems.

Conditions Treated by Cognitive Therapy

Cognitive therapy is effective for a wide range of psychological issues, including but not limited to:

- Depression
- Anxiety disorders (such as panic attacks, social anxiety, generalized anxiety disorder)
- Phobias
- Post-traumatic stress disorder (PTSD)
- Obsessive-compulsive disorder (OCD)
- Eating disorders
- Substance abuse and addiction
- Sleep disorders
- Personality disorders
- Chronic pain and illness-related stress

Approach and Techniques

- **Cognitive Restructuring:** Changing negative thought patterns.
- **Exposure Therapy:** Gradually exposing clients to feared situations to reduce anxiety.
- **Relaxation Techniques and Stress Management:** Teaching ways to calm the mind and body.
- **Mindfulness:** Focusing on the present moment to reduce rumination and worry.
- **Behavioral Experiments:** Testing out beliefs through real-life experiences.
- **Homework Assignments:** Practicing skills and techniques learned in therapy outside of sessions.

Efficacy and Duration

CBT is typically a short-term treatment, often lasting for a few weeks to several months, depending on the complexity of the issue. Its effectiveness is well-supported by research for many disorders. One of the key advantages of cognitive therapy is that it not only helps to alleviate symptoms in the short term but also equips individuals with skills that they can use throughout their lives to manage their mental health.

Conclusion

Cognitive therapy's focus on thought patterns and practical skills makes it a popular and effective form of psychotherapy. It empowers individuals to take an active role in their treatment, fostering self-awareness and resilience that can provide long-lasting benefits.

What are the steps in cognitive therapy?

Cognitive therapy, a form of cognitive-behavioral therapy (CBT), is structured and goal-oriented, involving a series of steps that are typically followed in the therapeutic process. Here is a general outline of these steps:

1. **Assessment and Relationship Building:**
   - **Initial Assessment:** The therapist conducts an initial assessment to understand the client's concerns, symptoms, and history.
   - **Therapeutic Relationship:** Establishing a strong, trusting relationship between the therapist and client is crucial for effective therapy.
2. **Identification of Problems and Goal Setting:**
   - **Problem Identification:** The therapist and client work together to identify specific problems or areas of concern.

- **Goal Setting:** They then set clear, achievable goals for therapy, which guide the treatment process.

3. **Education about Cognitive Model:**
   - **Understanding the Model:** The therapist explains how thoughts, emotions, and behaviors are interconnected.
   - **Psychoeducation:** This may include education about the client's specific condition and how CBT can help.
4. **Identification of Negative or Distorted Thinking:**
   - **Thought Monitoring:** Clients learn to observe and record their thoughts, particularly those that occur in response to specific situations.
   - **Recognizing Patterns:** The therapist helps the client identify patterns of negative or distorted thinking.
5. **Challenging and Reframing Thoughts:**
   - **Cognitive Restructuring:** Clients are taught how to challenge their negative thoughts and consider alternative interpretations.
   - **Reframing Thoughts:** The goal is to develop more balanced and realistic thoughts.
6. **Behavioral Techniques and Experiments:**
   - **Behavioral Experiments:** Testing out beliefs in real-world situations to see if they hold true.
   - **Skill Development:** Learning new coping skills and problem-solving strategies.
   - **Exposure Therapy:** Gradually facing fears in a controlled, safe manner (if applicable).
7. **Homework Assignments:**
   - **Practicing Skills:** Clients are often given tasks to practice outside of sessions to reinforce what they have learned.
   - **Journaling:** Keeping a diary of thoughts, feelings, and behaviors.
8. **Progress Review and Modification of Plan:**
   - **Regular Reviews:** Assessing progress towards goals and modifying the treatment plan as necessary.
   - **Adjustments:** Therapy is dynamic, and adjustments are made based on the client's progress and feedback.
9. **Development of Preventive Measures and Skills:**
   - **Relapse Prevention:** Developing strategies to maintain gains and handle future challenges.
   - **Skill Mastery:** Ensuring the client feels confident in using the skills independently.
10. **Termination and Follow-Up:**
    - **Review of Progress:** Reflecting on what has been learned and how the client has changed.
    - **Planning for the Future:** Discussing how to apply the skills going forward.
    - **Follow-Up Sessions:** Sometimes scheduled to check in on the client's progress post-therapy.

Throughout these steps, the therapist provides support, guidance, and feedback, helping the client to gain insight and build effective coping strategies. The exact nature and duration of these steps can vary depending on the individual's needs and the specific issues being addressed. The collaborative nature of cognitive therapy empowers clients, giving them an active role in their own treatment and fostering long-term, sustainable mental health improvements.

What is psychotherapy and how does it work?

Psychotherapy, often referred to as talk therapy, is a general term for treating mental health problems by talking with a mental health provider. It involves a range of techniques designed to improve the mental health of an individual, or to improve group relationships (as in family therapy).

How Psychotherapy Works:

1. **Understanding and Insight:** Psychotherapy helps individuals understand the causes of their problems by discussing their thoughts, feelings, and behaviors. This understanding can offer insight into how to better manage their life.
2. **Emotional Release:** It provides a safe environment to express and process emotions. Talking about one's problems with a therapist can provide a sense of relief and reduce feelings of isolation.
3. **Behavior and Thought Modification:** Psychotherapy often involves changing unhelpful or harmful thought patterns and behaviors. Therapists help individuals challenge these patterns and adopt healthier ways of thinking and acting.

4. **Skill Development:** It teaches coping and problem-solving skills to handle difficult situations more effectively.

5. **Support and Validation:** Psychotherapy provides support and validation. Having someone listen empathetically and acknowledge one's feelings can be profoundly healing.

6. **Relationship Improvement:** It can help improve communication skills and relationship dynamics, which is particularly important in couples or family therapy.

Types of Psychotherapy:

1. **Cognitive-Behavioral Therapy (CBT):** Focuses on identifying and changing negative thought patterns and behaviors.
2. **Psychodynamic Therapy:** Explores how past experiences and unconscious mind influence current behaviors and feelings.
3. **Humanistic Therapy:** Focuses on the individual's nature, emphasizing personal growth and self-actualization.
4. **Interpersonal Therapy (IPT):** Concentrates on improving interpersonal relationships and communication patterns.
5. **Family Therapy:** Involves treating a family system rather than an individual to improve the dynamics within the family.
6. **Group Therapy:** Provides a supportive environment where individuals with similar issues can share and work through problems.

How Effective is Psychotherapy?

- **Evidence-Based:** Many forms of psychotherapy, especially CBT, are evidence-based, meaning they have been scientifically tested and found effective.
- **Adaptability:** Different approaches may be more effective for certain types of problems. Therapists often adapt or combine approaches based on individual needs.
- **Individual Factors:** The effectiveness can also depend on factors such as the individual's situation, the therapist's skill, and the quality of the therapeutic relationship.

Conclusion

Psychotherapy can be a powerful intervention for a wide range of mental illnesses and emotional difficulties. Its effectiveness lies not only in the methods used but also in the therapeutic relationship that offers insight, support, and strategies for change. While it requires active participation and can be challenging, it is often a transformative process that enables individuals to live healthier, more adaptive, and fulfilling lives.

What is the difference between psychotherapy and therapy?

The terms "psychotherapy" and "therapy" are often used interchangeably, but they can have slightly different meanings depending on the context.

Psychotherapy

1. **Definition:** Psychotherapy, also known as "talk therapy" or psychological therapy, is a process where psychological problems are treated through communication and relationship factors between an individual and a therapist. It is primarily focused on achieving insight and change in behaviors, thoughts, emotions, and how these psychological factors interact.

2. **Approach:** Psychotherapy is usually more in-depth and long-term. It aims to understand and change complex behavioral patterns or emotional states. It often explores past experiences, subconscious thoughts, and deep-seated emotional issues.

3. **Types:** Includes specific types such as Cognitive Behavioral Therapy (CBT), Psychodynamic Therapy, Humanistic Therapy, and others.

4. **Professionals Involved:** Conducted by licensed professionals like psychologists, psychiatrists, psychotherapists, and some social workers and counselors who specialize in mental health.

Therapy

1. **Definition:** "Therapy" is a broader term that can refer to any treatment used to heal or relieve an illness or disability. It can encompass a wide range of treatments beyond just psychological issues, including physical therapy, occupational therapy, speech therapy, etc.

2. **Approach:** Depending on the type, therapy can be short-term or long-term and may focus on practical solutions to current problems, skill-building, rehabilitation, or physical healing processes.

3. **Types:** Includes psychotherapy, but also physical therapies (like physiotherapy), speech therapies, occupational therapies, and others.

4. **Professionals Involved:** Can be provided by a wide range of professionals, including but not limited to psychologists, physical therapists, occupational therapists, speech therapists, and counselors.

Key Differences

- **Scope:** Psychotherapy is a subset of therapy. All psychotherapies are therapies, but not all therapies are psychotherapies.
- **Focus:** Psychotherapy is specifically focused on mental health and emotional well-being, whereas therapy can refer to treatments for a variety of physical, emotional, and developmental issues.
- **Professionals:** Psychotherapy is provided by mental health professionals, while therapy can be provided by a broader range of healthcare professionals.

Conclusion

In casual conversation, "therapy" and "psychotherapy" are often used to mean the same thing, especially when referring to mental health treatment. However, when distinguishing between different types of treatments, "therapy" is a broader term that encompasses a variety of treatment modalities, of which psychotherapy is one specific type focused on mental and emotional health.

What are the types of psychology therapy?

Psychology therapy, more commonly known as psychotherapy or talk therapy, encompasses a variety of treatment techniques designed to help individuals overcome mental health issues, cope with difficult emotions, and make positive changes in their lives. There are several different types of psychotherapy, each with its own approach. Here are some of the most prominent ones:

1. **Cognitive Behavioral Therapy (CBT):**
   - Focuses on identifying and changing negative thinking patterns and maladaptive behaviors.
   - Often short-term and goal-oriented.
   - Effective for depression, anxiety, phobias, and other mental health disorders.
2. **Psychodynamic Therapy:**
   - Based on the principles of psychoanalysis, but typically less intensive and with a shorter duration.
   - Focuses on unconscious processes and how they affect current behavior.
   - Aims to help individuals gain insight into their lives and create change.
3. **Humanistic Therapy:**
   - Centers on the individual's nature and emphasizes personal growth and self-actualization.
   - Examples include client-centered therapy (or Rogerian therapy) and Gestalt therapy.
   - Focuses on the here and now, rather than past experiences.
4. **Dialectical Behavior Therapy (DBT):**
   - A form of CBT that combines standard cognitive-behavioral techniques with concepts of distress tolerance, acceptance, and mindfulness.
   - Originally developed to treat borderline personality disorder but is now used for a variety of conditions.
5. **Interpersonal Therapy (IPT):**
   - Focuses on improving interpersonal relationships and communication patterns.
   - Often used to treat depression.
6. **Family Therapy:**
   - Involves treating the family as a whole, rather than just the individual.
   - Useful for addressing family conflict, improving communication, and resolving issues within a family context.
7. **Group Therapy:**
   - Involves one or more therapists working with several people at the same time.
   - Beneficial for individuals who might gain insight and support from peers facing similar issues.
8. **Behavioral Therapy:**
   - Focuses on modifying harmful behaviors.
   - Uses conditioning techniques, such as positive/negative reinforcement, to encourage desired behaviors.
9. **Integrative or Holistic Therapy:**
   - Combines elements from different types of therapy.
   - Tailored to the individual's needs and personal circumstances.

10. **Art Therapy:**
    - Uses creative processes like painting, drawing, or sculpture as a therapeutic tool.
    - Helps individuals express themselves and explore their emotions.
11. **Narrative Therapy:**
    - Centers on the stories or narratives that people construct about their lives.
    - Aims to help people see themselves as separate from their problems and to rewrite their stories.
12. **Mindfulness-Based Therapies:**
    - Incorporate mindfulness practices to help individuals stay focused on the present.
    - Includes approaches like Mindfulness-Based Stress Reduction (MBSR) and Mindfulness-Based Cognitive Therapy (MBCT).

Each type of therapy has its strengths and is suited to specific kinds of issues or conditions. The effectiveness of therapy often depends on the individual's specific needs and the skill of the therapist. Many therapists use a blend of approaches to create a tailored treatment plan for their clients.

What are the different types of mental therapy?

Mental therapy, also known as psychotherapy or psychological therapy, encompasses a variety of approaches designed to help individuals deal with mental health issues, emotional challenges, and some psychiatric disorders. These therapies can vary widely in their methodologies and areas of focus. Here are some of the primary types of mental therapy:

1. **Cognitive Behavioral Therapy (CBT):**
    - Focuses on identifying and changing negative or unhelpful thought patterns and behaviors.
    - Effective for a range of issues including depression, anxiety, phobias, and stress management.
2. **Psychodynamic Therapy:**
    - Based on the principles of psychoanalysis.
    - Explores unconscious motivations and past experiences to understand current behavior.
    - Often used for long-term personal exploration and treating chronic psychological issues.
3. **Humanistic Therapies:**
    - Emphasizes the individual's capacity for self-realization and growth.
    - Includes approaches like Person-Centered Therapy (Rogerian Therapy) and Gestalt Therapy.
    - Focuses on the here and now, rather than on the unconscious or past experiences.
4. **Dialectical Behavior Therapy (DBT):**
    - A type of CBT that combines standard cognitive-behavioral techniques with concepts like mindfulness, emotional regulation, and distress tolerance.
    - Originally developed for borderline personality disorder but now used for various conditions.
5. **Interpersonal Therapy (IPT):**
    - Focuses on interpersonal relationships and communication skills.
    - Often used for depression and other mood disorders.
6. **Family and Couples Therapy:**
    - Involves treating relationships and dynamics within a family or couple.
    - Useful for addressing family conflicts, marital problems, and issues affecting family functioning.
7. **Group Therapy:**
    - Involves one or more therapists working with a group of clients at the same time.
    - Can provide support and perspective from peers dealing with similar issues.
8. **Behavior Therapy:**
    - Focuses on modifying harmful behaviors.
    - Utilizes principles of learning theory and conditioning.
9. **Integrative or Holistic Therapy:**
    - Combines elements from different therapeutic approaches.
    - Tailored to meet the individual needs of the client.

10. **Mindfulness-Based Therapies:**
    - Includes practices like Mindfulness-Based Stress Reduction (MBSR) and Mindfulness-Based Cognitive Therapy (MBCT).
    - Helps individuals focus on the present moment and develop a non-judgmental awareness of their thoughts and feelings.
11. **Art and Creative Therapies:**
    - Uses creative processes (art, music, drama, etc.) as a therapeutic tool.
    - Helps in expressing emotions and dealing with psychological issues.
12. **Narrative Therapy:**
    - Focuses on the stories people construct about their lives.
    - Aims to help clients view their problems in a separate narrative and rewrite their story.
13. **Exposure Therapy:**
    - Commonly used for treating phobias and anxiety disorders.
    - Involves controlled exposure to the feared object or context without any danger, to help overcome fears.

Each type of therapy has its own unique methods and areas of focus, and some types may be more effective for certain conditions than others. Therapists often tailor their approach to the specific needs and circumstances of their clients, sometimes combining elements from different approaches. The choice of therapy depends on the individual's particular issues, their personal preferences, and the therapist's expertise.

How psychotherapy is used to treat depression?

Psychotherapy is a key component in the treatment of depression, offering a supportive environment where individuals can explore their feelings, thoughts, and behaviors, and learn strategies to cope with and alleviate depressive symptoms. Here is how psychotherapy is typically used to treat depression:

1. **Understanding and Identifying Issues:**
    - Psychotherapy helps individuals understand the underlying issues contributing to their depression, such as relationship problems, grief, stress, or unresolved past events.
    - Therapists work with clients to identify patterns of negative thinking or behavior that exacerbate depressive symptoms.
2. **Cognitive Behavioral Therapy (CBT):**
    - CBT is one of the most effective forms of psychotherapy for depression.
    - It involves identifying and challenging negative thought patterns and beliefs, and replacing them with more balanced and constructive ones.
    - CBT also focuses on changing behaviors that contribute to depression, such as withdrawing from activities and social isolation.
3. **Interpersonal Therapy (IPT):**
    - IPT focuses on the individual's relationships with others and aims to improve interpersonal skills.
    - It helps in understanding and managing relationship problems, which can be a significant factor in depression.
4. **Psychodynamic Therapy:**
    - This approach involves exploring past experiences and emotions to understand current depressive symptoms.
    - It helps in identifying and resolving conflicts from past relationships that may be affecting the individual's current mental state.
5. **Behavioral Activation:**
    - Encourages clients to engage in activities they find enjoyable or fulfilling.
    - Helps to break the cycle of inactivity and avoidance behaviors that can worsen depression.
6. **Problem-Solving Therapy:**
    - Focuses on improving an individual's ability to cope with stressful life experiences.
    - It involves identifying problems and developing practical solutions.
7. **Mindfulness-Based Cognitive Therapy (MBCT):**
    - Combines cognitive therapy with mindfulness techniques.
    - Helps individuals to focus on the present moment and become aware of their thoughts and feelings without becoming overwhelmed by them.
8. **Supportive Counseling:**
    - Provides emotional support and validation.

- Helps clients feel heard and understood, which is crucial for individuals with depression.

9. **Learning Coping Strategies:**

   - Psychotherapy teaches various coping mechanisms and skills to manage symptoms of depression.
   - Includes stress management, relaxation techniques, and coping with negative thoughts.

10. **Homework Assignments:**

    - Many therapists assign homework to help clients practice the skills learned in therapy sessions.
    - These might include journaling, practicing relaxation techniques, or engaging in specific activities.

11. **Combination with Medication:**

    - In some cases, psychotherapy is combined with antidepressant medication, especially for moderate to severe depression.
    - The combination can be more effective than either treatment alone.

12. **Long-term Benefits:**

    - Psychotherapy not only addresses the current episode of depression but also equips individuals with tools and skills to prevent future episodes.

13. **Personalized Approach:**

    - Therapy is tailored to the individual's specific needs, symptoms, and circumstances.

Psychotherapy provides a safe space for individuals to explore their emotions and thoughts, understand their condition better, and develop strategies to cope with depression. It is about empowering the individual to take control of their mental health and make positive changes in their life.

How effective is Gestalt therapy?

Gestalt therapy, developed by Fritz and Laura Perls in the 1940s, is a form of psychotherapy that emphasizes personal responsibility and focuses on the individual's experience in the present moment, the therapist-client relationship, the environmental and social contexts of a person's life, and the self-regulating adjustments people make as a result of their overall situation. Its effectiveness, like many therapeutic approaches, can vary depending on several factors:

1. **Nature of the Issue:** Gestalt therapy has been found effective for a range of issues, particularly those involving self-awareness, relationship problems, and personal growth. It may be less suitable for severe mental health conditions like schizophrenia or bipolar disorder.
2. **Client Engagement:** The effectiveness of Gestalt therapy largely depends on the client's willingness to engage actively in the process. This therapy requires clients to explore their feelings and take responsibility for their thoughts and actions.
3. **Therapist Skill and Experience:** As with any therapy, the skill, experience, and approach of the therapist play a crucial role in the effectiveness of Gestalt therapy.
4. **Client-Therapist Relationship:** A strong therapeutic alliance, which is central in Gestalt therapy, can significantly enhance its effectiveness.
5. **Research and Evidence:** Compared to therapies like Cognitive Behavioral Therapy (CBT), there is less empirical research available on the effectiveness of Gestalt therapy. However, the research that does exist generally supports its efficacy, particularly in improving self-awareness and enhancing the quality of interpersonal relationships.
6. **Short-term vs. Long-term Issues:** Gestalt therapy is often considered effective for short-term therapy goals, such as addressing specific interpersonal issues or enhancing self-awareness. Its effectiveness in treating chronic mental health conditions over the long term is less clear and often requires an integrated approach with other therapies.
7. **Adaptability and Integration:** Gestalt therapy techniques and principles are often integrated into other types of therapy, which can enhance overall therapeutic effectiveness.
8. **Personal Compatibility:** As with any therapeutic approach, individual preferences and compatibility with the therapy's style and approach are crucial. Some clients resonate more with the experiential and present-focused approach of Gestalt therapy, while others may not find it as beneficial.

In conclusion, while Gestalt therapy can be effective for many individuals, its success largely depends on the specific circumstances of the client, including their particular issues, their engagement with the therapy, and the skill of the therapist. It is always recommended to consult with a mental health professional to determine the most appropriate therapeutic approach for an individual's needs.

What are the different types of counselling approaches?

Counseling is a diverse field with various approaches designed to support individuals in understanding and overcoming challenges in their lives. These approaches differ in their theories about human behavior, emotions, and thought processes. Here are some of the major types of counseling approaches:

1. **Cognitive Behavioral Therapy (CBT):**
   - Focuses on identifying and changing negative thought patterns and behaviors.
   - Employs techniques to challenge irrational beliefs and develop more rational, adaptive thinking.
   - Often used for anxiety, depression, and other mental health disorders.
2. **Psychodynamic Counseling:**
   - Based on psychoanalytic theories, it explores how unconscious processes and past experiences shape current behavior.
   - Aims to increase self-awareness and understanding of the influence of the past on present behavior.
3. **Humanistic Counseling:**
   - Focuses on the individual's unique nature and capacity for self-growth and self-actualization.
   - Includes approaches like Person-Centered Therapy (developed by Carl Rogers) and Gestalt Therapy.
4. **Integrative Counseling:**
   - Combines elements from different counseling approaches tailored to the client's individual needs.
   - Allows flexibility and creativity in the therapeutic process.
5. **Solution-Focused Brief Therapy (SFBT):**
   - Concentrates on finding solutions in the present time and exploring one's hope for the future.
   - Focuses on what the client wants to achieve rather than on the problem(s) that made them seek help.
6. **Narrative Therapy:**
   - Sees people as separate from their problems.
   - Encourages clients to rely on their own skill sets to minimize the problems that exist in their everyday lives.
7. **Couples and Family Counseling:**
   - Focuses on improving communication within relationships and resolving conflicts.
   - Family therapy views problems within the context of family systems theory.
8. **Group Counseling:**
   - Involves one or more therapists working with a group of clients.
   - Useful for individuals who can benefit from peer support and interaction.
9. **Existential Counseling:**
   - Focuses on issues related to existence, such as the meaning of life, death, freedom, and responsibility.
   - Aims to help clients face these challenges and make meaningful, authentic life choices.
10. **Mindfulness-Based Therapies:**
    - Includes practices like Mindfulness-Based Stress Reduction (MBSR) and Mindfulness-Based Cognitive Therapy (MBCT).
    - Emphasizes being fully present in the moment and developing an awareness of thoughts and feelings without attachment.
11. **Art Therapy**:
    - Uses creative processes (like drawing, painting, or sculpture) to help clients explore and express feelings that may be difficult to articulate verbally.
12. **Behavioral Therapy:**
    - Focuses on changing unhealthy or destructive behaviors through behavior modification techniques.

Each counseling approach has its unique strengths and is suited to different types of issues or client preferences. A counselor might use a combination of approaches depending on the situation and the needs of the client. The effectiveness of counseling often depends on the relationship between the counselor and the client, the specific needs of the client, and the skill and approach of the counselor.

What are the personality traits of a physical therapist?

Physical therapists, also known as physiotherapists, are healthcare professionals who help patients reduce pain and improve or restore mobility. To be effective in their role, physical therapists often possess a combination of personal and professional traits that enable them to provide high-quality care and support to their patients. Some key personality traits of a successful physical therapist include:

1. **Empathy and Compassion:** Understanding and sharing the feelings of others is crucial. Physical therapists often work with patients who are in pain or are experiencing frustrating physical limitations.
2. **Strong Communication Skills:** They must be able to explain complex medical information in understandable terms, listen effectively to patient concerns, and communicate with other healthcare professionals.
3. **Patience and Perseverance:** Physical therapy can be a slow process, and patients may progress at different rates. Patience is key in guiding patients through gradual progress and setbacks.
4. **Problem-Solving Skills:** Physical therapists must assess each patient's unique situation and devise and adapt treatment plans accordingly.
5. **Physical Stamina and Dexterity:** The job can be physically demanding, involving standing for long periods and sometimes assisting or lifting patients.
6. **Detail-Oriented:** Paying close attention to detail is important in diagnosing a patient's issue and creating an effective treatment plan.
7. **Organizational Skills:** Managing multiple patients, treatment plans, and administrative tasks requires good organization.
8. **Interpersonal Skills:** Building rapport and trust with patients is essential, as is the ability to work collaboratively with other healthcare providers.
9. **Adaptability and Flexibility:** Being open to change and adaptable is important, especially when working with a diverse patient population and in different healthcare settings.
10. **Enthusiasm and Motivation:** A positive attitude can be infectious, especially in encouraging patients to adhere to their treatment plans and exercise routines.
11. **Professionalism and Ethics:** Maintaining professionalism in all interactions and adhering to ethical standards of practice is paramount in healthcare.
12. **Lifelong Learner:** The field of physical therapy is constantly evolving, so a commitment to ongoing education and staying updated with the latest in medical research and techniques is important.

These traits not only aid physical therapists in providing effective treatment but also in building strong therapeutic relationships with their patients, which can significantly impact the effectiveness of the therapy.

What is placebo?

A placebo is a substance or treatment that has no therapeutic effect and is typically used in clinical trials as a control to test the efficacy of a new medication or treatment. The key characteristics of a placebo are that it is inert and does not contain any active ingredients that are intended to affect health.

Key Aspects of Placebos:

1. **Appearance and Form:** Placebos often look identical to the actual medication being tested but do not contain the active substance. This can include sugar pills, saline injections, or even sham surgeries in some cases.
2. **Placebo Effect:** The placebo effect is a significant psychological phenomenon where a patient experiences a perceived improvement in their condition despite having received an inactive treatment. This effect is believed to result from the patient's expectations of the treatment, suggesting that the mind can sometimes influence the body's response to treatment.
3. **Use in Clinical Trials:** In clinical research, placebos are used as a benchmark to measure the effectiveness of new drugs. Patients are randomly assigned to a placebo group or the treatment group, and neither the patients nor the researchers know who is receiving the real treatment (a method known as double-blinding). This helps to ensure that the results are due to the treatment itself and not to the patients' or researchers' expectations or biases.

4. **Ethical Considerations:** The use of placebos in clinical trials has ethical implications, especially in cases where effective standard treatment is already available. In such cases, using a placebo would mean withholding effective treatment from patients, which might be unethical. Therefore, the use of placebos is typically governed by strict ethical guidelines.

5. **Nocebo Effect:** Similar to the placebo effect, the nocebo effect occurs when negative expectations or beliefs about an inert substance or treatment lead to adverse effects.

The concept of the placebo is fundamental in clinical research as it helps to establish the efficacy and safety of new treatments. While placebos are not designed to have a therapeutic effect, their role in demonstrating the effectiveness of medical treatments is invaluable. The placebo effect itself, a topic of much interest, highlights the complex relationship between the mind and body in health and healing.

Why do placebos work?

The placebo effect, where a patient experiences a perceived or actual improvement in their medical condition after receiving a placebo, an inactive substance or treatment, is a fascinating and complex phenomenon. The exact reasons why placebos work are not entirely understood and are a subject of ongoing research, but several theories and factors contribute to this effect:

1. **Expectation Theory:** One of the main theories is that the placebo effect is driven by the patient's expectations. If a person expects a treatment to work, they may perceive an improvement in their symptoms. This expectation can trigger various physiological responses in the brain and body that produce real symptom relief.

2. **Conditioning:** Placebo effects can also occur through classical conditioning. If a person has previously experienced relief from a particular treatment, they might respond positively to a placebo that looks or feels like the original treatment, due to conditioned responses.

3. **Psychological Response:** The act of receiving treatment can be reassuring and reduce anxiety and stress, which can in turn reduce symptoms or make them more manageable. This is especially true for conditions that are influenced by psychological factors, such as pain, mood disorders, and stress-related symptoms.

4. **Endorphin Release:** Some studies suggest that placebos can trigger the release of endorphins, the body's natural painkillers. This can lead to a real, physiological reduction in pain.

5. **Brain Chemistry and Function Changes:** Neuroimaging studies have shown that placebos can lead to changes in brain activity and chemistry, similar to those caused by active drugs. For instance, in pain treatment, placebos can activate the brain regions involved in pain perception and relief.

6. **Mind-Body Connection:** The placebo effect is a clear example of the mind-body connection, where psychological factors can influence physical health. It underscores the role of mental states in physical healing.

7. **Natural Fluctuation of Symptoms:** In some cases, the perceived improvement might not be directly due to the placebo effect, but rather a natural progression of the illness or condition. Many medical conditions have periods of worsening and improvement, which can coincide with placebo administration.

8. **Reporting Bias:** Sometimes, patients may report improvements in symptoms because they believe they are expected to feel better after receiving what they think is a treatment, rather than an actual improvement in their condition.

The placebo effect highlights the importance of psychological and contextual factors in medical treatment and the perception of health. It is a reminder that the way patients perceive and react to treatments is a critical component of the therapeutic process. Understanding and harnessing the placebo effect can be a powerful tool in improving healthcare outcomes, although it is crucial to approach it ethically and transparently.

What are the advantages of placebos?

The use of placebos in medical research and practice offers several advantages, mainly in the context of clinical trials and understanding patient responses to treatments. Here are some of the key benefits:

1. **Determining Drug Efficacy:** In clinical trials, placebos are essential for establishing the effectiveness of a new drug. By comparing the effects of the drug to a placebo, researchers can determine whether the drug's effects are due to its active ingredients or to psychological factors.

2. **Controlling for Psychological Factors:** The placebo effect highlights the impact of psychological factors on physical health. Using a placebo control helps to isolate the psychological influences from the physiological effects of the treatment.
3. **Reducing Medication Use:** In some cases, particularly where medication might pose a risk of side effects, a placebo can offer a safer alternative. If a patient responds well to a placebo, they might avoid unnecessary medication use.
4. **Ethical Treatment Option:** In situations where no known effective treatment exists, a placebo may ethically be used to provide some relief, provided that there is no deception involved and it is done with informed consent.
5. **Understanding Patient Perception and Expectation:** Placebos help in understanding how patient expectations and beliefs affect the perception of symptoms and treatment outcomes. This can be valuable in enhancing patient care and developing more effective treatment approaches.
6. **Mind-Body Interaction Insight:** Research on placebos contributes to our understanding of the mind-body interaction, particularly how mental and emotional states can physically influence the body.
7. **Managing Certain Conditions:** For some conditions, especially those with a significant psychological component (like certain types of pain or depression), placebos can sometimes lead to symptom relief.
8. **Reducing Costs:** In research, using placebos can be more cost-effective than using the actual drug, especially in the preliminary stages of a study.
9. **No Drug Side Effects:** Since placebos do not contain active ingredients, they do not carry the risk of side effects associated with many medications. This can be particularly advantageous in the context of clinical trials.
10. **Improving Doctor-Patient Relationship:** The act of receiving treatment, even if it is a placebo, can improve the doctor-patient relationship, fostering a sense of being cared for and taken seriously.

It is important to note that while placebos have these advantages, their use in clinical practice is subject to ethical considerations. Placebos should not replace effective treatments, and their use must always consider patient welfare and informed consent. Understanding and harnessing the placebo effect can lead to more comprehensive and patient-centered approaches to treatment.

What is the purpose of a placebo?

The purpose of a placebo in medical research and practice can be multifaceted, primarily serving as a tool in clinical trials and understanding the impact of treatment beyond the pharmacological effects. Here are the main purposes of using a placebo:

1. **Establishing Efficacy in Clinical Trials:** In clinical trials, the primary purpose of a placebo is to serve as a control to determine the efficacy of a new drug or treatment. By comparing the effects of the active treatment with the placebo, researchers can assess whether the treatment's effects are due to its specific action or to other factors like patient expectations.
2. **Controlling for the Placebo Effect:** The placebo effect can be powerful, and using a placebo control helps to isolate this psychological or psychosomatic component from the actual physiological effects of the treatment being tested. This is crucial for obtaining accurate and reliable results in clinical research.
3. **Ethical Use in Practice:** In some clinical settings, particularly when no known effective treatment exists, or when administering a non-active treatment is considered safe and ethical, placebos might be used to provide psychological relief to patients. This must be done under strict ethical guidelines and with informed consent.
4. **Understanding Patient Responses:** Placebos help in understanding how patient beliefs, expectations, and psychological states influence their perception of symptoms and treatment outcomes. This insight can inform clinical practice and enhance patient care.
5. **Reduction of Medication Use:** For some conditions, particularly those with a significant psychological component, a placebo can lead to symptom relief without the need for medication, thereby avoiding potential side effects and interactions associated with pharmaceuticals.
6. **Investigating Mind-Body Interactions:** Placebo research provides valuable information on the mind-

body connection, offering insights into how psychological factors can influence physical health and healing processes.

7. **Training and Education:** In medical training and education, understanding the placebo effect and its implications helps future healthcare providers in comprehensively managing patient care.

8. **Cost-Effective Research:** In some cases, using placebos can reduce the costs associated with clinical trials, especially in the early stages of research.

While placebos have these diverse purposes, their use, particularly in clinical practice, must be approached with caution and ethical consideration. Placebos are not meant to replace effective treatments but can be a valuable tool in understanding and enhancing the therapeutic process. Their use should always prioritize patient welfare, informed consent, and transparent communication.

How effective are placebos?

The effectiveness of placebos can vary significantly depending on various factors. The "placebo effect" – where a patient experiences a perceived or actual improvement in their condition after receiving a placebo – is a well-documented phenomenon, but its strength and impact can differ from person to person and condition to condition. Here are some key points about the effectiveness of placebos:

1. **Condition Specific:** The effectiveness of a placebo tends to vary depending on the type of condition being treated. Placebos are often more effective for conditions with subjective symptoms, such as pain, fatigue, or depression, where the patient's perception plays a large role.

2. **Psychological Factors:** A significant part of the placebo effect is psychological. Patients who believe they are receiving an effective treatment often experience a greater placebo effect. This effect is influenced by expectations, beliefs, the patient's previous experiences with treatments, and the perceived credibility of the treatment.

3. **Neurobiological Responses:** Research shows that placebos can trigger real physiological responses in the brain and body. For instance, in pain treatment, placebos can activate endorphin release, which can genuinely reduce pain.

4. **Patient-Provider Relationship:** The interaction between a healthcare provider and a patient can also influence the effectiveness of a placebo. A positive, supportive relationship can enhance the placebo effect.

5. **Context and Presentation:** How a placebo is presented (e.g., as a pill or injection) and the environment in which it is given can affect its effectiveness. More "impressive" interventions, such as injections, may have a stronger placebo effect than simpler ones like pills.

6. **Variable Outcomes:** Not everyone responds to placebos, and the degree of response can vary greatly. Some people may experience significant improvement in their symptoms, while others may not notice any change.

7. **Ethical Considerations:** While the placebo effect can be significant, it is essential to consider the ethics of using placebos in clinical practice. Deceiving patients by presenting placebos as active treatments raises ethical concerns.

8. **Limitations in Severe Conditions:** Placebos generally have limited effectiveness in treating severe or life-threatening conditions, such as cancer or heart disease, where objective measures (like tumor size or cholesterol levels) are used to assess treatment efficacy.

9. **Research Tool:** In clinical trials, placebos are invaluable for determining the efficacy of new treatments. They help to distinguish the specific effects of the treatment from psychological or other non-specific effects.

10. **Long-term Effectiveness:** While placebos can provide temporary relief or improvement in symptoms, they do not typically provide a long-term cure, especially for chronic or progressive conditions.

In summary, while placebos can be surprisingly effective in certain situations, largely due to psychological factors and the body's own ability to mimic responses to real treatments, their use as a therapeutic tool is limited and must be approached with ethical consideration. They are most valuable as a control in clinical research.

What is a Nocebo?

The term "nocebo" refers to a phenomenon that is essentially the opposite of the placebo effect. While a placebo involves health improvements or beneficial responses following a treatment that has no therapeutic value, a nocebo effect occurs when negative expectations or beliefs about a harmless or inert treatment or substance lead to adverse side effects or a worsening of symptoms. Here are key aspects of the nocebo effect:

1. **Negative Expectations:** The nocebo effect arises from a person's belief or expectation that a treatment will cause harm or discomfort. For instance, if a patient believes that a medication (even if it is a placebo) will cause side effects, they might actually experience those negative effects.
2. **Psychological Basis:** Like the placebo effect, the nocebo effect is primarily psychological. It demonstrates the power of the mind to influence bodily responses, even in the absence of an active pharmaceutical agent.
3. **Physical Manifestations:** The nocebo effect can produce real, physical symptoms, such as pain, nausea, headaches, or other bodily responses. These symptoms are not due to any direct physiological effect of a treatment but are instead triggered by the person's psychological state.
4. **Communication and Context:** The way in which medical information is communicated can contribute to the nocebo effect. For example, a healthcare provider discussing potential side effects in a way that emphasizes their severity or likelihood can inadvertently contribute to the nocebo effect.
5. **Anxiety and Fear:** Anxiety and fear about treatment outcomes can significantly contribute to the nocebo effect. Individuals who are more anxious or fearful about medical treatments or their health in general may be more susceptible to experiencing nocebo responses.
6. **Ethical Implications:** The nocebo effect raises important ethical considerations in clinical practice and research. It underscores the need for healthcare providers to communicate effectively and empathetically, balancing the need for informed consent with the potential for inducing nocebo responses.
7. **Clinical Trials and Research:** In clinical trials, the nocebo effect can complicate the interpretation of data. Participants who experience negative side effects in the placebo arm of a study may be experiencing the nocebo effect.
8. **Treatment Adherence:** The nocebo effect can impact treatment adherence, as patients may discontinue or avoid beneficial treatments due to fear of side effects, which they might actually be experiencing due to their negative expectations rather than the treatment itself.

In summary, the nocebo effect is a fascinating illustration of the mind-body connection, showing how negative expectations or beliefs can result in adverse health outcomes. It highlights the importance of considering psychological factors in medical treatment and the way information is conveyed to patients.

What is the difference between placebo and nocebo?

The placebo and nocebo effects are two sides of the same coin, both demonstrating the powerful influence of the mind on the body, particularly in the context of medical treatment. However, they differ fundamentally in their outcomes and the mechanisms that drive them. Here is a comparison:

Placebo Effect

1. **Definition:** A placebo effect occurs when a patient experiences a positive outcome, such as pain relief or improvement in symptoms, after receiving an inert or inactive treatment, due to their belief in the treatment's efficacy.
2. **Mechanism:** This effect is driven by positive expectations. If a person believes a treatment will help them, this can lead to real changes in their health.
3. **Outcomes:** The outcomes are generally beneficial, such as reduced pain, alleviation of symptoms, or even improvement in a disease condition.
4. **Examples:** A sugar pill improving headaches, or a saline injection reducing joint pain.
5. **Psychological Basis:** Often based on optimism, belief, and expectation of benefit.

Nocebo Effect

1. **Definition:** The nocebo effect occurs when negative expectations or beliefs about an inert or inactive treatment lead to adverse side effects or a worsening of symptoms.
2. **Mechanism:** Driven by negative expectations or fear. The anticipation of negative outcomes can cause a person to experience those negative effects.

3. **Outcomes:** The outcomes are detrimental, such as increased pain, development of symptoms, or perceived worsening of a condition.

4. **Examples:** A person experiencing side effects like nausea after taking a sugar pill because they were told the pill might cause such effects.

5. **Psychological Basis:** Often based on fear, anxiety, and expectation of harm.

Common Ground

- **Influence of Perception:** Both are influenced by how a treatment is perceived, rather than any pharmacological action of the treatment itself.

- **Psychosomatic Response:** Both demonstrate the ability of the mind to influence physical health - the body's physiological response to psychological stimuli.

Key Differences

- **Nature of Effect:** Placebo effects are positive and beneficial, while nocebo effects are negative and harmful.

- **Expectation:** Placebo effects stem from positive expectations, whereas nocebo effects are the result of negative expectations.

In both cases, these phenomena underscore the complex interaction between the mind, body, and the external factors influencing health perceptions. They highlight the importance of psychological factors in medical treatments and the need for mindful communication in healthcare settings to maximize therapeutic outcomes and minimize potential harm.

What is placebo surgery?

Placebo surgery, also known as sham surgery, is a procedure used in clinical trials to test the efficacy of surgical interventions. It involves performing a fake surgical procedure on a group of study participants, mimicking all aspects of the actual surgery without actually performing the therapeutic part of the operation. This method is used to create a control group that is subjected to the same experience as the group undergoing the real surgery, minus the critical surgical element believed to be therapeutic.

Key Aspects of Placebo Surgery:

1. **Mimicking Real Surgery:** In placebo surgery, patients are treated as if they are receiving actual surgery. This includes preparation for surgery, anesthesia, making incisions, and sometimes even mimicking the sounds and sensations of the real procedure.

2. **Blinding:** Both the patients and the researchers assessing the outcomes are often blinded to who received the actual surgery and who received the placebo surgery. This is done to prevent bias in the reporting and assessment of results.

3. **Ethical Considerations:** Placebo surgery raises significant ethical concerns, primarily because it involves subjecting patients to potentially unnecessary risks associated with surgery, such as infection, anesthesia complications, and the psychological impact of undergoing a surgical procedure. Consequently, the use of placebo surgery is highly regulated and is considered ethical only under strict conditions.

4. **Conditions for Use:** It is typically used in situations where there is uncertainty about the efficacy of a surgical procedure, and where the risks of the placebo surgery are justified by the potential benefits of the knowledge to be gained.

5. **Informed Consent:** Patients must give informed consent to participate in such trials, with full knowledge that they might receive the placebo surgery.

6. **Purpose in Research:** Placebo surgery helps to determine whether the benefits of a surgical procedure are due to the actual surgical intervention or to the placebo effect, which can include the patient's belief in the efficacy of the surgery or the natural course of the disease.

7. **Historical Examples:** There have been notable instances where placebo surgeries have led to surprising findings, such as in the case of certain knee surgeries, where placebo surgeries performed as well as actual surgeries in improving patient outcomes.

8. **Outcome Assessment:** The outcomes of both the real and placebo surgeries are compared to evaluate the effectiveness of the surgical intervention.

Placebo surgery is a powerful tool in medical research but is used sparingly due to the ethical complexities involved. When conducted, it provides valuable insights into the effectiveness of surgical procedures and the extent to which the benefits of surgery might be attributed to the placebo effect.

What is a placebo procedure?

A placebo procedure, similar to placebo surgery, is a medical intervention that mimics an actual therapeutic procedure but does not contain an active therapeutic element. It is primarily used in clinical research to test the efficacy of a new treatment or procedure. The placebo procedure is designed to appear identical to the real treatment in every way, except that it lacks the key therapeutic component. This approach helps to isolate the effects of the treatment itself from other factors, such as patient expectations or the natural progression of a disease.

Key Features of Placebo Procedures:

1. **Mimicry of Actual Treatment:** The placebo procedure closely imitates the real treatment in appearance and process, creating the impression that a legitimate medical intervention is being carried out.
2. **Lack of Active Therapeutic Elements:** Although it mimics the real treatment, the placebo procedure does not contain any active therapeutic agents or elements that are expected to affect the condition being treated.
3. **Blinding:** In clinical trials, both the patients and the researchers are often unaware of who receives the actual treatment and who receives the placebo. This method, known as "double-blinding," helps to prevent bias in the results.
4. **Use in Clinical Trials:** Placebo procedures are commonly used in clinical trials to test the efficacy and safety of new treatments. By comparing outcomes between the placebo group and the group receiving the actual treatment, researchers can determine the true effect of the treatment.
5. **Ethical Considerations:** Like placebo surgery, placebo procedures raise important ethical questions, especially regarding subjecting patients to potentially unnecessary procedures. Informed consent is critical, where participants must be fully aware that they might receive a placebo as part of the study.
6. **Patient Expectation and Psychological Effects:** One of the purposes of a placebo procedure is to account for the psychological effects that the act of receiving treatment can have on a patient's perception of their symptoms and overall health.
7. **Reducing Bias:** Placebo procedures help in reducing the placebo effect's bias in the assessment of a new treatment's efficacy. This is particularly important for conditions that are subjective and can be influenced by the patient's mindset, like pain or depression.
8. **Control Group in Research:** In a clinical trial, the group receiving the placebo procedure serves as a control group, providing a baseline to compare the effects of the actual treatment.

Conclusion

Placebo procedures are a valuable tool in medical research, allowing for more accurate assessment of a treatment's true effects. However, their use must be carefully considered and ethically justified, ensuring that the potential benefits of the knowledge gained outweigh the risks to the participants.

What is a placebo investigation?

A placebo investigation, commonly known as a placebo-controlled study, is a type of clinical research designed to evaluate the effectiveness and safety of a medical treatment, drug, or therapeutic procedure. In these studies, the investigational treatment is compared against a placebo – an inactive substance or sham procedure that has no therapeutic effect. This comparison is crucial for determining the true efficacy of the treatment being tested, as it helps to isolate the specific effects of the treatment from other factors.

Key Features of Placebo Investigations:

1. **Control Group:** In a placebo investigation, one group of participants receives the actual treatment, while a control group receives a placebo. The placebo is designed to look, feel, or taste like the actual treatment but lacks the active therapeutic component.
2. **Blinding:** To minimize bias, placebo investigations often employ blinding. In a single-blind study, the participants don't know whether they're receiving the real treatment or a placebo. In a double-blind study, neither the participants nor the researchers know who is receiving which until the study is completed.
3. **Objective Evaluation:** Comparing the outcomes of the treatment group and the placebo group allows researchers to objectively assess the treatment's effectiveness. Any difference in outcomes can be attributed to the treatment itself, rather than to participants' expectations or other external factors.
4. **Psychological Effects:** Placebo investigations account for the "placebo effect," where participants may experience a perceived or actual improvement in their condition simply because they believe they are receiving an effective treatment.

5. **Standard in Clinical Trials:** Placebo-controlled studies are considered a gold standard in clinical trials, especially in the development and testing of new drugs, as they provide a clear measure of a treatment's efficacy over and above the placebo effect.
6. **Ethical Considerations:** The use of placebos raises ethical issues, particularly in cases where withholding an effective treatment could harm participants. Therefore, placebo investigations are carefully designed to ensure ethical standards are met, often used when no current effective treatment is available or as an addition to standard treatment.
7. **Statistical Reliability:** These studies are designed to provide statistically reliable data, helping researchers determine if the effects of the treatment are clinically significant and not just due to chance.
8. **Informed Consent:** Participants in placebo-controlled studies are typically required to give informed consent, acknowledging that they may receive a placebo instead of the active treatment.

Conclusion

Placebo investigations are a fundamental part of clinical research, providing a rigorous method for testing the efficacy and safety of new treatments. By controlling for factors like participant expectations and the natural progression of disease, these studies help ensure that the benefits of a new treatment are accurately understood and scientifically validated.

What is the process of meditation?

Meditation is a mental exercise that involves focusing and quieting the mind, often for the purposes of achieving a state of relaxation, heightened awareness, or some kind of spiritual insight or experience. While there are many styles and techniques of meditation, most share some common elements in their process. Here is a generalized outline of the meditation process:

1. **Preparation:**
   - **Choosing a Quiet Location:** Find a quiet and comfortable place where you won't be disturbed.
   - **Setting a Time Limit:** Especially for beginners, it is helpful to choose a short time, like 5 or 10 minutes.
   - **Comfortable Position:** Sit or lie in a comfortable position. You can sit on a chair, on the floor, or on a cushion. Keep your back straight to prevent drowsiness.
2. **Body Relaxation:**
   - Take a few deep breaths to relax your body.
   - Do a quick body scan mentally from head to toe, relaxing each part of the body.
3. **Focus on the Breath:**
   - Focus your attention on your breath, the inhalation and exhalation.
   - Feel the air entering your nostrils, filling your lungs, and then leaving your body.
   - This focus on breathing helps anchor the mind in the present moment.
4. **Mindfulness:**
   - As you meditate, you will notice your mind wandering to other thoughts.
   - When you realize your mind has wandered, gently redirect your focus back to your breathing.
   - The key is to observe these wandering thoughts without judgment and then return to your breath.
5. **Deeper Focus or Visualization (Optional):**
   - Depending on the type of meditation, you might engage in visualization, repeating a mantra, or focusing on a particular concept like love or compassion.
6. **Maintaining Stillness:**
   - Try to stay still during your meditation, resisting the urge to itch, fidget, or adjust your position too frequently.
7. **Gentle Return:**
   - When your time is up, don't stand up immediately.
   - Open your eyes slowly and give yourself a moment to become aware of your surroundings and body.
   - Gradually allow yourself to transition from the meditative state back to a normal state of consciousness.
8. **Reflection:**
   - After the session, spend a few minutes reflecting on the experience. Notice any changes in your mood, thoughts, or feelings.

9. **Consistency:**
   - Regular practice enhances the benefits of meditation. Try to meditate daily, even if it is for a short period.

Types of Meditation:

- **Mindfulness Meditation:** Focuses on being intensely aware of what you are sensing and feeling in the moment.
- **Transcendental Meditation:** Involves silently repeating a mantra to yourself to focus your mind.
- **Guided Meditation:** Uses guided imagery or visualization led by a teacher or an audio guide.
- **Loving-kindness Meditation (Metta):** Involves mentally sending goodwill, kindness, and warmth towards others.

Benefits:

Meditation is known for its stress-reducing benefits, but it also improves concentration, increases self-awareness, and can contribute to a greater sense of overall well-being.

Remember, meditation is a skill that takes practice. Be patient with yourself, and don't be discouraged if your mind wanders or if you find it challenging initially. With time and practice, meditation typically becomes easier and more effective.

What is mindfulness?

Mindfulness is a mental state achieved by focusing one's awareness on the present moment, while calmly acknowledging and accepting one's feelings, thoughts, and bodily sensations. It is a therapeutic technique rooted in mindfulness meditation, a practice derived from Buddhist traditions. Over the past few decades, mindfulness has been increasingly incorporated into Western psychology and healthcare as a means of helping people manage a variety of mental and physical conditions.

Key Elements of Mindfulness:

1. **Present Moment Awareness:** Mindfulness involves being fully present in the moment, paying attention to what's happening right now – not in the past or the future.
2. **Non-judgmental Observation:** This means observing thoughts, feelings, and sensations without labeling them as good or bad, right or wrong. It is about accepting whatever arises in your awareness at each moment.
3. **Acceptance:** Mindfulness encourages acceptance of whatever is happening in your internal or external environment. This does not mean resignation or giving up, but rather acknowledging the reality of the situation.
4. **Mind-Body Connection:** Mindfulness fosters a heightened awareness of the connection between the mind and body. Practitioners often report feeling more attuned to physical sensations and emotions.

Practices and Techniques:

1. **Mindfulness Meditation:** Sitting quietly and focusing on your natural breathing or on a word or phrase. You observe the thoughts, emotions, and sensations that arise, acknowledging them without judgment and returning to your focus.
2. **Body Scan Meditation:** Paying attention to different parts of the body, noticing any physical sensations, pain, or discomfort.
3. **Mindful Breathing:** Focusing solely on the breath, observing each inhale and exhale without trying to change it.
4. **Mindful Observation:** Focusing on an object or a process (like eating or walking) and observing it in a detailed way.
5. **Mindful Listening:** Listening without judgment, staying present and fully engaging with what is being heard.

Applications of Mindfulness:

1. **Stress Reduction:** One of the most common reasons people try mindfulness is to reduce stress.
2. **Managing Anxiety and Depression:** Mindfulness can help break the cycle of chronic negative thoughts.
3. **Chronic Pain Management:** It helps in altering the perception of pain and can improve quality of life.
4. **Improving Focus and Concentration:** Regular mindfulness practice can enhance attention and focus.
5. **Enhancing Emotional Regulation:** It aids in recognizing and accepting complex emotions, thereby facilitating better emotional regulation.
6. **Coping with Illness:** Mindfulness can be a tool to help people deal with serious illness and the anxiety and depression that can accompany it.

7. **Preventing Relapse of Mental Health Issues:** It is used in therapies like Mindfulness-Based Cognitive Therapy (MBCT) to help prevent the relapse of depression.

Mindfulness is adaptable and can be practiced by anyone, regardless of age or background. While it has its roots in Buddhist meditation, a secular practice of mindfulness has entered the mainstream as a respected and recommended therapy. It is a versatile tool, beneficial not only for mental health issues but also for enhancing overall well-being and quality of life.

What are the benefits of mindfulness?

Mindfulness, a practice of focusing one's attention on the present moment and accepting it without judgment, offers a wide array of benefits for mental, emotional, and physical health. These benefits have been increasingly recognized and supported by scientific research. Here are some of the key benefits of mindfulness:

1. **Stress Reduction:** Mindfulness is highly effective in reducing stress. It helps in managing and responding to stressful situations more calmly and effectively.
2. **Enhances Emotional Well-being:** Regular mindfulness practice can lead to a decrease in depressive symptoms, anxiety, and negative emotions. It also increases positive emotions and leads to a more optimistic outlook on life.
3. **Improves Focus and Concentration:** Practicing mindfulness can improve the ability to concentrate and focus. It helps in reducing mind-wandering and improves cognitive performance.
4. **Increases Resilience:** Mindfulness enhances the ability to deal with adverse events and challenges, fostering resilience.
5. **Improves Relationships:** By increasing empathy and compassion, mindfulness can improve relationships with others. It helps in understanding others' perspectives and responding to relationship stress more constructively.
6. **Reduces Rumination:** Mindfulness practice can help in reducing the tendency to ruminate on negative thoughts, a habit that is often linked with depression and anxiety.
7. **Enhances Self-Awareness:** Mindfulness increases self-awareness, helping individuals to understand themselves better and make more aligned choices.
8. **Better Sleep Quality:** Mindfulness can contribute to a better quality of sleep, as it helps in calming the mind and reducing the occurrence of racing thoughts that can interfere with falling and staying asleep.
9. **Pain Management:** It can alter the perception of pain and is often used as a part of the treatment plan for chronic pain management.
10. **Boosts Immune System:** Regular mindfulness practice can have a positive impact on the immune system, making the body better at fighting off illnesses.
11. **Lowers Blood Pressure:** Mindfulness meditation can lead to a reduction in blood pressure, which is beneficial for heart health.
12. **Decreases Cognitive Decline from Aging or Alzheimer's:** Some studies suggest that mindfulness can help slow the progression of cognitive decline in the elderly, including those with Alzheimer's disease.
13. **Improves Mental Health:** In clinical settings, mindfulness forms the basis of therapies like Mindfulness-Based Stress Reduction (MBSR) and Mindfulness-Based Cognitive Therapy (MBCT), which are effective for a range of mental health issues.
14. **Helps with Substance Abuse and Recovery:** Mindfulness training can be an effective tool in the treatment of substance abuse and in managing cravings and preventing relapse.
15. **Increases General Health and Well-being:** Overall, mindfulness contributes to a greater sense of well-being and encourages a healthy lifestyle.

While mindfulness has many benefits, it is important to note that it is not a panacea and should not replace medical treatment where necessary. It is, however, a valuable tool that can complement other treatment approaches and is accessible to most people.

What is the difference between meditation and mindfulness?

Meditation and mindfulness are closely related concepts and practices, but they are not exactly the same. Understanding their differences can help in choosing the right practice for personal needs and goals.

Meditation:

1. **Broad Practice:** Meditation is a broad term that encompasses various techniques of focus, concentration, and mental discipline designed to calm the mind and achieve a state of relaxed awareness or contemplation. It is a deliberate practice.
2. **Different Forms:** There are many forms of meditation, including mindfulness meditation, transcendental meditation, loving-kindness meditation, concentrative meditation, etc., each with different techniques and goals.
3. **Dedicated Time and Space:** Meditation typically involves setting aside specific time and finding a quiet space to practice these techniques. It often requires a posture like sitting, though there are moving meditations like walking meditation.
4. **Variety of Goals:** The goals of meditation can vary widely, from achieving a sense of peace and relaxation to spiritual enlightenment. It often involves going beyond or detaching from the immediate sensory experience.

Mindfulness:

1. **Specific Type of Meditation:** Mindfulness is a type of meditation focused on the awareness and acceptance of the present moment. It is about being fully engaged with whatever is happening, without judgment or distraction.
2. **Everyday Practice:** Mindfulness can be practiced at any moment of the day, not just during a dedicated meditation session. It is about bringing a mindful approach to everyday activities like eating, walking, or listening.
3. **Focus on the Present Moment:** The key aspect of mindfulness is the emphasis on being present and fully engaged with the current experience – acknowledging and accepting thoughts, feelings, and sensations as they arise.
4. **Therapeutic Tool:** Mindfulness is widely used in mental health and therapy settings, particularly in approaches like Mindfulness-Based Stress Reduction (MBSR) and Mindfulness-Based Cognitive Therapy (MBCT).

Key Differences:

- **Scope:** Meditation is a broader concept that includes various practices, of which mindfulness is one. Mindfulness is a form of meditation focused specifically on the present moment and awareness.
- **Application:** Meditation often requires dedicated time and space and is practiced for specific durations. Mindfulness, on the other hand, can be incorporated into daily life at any moment.
- **Techniques and Goals:** While meditation can have a variety of techniques and goals (including transcendental experiences or deep contemplation), mindfulness specifically aims at being present and fully experiencing the current moment without judgment.

In summary, while all mindfulness can be considered meditation, not all meditation is mindfulness. Mindfulness is a specific kind of meditation practice with a particular focus on the present moment, awareness, and acceptance, and it can be practiced both as a formal meditation and as a way of life.

Why is meditation beneficial?

Meditation, a practice with ancient roots in various cultural and spiritual traditions, has gained widespread acceptance in the modern world for its numerous mental, emotional, and physical health benefits. These benefits have been supported by a growing body of scientific research. Here are some of the key reasons why meditation is beneficial:

1. **Reduces Stress:** Meditation is well-known for its ability to reduce stress. It lowers levels of cortisol, the body's stress hormone, which helps reduce symptoms associated with stress such as anxiety, high blood pressure, and insomnia.
2. **Improves Emotional Well-being:** Regular meditation can lead to an improved self-image and a more positive outlook on life. It can also decrease symptoms of depression and anxiety.
3. **Enhances Attention and Concentration:** Certain types of meditation, like mindfulness, can train the brain to focus better, increase the strength and endurance of your attention, and may even improve memory.
4. **Promotes Mindfulness:** By encouraging present-moment awareness, meditation helps cultivate mindfulness, which can improve your quality of life and how you engage with others.
5. **Helps with Sleep:** Meditation can help relax the body, releasing tension and placing you in a peaceful state in which you are more likely to fall asleep.

6. **Can Decrease Blood Pressure:** Meditation can improve physical health by reducing strain on the heart. Over time, high blood pressure makes the heart work harder to pump blood, which can lead to poor heart function.

7. **Improves Emotional Health:** Some forms of meditation can lead to an improved self-image and more positive outlook on life. It can also decrease symptoms of depression.

8. **Can Help with Pain Management:** The mental discipline developed through meditation can help break the cycle of chronic pain where pain increases stress and fatigue, which in turn increases pain.

9. **Enhances Self-Awareness:** Some forms of meditation can help you develop a stronger understanding of yourself, helping you grow into your best self.

10. **Reduces Age-Related Memory Loss:** The enhanced focus and clarity gained through regular meditation may increase memory and mental clarity. These benefits can help fight age-related memory loss and dementia.

11. **May Help Fight Addictions:** Meditation can develop mental discipline and willpower, which can help you avoid triggers for unwanted impulses and potentially aid in recovering from addiction.

12. **Increases Kindness:** Some types of meditation, like Metta (a type of loving-kindness meditation), increase positive feelings and actions toward oneself and others.

13. **Can Help Reduce Symptoms in People with Chronic Diseases:** For some chronic diseases like heart disease, meditation can be a part of the treatment plan to help manage symptoms and improve overall quality of life.

It is important to note that while meditation can be a powerful tool for health and well-being, it is not a standalone cure or treatment. It is often most effective when used in conjunction with other forms of therapy and medical treatment, especially for more serious conditions. Additionally, the benefits of meditation can vary greatly from person to person and depend on regular practice.

What are the best meditation techniques?

The "best" meditation techniques vary depending on individual preferences, goals, and needs. Different techniques offer different benefits and experiences. Here are some widely practiced and effective meditation techniques:

1. **Mindfulness Meditation:**
   - **Origin:** Rooted in Buddhist meditation practices.
   - **Technique:** Involves paying attention to your thoughts as they pass through your mind. The aim is not to judge the thoughts or become involved with them but simply to be aware of each mental note as it arises.
   - **Benefits:** Increases moment-to-moment awareness, reduces stress, enhances personal insight and emotional intelligence.

2. **Focused Attention Meditation:**
   - **Technique:** Involves concentrating on a single object, thought, sound, or visualization. It emphasizes ridding your mind of distraction. Common focuses include breathing, a mantra, or a calming sound.
   - **Benefits:** Enhances concentration, reduces random mental activity, increases mental clarity.

3. **Transcendental Meditation:**
   - **Technique:** Practiced for 20 minutes twice daily while sitting comfortably with the eyes closed. It involves silently repeating a specific mantra given by a trained teacher.
   - **Benefits:** Reduces stress and anxiety, improves heart health, enhances clarity of thought.

4. **Body Scan or Progressive Relaxation:**
   - **Technique:** Involves scanning your body for areas of tension. The goal is to notice tension and to allow it to release.
   - **Benefits:** Promotes body awareness, relaxation, and stress reduction.

5. **Loving-kindness Meditation (Metta Meditation):**
   - **Technique:** Involves mentally sending kindness, love, and well-wishes to yourself and others. It starts with self-compassion, then expands to others.
   - **Benefits:** Increases feelings of compassion and love, decreases negative emotions toward oneself and others.

6. **Movement Meditation:**
   - **Technique:** Movement meditation is an active form of meditation where movement guides you. Examples include yoga, walking meditation, Tai Chi, or Qigong.
   - **Benefits:** Good for those who find peace in action and prefer to let their minds wander.
7. **Visualization Meditation:**
   - **Technique:** Involves visualizing a scene, image, or journey with a specific goal in mind. The visualization should be as vivid and detailed as possible.
   - **Benefits:** Promotes relaxation, calmness, and can be motivational.
8. **Chakra Meditation:**
   - **Technique:** Focuses on cleansing and opening the body's chakras or energy centers. Often involves visualization or guided imagery.
   - **Benefits:** Promotes healing and spiritual development.
9. **Guided Meditation:**
   - **Technique:** Involves meditating with the help of a guided recording led by a narrator or teacher.
   - **Benefits:** Easier for beginners as it requires less effort in terms of concentration.
10. **Zen Meditation (Zazen):**
    - **Origin:** Rooted in Buddhist practice.
    - **Technique:** Involves specific steps and postures and is usually practiced under the guidance of a teacher.
    - **Benefits:** Increases mindfulness, focus, and presence.

It is important to experiment with different techniques to see which one resonates with you the most. For beginners, guided meditations or apps can be a helpful start. Consistency is key to reaping the benefits of meditation, so choosing a practice that you can incorporate into your daily routine is crucial.

What is neuroplasticity and how does it help?

Neuroplasticity refers to the brain's ability to change and adapt as a result of experience. It is a fundamental property of the nervous system that enables learning and memory, and it plays a crucial role in the brain's capacity to recover from injury. Neuroplasticity can occur at various levels, ranging from cellular changes due to learning, to large-scale cortical remapping in response to injury.

How Neuroplasticity Works:

1. **Synaptic Plasticity:** This is the ability of synapses (the connections between neurons) to strengthen or weaken over time in response to increases or decreases in their activity. It underlies learning and memory.
2. **Cortical Remapping:** In response to injury, the brain can reorganize itself by forming new neural connections. For instance, if one part of the brain is damaged, another part may take over some of its functions.
3. **Neurogenesis:** Although once believed impossible, it is now known that the brain can generate new neurons (neurogenesis), albeit to a limited extent and primarily in certain brain regions.

How Neuroplasticity Helps:

1. **Learning and Memory:** Neuroplasticity is essential for learning new information and skills, and for forming memories. When we learn something new, the connections between neurons in our brain change, which reflects that new learning.
2. **Recovery from Brain Injuries:** After a brain injury, such as a stroke, the brain can partly rewire itself. While the damaged area may not fully recover, other parts of the brain can adapt to take over some of its functions, aiding in rehabilitation.
3. **Adapting to New Situations or Changes in the Environment:** Neuroplasticity allows the brain to adapt to new situations or changes in the environment, improving the individual's ability to cope with new challenges.
4. **Overcoming Mental Health Issues:** Treatments for mental health issues, such as cognitive behavioral therapy, exploit neuroplasticity to change maladaptive thought patterns and behaviors.
5. **Age-Related Cognitive Decline:** Engaging in mentally stimulating activities can harness neuroplasticity to maintain and even improve cognitive functioning in older adults, helping to delay or mitigate age-related cognitive decline.

Enhancing Neuroplasticity:

Certain activities and lifestyle choices can enhance neuroplasticity:

- **Continuous Learning:** Engaging in new learning activities and hobbies.
- **Physical Exercise:** Regular physical activity is known to boost neurogenesis and improve brain health.
- **Mindfulness and Meditation:** These practices have been shown to change brain structures and improve areas related to attention, emotion regulation, and mental flexibility.
- **Healthy Diet:** Nutrition plays a role in brain health, with certain diets (like those rich in omega-3 fatty acids) promoting brain plasticity.
- **Adequate Sleep:** Quality sleep is crucial for consolidating learning and memory, processes that are intimately tied to neuroplasticity.

In conclusion, neuroplasticity is a powerful attribute of the brain, enabling it to learn from experiences, adapt to changes, and recover from injuries. Understanding and harnessing neuroplasticity can have profound implications for education, rehabilitation, and mental health treatment.

What are tremors?

Tremors are involuntary, rhythmic muscle movements involving to-and-fro movements (oscillations) of one or more parts of the body. They are the most common of all involuntary movements and can affect various parts of the body, such as the hands, arms, head, face, voice, trunk, and legs. Tremors can occur in anyone, but they are more common in middle-aged and older people.

Types of Tremors:

1. **Resting Tremors:** Occur when the muscle is at rest and not doing any work. They often affect the hands and fingers and are characteristic of Parkinson's disease.
2. **Action Tremors:** Occur with the voluntary movement of a muscle. Most tremors are considered action tremors. Action tremors are further divided into several subtypes:
   - **Postural Tremors:** Occur when holding a position against gravity, such as holding your arms outstretched.
   - **Kinetic Tremors:** Occur during movement of a body part, like moving your wrist up and down.
   - **Intention Tremors:** Occur during targeted movement, such as touching your finger to your nose. They are often associated with cerebellar disorders.
   - **Task-Specific Tremors:** Appear when performing highly skilled, goal-oriented tasks like writing or speaking.
   - **Isometric Tremors:** Occur during a voluntary muscle contraction that is not accompanied by any movement, such as holding an object still.
3. **Physiological Tremors:** These are normal tremors that everyone has and are not usually noticeable. They can be exacerbated by stress, extreme emotions, fatigue, caffeine, or temperature extremes.

Causes of Tremors:

- **Neurological Disorders:** Such as Parkinson's disease, multiple sclerosis, stroke, and traumatic brain injury.
- **Metabolic and Degenerative Conditions:** Like hyperthyroidism or liver failure.
- **Alcohol Abuse or Withdrawal**
- **Certain Medications:** Such as certain anti-depressants, lithium, and certain asthma medications.
- **Stress and Anxiety**
- **Genetic Factors:** Some forms of tremor are inherited.

Diagnosis and Treatment:

- **Medical Evaluation:** Diagnosis typically involves a neurological examination and review of medical history. In some cases, tests like blood tests or brain imaging may be used to identify underlying conditions.
- **Treatment:** Depends on the type of tremor and its cause. It may include medications, physical therapy, lifestyle changes (like reducing caffeine and managing stress), and in severe cases, surgical interventions such as deep brain stimulation.
- **Lifestyle Modifications:** Techniques for relaxation and stress management can be beneficial for some people.

It is important to note that while tremors can be a symptom of a neurological disorder, they are often benign (known as benign essential tremor) and not indicative of a serious disease. However, anyone experiencing unexplained tremors should consult a healthcare provider for a proper diagnosis and appropriate treatment.

What are essential tremors?

Essential tremor is a neurological disorder that causes involuntary and rhythmic shaking. It can affect almost any part of your body, but the trembling occurs most often in your hands — especially when you do simple tasks, such as drinking from a glass or tying shoelaces. Essential tremor is usually not a dangerous condition, but it typically worsens over time and can be severe in some people.

Other characteristics of essential tremor include:

1. **Tremor that worsens with action:** The condition is marked by tremors that become more pronounced during movement or when attempting to use the affected muscles.
2. **Upper body involvement:** Essential tremor usually affects the hands, arms, head, and voice. It may also affect the legs and trunk in less common cases.
3. **Mild at first:** It often starts mildly and progresses gradually.
4. **May affect one or both sides of the body:** It is common for the tremor to affect both sides of the body, but it may be more noticeable in one limb.
5. **Family history:** Many people with essential tremor have a family history of the condition, suggesting a genetic component.

The exact cause of essential tremor is unknown, but it is believed to involve abnormal electrical brain activity. The condition is often confused with Parkinson's disease, but they are distinct disorders. Unlike Parkinson's, essential tremor does not lead to other health problems, and it does not affect life expectancy. However, it can be a significant cause of discomfort and embarrassment and can interfere with daily activities.

Treatment for essential tremor may include medications or, in severe cases, surgical procedures. Lifestyle adjustments and physical therapy can also help manage symptoms.

What are Parkinson's tremors?

Parkinson's tremors are a well-known symptom of Parkinson's disease, a progressive neurological disorder. These tremors are distinct in several ways from those seen in other conditions, like essential tremor. Key characteristics of Parkinson's tremors include:

1. **Resting Tremors:** The tremors of Parkinson's disease are primarily resting tremors, which means they occur when a muscle is relaxed and at rest. For example, a person with Parkinson's might have a tremor in their hands when it is resting in their lap, but it might decrease or stop when they start using the hand.
2. **"Pill-Rolling" Tremor:** A common type of Parkinson's tremor is the so-called "pill-rolling" tremor, where the thumb and fingers move in a circular motion, as if rolling a small pill between them.
3. **Unilateral Onset:** Parkinson's tremors usually begin on one side of the body (unilaterally) and may remain worse on that side even as the disease progresses.
4. **Slowness of Movement (Bradykinesia):** In addition to tremors, Parkinson's disease is often accompanied by a general slowing of movement.
5. **Muscle Stiffness and Postural Instability:** Individuals with Parkinson's disease may also experience rigidity in the muscles and problems with balance and coordination.
6. **Other Non-Motor Symptoms:** Parkinson's disease can also include symptoms unrelated to movement, such as sleep disturbances, mood changes, and cognitive impairment.

The tremors of Parkinson's disease result from a decline in dopamine-producing cells in the brain. Dopamine is a neurotransmitter that plays a key role in controlling movement, and its reduced levels lead to the symptoms of Parkinson's.

Parkinson's disease is a chronic and progressive condition, meaning that its symptoms worsen over time. While there is no cure, medications can significantly reduce symptoms, and in some cases, surgical therapies may be beneficial. Lifestyle modifications, including regular exercise and physical therapy, can also help manage symptoms and improve quality of life.

What are enhanced physiological tremors?

Enhanced physiological tremor is a type of involuntary shaking movement. It is an exaggerated form of a normal tremor that everyone has to some degree, which is usually not perceptible to the naked eye. This type of tremor becomes more noticeable and may become a concern for the affected person. Key aspects of enhanced physiological tremors include:

1. **Exacerbated by Physical Factors:** This tremor is often brought on or intensified by physical exhaustion, stress, intense emotion, extreme temperatures, caffeine, and certain medications.
2. **General Characteristics:** Enhanced physiological tremors are usually fine, rapid tremors that primarily affect the hands but can also involve other parts of the body.
3. **Reversible:** Unlike tremors associated with neurodegenerative disorders, enhanced physiological tremors are typically reversible. They often reduce or disappear when the underlying cause (like stress or caffeine consumption) is removed or managed.
4. **Impact on Daily Activities:** While they can be bothersome, these tremors usually don't indicate a serious underlying medical condition and typically don't interfere significantly with daily tasks.
5. **Differential Diagnosis:** It is important to distinguish enhanced physiological tremor from other types of tremor, such as those caused by Parkinson's disease or essential tremor. This differentiation is usually done based on clinical examination and the patient's history.
6. **Management:** Treatment is not always necessary, particularly if the tremor is mild. If treatment is required, it may involve lifestyle changes, such as reducing caffeine intake and managing stress. In some cases, medications may be used.

Because enhanced physiological tremors are often a response to specific stimuli or circumstances, addressing these factors can be an effective way to manage the condition. However, if someone experiences a significant or persistent tremor, it is advisable to seek medical advice to rule out other causes.

What are drug and metabolite induced tremors?

Drug and metabolite-induced tremors are involuntary shaking movements that occur as a side effect of certain medications or substances. These tremors can arise from the direct effects of a drug on the nervous system or from metabolic changes caused by the drug. They are often reversible and may decrease or disappear once the offending medication is discontinued or its dosage is adjusted. Key aspects of drug and metabolite-induced tremors include:

1. **Wide Range of Medications:** Many different types of medications can cause tremors, including but not limited to antidepressants, mood stabilizers, stimulants, and drugs used to treat asthma or other respiratory conditions.
2. **Variable Characteristics:** The characteristics of the tremor can vary depending on the drug involved. They are commonly action tremors, occurring during voluntary movement, but they can also be resting tremors.
3. **Association with Dosage:** The severity of the tremor may correlate with the dosage of the medication; higher doses are more likely to cause tremors or increase their severity.
4. **Potential for Onset After Long-Term Use:** Some drug-induced tremors only appear after long-term use of a medication, while others might occur shortly after starting the drug.
5. **Metabolic Causes:** In addition to direct drug effects, tremors can be caused by metabolic changes induced by drugs, such as alterations in blood sugar levels or thyroid function.
6. **Management and Treatment:** The primary approach to managing drug-induced tremors is to adjust the medication causing the problem, either by reducing the dosage or switching to an alternative drug. In some cases, additional medications may be prescribed to help control the tremors.
7. **Importance of Medical Supervision:** It is essential to manage these tremors under medical supervision. Patients should not stop or alter their medication regimen without consulting their healthcare provider, as abrupt changes can have serious health consequences.

Understanding the potential side effects of medications, including the possibility of tremors, is an important aspect of managing any treatment plan. If a patient suspects that their tremor is related to a medication, they should consult with their healthcare provider for an assessment and potential adjustment of their treatment.

What are cerebellar tremors?

Cerebellar tremors are a type of tremor that originate from damage or dysfunction in the cerebellum, the part of the brain that is involved in the coordination of movement. These tremors are distinct from other forms of tremor, such as those caused by Parkinson's disease or essential tremor. Key characteristics of cerebellar tremors include:

1. **Intention Tremor:** Cerebellar tremors are primarily intention tremors, meaning they are most evident when a person attempts a voluntary movement, such as reaching for an object. The tremor typically gets worse as the person gets closer to the target.
2. **Cause:** They are often caused by conditions that damage the cerebellum, such as stroke, multiple sclerosis, brain tumor, chronic alcoholism, or a degenerative disease like spinocerebellar ataxia.
3. **Unilateral or Bilateral:** These tremors can affect either one side of the body (unilateral) or both sides (bilateral), depending on the extent and location of cerebellar damage.
4. **Other Cerebellar Symptoms:** Individuals with cerebellar tremors may also exhibit other signs of cerebellar dysfunction, such as uncoordinated movement (ataxia), difficulty with precise movements, and problems with balance and gait.
5. **Posture and Gait Issues:** Patients might have difficulty with maintaining a steady posture and may have an unsteady, wide-based walk.
6. **Severity and Progression:** The severity of cerebellar tremors can vary widely. They may remain relatively stable over time, or they can worsen, especially if the underlying neurological condition progresses.
7. **Treatment:** Managing cerebellar tremors typically focuses on treating the underlying cause, if possible. Medications may help to reduce the tremor, and physical therapy can be beneficial in improving coordination and balance. In some severe cases, surgical interventions like deep brain stimulation (DBS) might be considered.

Cerebellar tremors can significantly impact a person's ability to perform daily activities, especially tasks that require fine motor skills. As such, a comprehensive approach that includes medical treatment, physical therapy, and adaptive devices can be important for maintaining independence and quality of life.

What are psychogenic tremors?

Psychogenic tremors, also known as functional tremors, are a type of movement disorder that is thought to have a psychological origin. These tremors are part of a group of symptoms known as functional movement disorders, which are physical manifestations of psychological distress. Characteristics of psychogenic tremors include:

1. **Variable Symptoms:** Psychogenic tremors often vary in their frequency, amplitude, and location. They can change or disappear with distraction or when the individual's attention is directed away from the tremor.
2. **Sudden Onset:** These tremors often begin suddenly and can sometimes be traced back to a traumatic or stressful event.
3. **Inconsistency and Coactivation Sign:** The tremor may change in terms of its characteristics (such as direction, amplitude, or frequency) over time or even during a single examination. A "coactivation sign" is a typical feature, where increased tremor intensity is seen when an opposing muscle group is activated.
4. **Presence of Other Psychiatric Symptoms:** Patients with psychogenic tremors often have a history of psychiatric illness or psychological stressors. Conditions such as anxiety, depression, or post-traumatic stress disorder (PTSD) are commonly associated.
5. **Response to Placebo or Suggestion:** These tremors may improve with placebo treatment or through suggestion during a clinical examination.
6. **Absence of Neurological Disorder:** Psychogenic tremors usually occur in the absence of an identifiable neurological disorder that could explain the symptoms.
7. **Functional Disability:** Despite the absence of an organic cause, the tremor can be disabling and significantly interfere with daily activities.
8. **Diagnosis and Treatment:** Diagnosing psychogenic tremors typically involves ruling out other medical causes. Treatment often requires a multidisciplinary approach, including psychological therapy, physical therapy, and sometimes medication to manage associated psychiatric symptoms.

It is important to note that psychogenic tremors are a real and disabling condition. They are not "made up" by the patient. The psychological distress causing these tremors is genuine, and effective treatment usually requires addressing the underlying psychological factors.

What are tremors in children?

Tremors in children can be a cause for concern, but they can also be a part of normal development or due to benign conditions. It is important to understand the various causes and characteristics of tremors in children. Here is an overview:

1. **Physiological Tremors:** These are fine, rapid tremors that are a normal part of motor development in children. They are usually most noticeable when the child is stressed or anxious.
2. **Enhanced Physiological Tremors:** Similar to adults, children may experience enhanced physiological tremors due to stress, fatigue, or certain medications.
3. **Essential Tremor:** Although more common in adults, essential tremor can also occur in children. It is often characterized by tremors during voluntary movements, like eating or writing, and may have a genetic component.
4. **Cerebellar Tremors:** These are intention tremors that worsen as the child reaches towards an object. They can be due to cerebellar disorders, which may be congenital or acquired.
5. **Neonatal Tremors:** Newborns, especially preterm infants, may exhibit tremors due to immature nervous system development. These usually resolve as the child grows.
6. **Drug-Induced Tremors:** Certain medications can cause tremors in children, similar to how they affect adults.
7. **Neurological Disorders:** Conditions like multiple sclerosis, brain injury, or neurodegenerative diseases, though rare in children, can cause tremors.
8. **Psychogenic Tremors:** In some cases, tremors in children might be psychogenic, related to psychological factors or stress.
9. **Metabolic and Genetic Disorders:** Metabolic imbalances or genetic conditions can present with tremors among other symptoms.
10. **Infectious Diseases:** Certain infections affecting the nervous system might cause tremors in children.

When evaluating tremors in children, it is important to consider the context, associated symptoms, family history, and any other health issues. In many cases, tremors in children are benign and may resolve on their own. However, if tremors are persistent, worsening, or accompanied by other neurological symptoms (like weakness, difficulty walking, or speech problems), it is important to seek medical evaluation to rule out more serious conditions. Treatment and management depend on the underlying cause, and may range from simple observation to medication and therapy.

What is the treatment of tremors?

The treatment of tremors depends on their type, severity, underlying cause, and the impact they have on the patient's life. There is no one-size-fits-all approach, and treatment strategies can range from lifestyle modifications to medication and, in some cases, surgical interventions. Here is a general overview:

1. **Lifestyle Modifications:** For mild tremors, especially those exacerbated by stress or stimulants, lifestyle changes can be beneficial. These might include stress reduction techniques, avoiding caffeine and other stimulants, and reducing alcohol intake.
2. **Physical Therapy:** Exercises to improve muscle strength, control, and coordination can be helpful, especially for those with essential tremor or cerebellar tremors.
3. **Medications:** Various medications can be used to reduce the severity of tremors, depending on the type of tremor:
   - **Essential Tremor:** Beta-blockers (like propranolol) and anticonvulsant drugs (like primidone) are commonly used.
   - **Parkinson's Disease Tremors:** Medications that increase or mimic dopamine, such as levodopa and dopamine agonists, are typically prescribed.
   - **Cerebellar Tremors:** Medications like gabapentin, topiramate, or clonazepam may be used.
   - **Psychogenic Tremors:** Treatment may involve psychiatric medications if there are underlying mental health conditions.
4. **Botulinum Toxin Injections:** For tremors that affect specific parts of the body, such as the hands or head, botulinum toxin injections can sometimes be effective.
5. **Surgical Options:** In severe cases where tremors do not respond to medication, surgical interventions might be considered:
   - **Deep Brain Stimulation (DBS):** This involves implanting a device that sends electrical signals to specific parts of the brain.

- **Thalamotomy:** A surgical procedure that involves creating a lesion in parts of the thalamus, a brain region involved in movement control.

6. **Assistive Devices:** For some patients, especially those with essential tremor, assistive devices like weighted utensils can make daily tasks easier.
7. **Treatment of Underlying Conditions:** If the tremor is a symptom of an underlying condition (like hyperthyroidism), treating that condition can reduce or eliminate the tremor.
8. **Avoidance of Triggering Medications:** If a medication is causing the tremor, adjusting the dose or switching to an alternative medication might help.
9. **Psychological Therapies:** For psychogenic tremors, psychological counseling, cognitive-behavioral therapy, and stress management strategies can be effective.

It is important for patients with tremors to work closely with their healthcare provider to determine the most appropriate treatment plan based on their specific circumstances. In many cases, a multidisciplinary approach involving neurologists, psychiatrists, physical therapists, and other specialists is optimal. Regular follow-up is essential to monitor the effectiveness of the treatment and make adjustments as needed.

What is delirium?

Delirium is a serious disturbance in mental abilities that results in confused thinking and reduced awareness of the environment. It is a rapid-onset condition that can fluctuate in severity over a short period of time, such as hours or days. Delirium is particularly common in older adults, especially those who are hospitalized or living in long-term care facilities, but it can affect people of any age. Key aspects of delirium include:

1. **Rapid Onset:** Unlike many other cognitive disorders, delirium develops quickly, often within hours or a few days.
2. **Fluctuating Symptoms:** Symptoms can fluctuate significantly throughout the day. A person with delirium may have periods of lucidity followed by increased confusion.
3. **Reduced Awareness:** Individuals with delirium may seem less aware of their environment. They might have trouble focusing, sustaining or shifting attention.
4. **Confusion and Disorientation:** People experiencing delirium often feel disoriented and may not know where they are, what time it is, or even their own identity.
5. **Memory Problems:** Short-term memory may be impaired, while long-term memory remains intact.
6. **Hallucinations and Delusions:** Some individuals with delirium experience hallucinations, delusions, or paranoia.
7. **Altered Sleep Patterns:** Changes in sleep patterns, such as sleepiness during the day and restlessness at night, are common.
8. **Emotional Disturbances:** Mood swings, anxiety, agitation, irritability, or apathy can occur.
9. **Causes:** Delirium can be triggered by a wide range of factors, including infections, surgery, medication side effects, drug or alcohol withdrawal, certain medical conditions, or anything that disrupts the normal functioning of the brain.
10. **Risk Factors:** Older age, pre-existing brain disorders (like dementia), severe illness, and polypharmacy (taking multiple medications) are risk factors.
11. **Diagnosis:** Delirium is diagnosed based on clinical observation and a thorough assessment of the patient's medical history, symptoms, and potentially, laboratory tests to identify underlying causes.
12. **Treatment:** Addressing the underlying cause of delirium is the primary approach to treatment. This may involve adjusting medications, treating infections, or addressing other medical issues. Supportive care to prevent complications, ensuring safety, and helping with orientation and mobility are also important.
13. **Prevention and Management:** Strategies like maintaining hydration, ensuring adequate nutrition, managing pain, promoting good sleep habits, and providing a calm and orienting environment can help prevent delirium or reduce its severity.

Delirium is a medical emergency, as it can signal a serious underlying health issue. It is important for it to be recognized and treated promptly. Additionally, delirium can have lasting effects on cognitive and physical functioning, especially in older adults, making early intervention crucial.

What are other commonly associated features of delirium?

Delirium, a complex and multifaceted condition, can manifest with a variety of features beyond the core symptoms of confusion, altered consciousness, and cognitive impairment. Some commonly associated features include:

1. **Psychomotor Changes:** These can range from hyperactivity (agitation, restlessness) to hypoactivity (lethargy, reduced motor activity), and some patients may alternate between these states.
2. **Speech and Language Disturbances:** Difficulty in articulating thoughts, rambling or incoherent speech, and problems with understanding or following conversations.
3. **Disrupted Sleep-Wake Cycle:** This includes insomnia, daytime sleepiness, night time agitation, and a complete reversal of the normal sleep-wake pattern.
4. **Emotional Lability:** Rapid and unpredictable changes in emotion, such as sudden tears or laughter, anxiety, fear, irritability, or anger.
5. **Altered Perception:** This can involve misinterpretations (misunderstanding objects or events), illusions (distorted perception of real stimuli), and hallucinations (perceiving things that are not present), often of a visual nature.
6. **Fluctuation of Symptoms:** The severity and nature of symptoms can change over the course of the day, often worsening at night (a phenomenon known as "sundowning").
7. **Impaired Attention and Concentration:** Difficulty focusing, being easily distractible, or having trouble keeping track of what is being said or done.
8. **Physical Symptoms:** Such as changes in appetite or eating patterns, dehydration, incontinence, and changes in vital signs (like heart rate, blood pressure, and temperature).
9. **Behavioral Changes:** Uncharacteristic behavior such as suspicion, paranoia, or resistance to care.
10. **Cognitive Fluctuations:** Varying levels of consciousness, ranging from hyperalertness to stupor.

These features can make delirium particularly challenging to diagnose and manage, especially in patients who are unable to communicate effectively, such as those with pre-existing cognitive impairments or severe illnesses. The presence and severity of these features can also provide insights into the underlying cause of delirium and guide treatment strategies. Early recognition and comprehensive management of these features are crucial in the care of patients with delirium to improve outcomes and reduce the potential for long-term consequences.

What are subtypes of delirium?

Delirium can be classified into several subtypes based on the clinical presentation and predominant features. Understanding these subtypes is important for accurate diagnosis and effective management. The main subtypes of delirium are:

1. **Hyperactive Delirium:** This is the most easily recognized form. Patients with hyperactive delirium are typically agitated, restless, or even combative. They may experience hallucinations, delusions, and severe mood swings. This subtype is often associated with high levels of anxiety and paranoia.
2. **Hypoactive Delirium:** Patients with hypoactive delirium present with lethargy, reduced motor activity, and sluggishness. They may appear drowsy or sedated. This subtype can be particularly challenging to diagnose because it can be mistaken for depression or fatigue. Hypoactive delirium is often underdiagnosed because its symptoms are less overt than those of hyperactive delirium.
3. **Mixed Delirium:** This subtype involves a combination of hyperactive and hypoactive features. Patients may fluctuate between states of agitation and inactivity. The mixed form of delirium is common, and its fluctuating nature can complicate the diagnosis and management.
4. **Normal Psychomotor Delirium:** In this rare subtype, psychomotor activity appears normal, yet there are significant alterations in cognition and consciousness. This form of delirium can be particularly difficult to identify, as the usual motoric clues are absent.

The subtype of delirium can be influenced by several factors, including the underlying cause, patient's age, pre-existing cognitive or physical health, and environmental factors. For instance, delirium due to withdrawal from alcohol or drugs is often hyperactive, whereas delirium associated with metabolic disorders may be hypoactive.

Early recognition and accurate identification of the delirium subtype are crucial for effective treatment. Each subtype may respond differently to interventions, and treatment should be tailored to the individual's specific symptoms and needs. Additionally, understanding the subtype can help in predicting the course of the condition and potential complications.

How must delirium be managed?

Managing delirium involves a multifaceted approach that addresses both the underlying cause and the symptoms. The approach should be individualized, taking into account the patient's medical history, the severity of the delirium, and the specific symptoms they are experiencing. Here are key components of delirium management:

1. **Identify and Treat the Underlying Cause:** This is the most crucial step. Common causes include infections, dehydration, metabolic imbalances, medication side effects, substance withdrawal, and acute medical illnesses. Appropriate tests should be conducted to identify and treat these underlying issues.
2. **Medication Review and Management:** Review the patient's medications to identify any that could contribute to delirium. Adjusting, stopping, or changing medications can often improve symptoms.
3. **Environmental Modifications:** Creating a calm, comfortable, and safe environment can help. This includes ensuring good lighting, reducing noise, providing clocks and calendars for orientation, and allowing personal items that the patient recognizes.
4. **Supportive Care:** Ensure adequate hydration and nutrition, manage pain effectively, and assist with personal needs. Monitor vitals regularly.
5. **Minimize Use of Restraints and Sedatives:** Physical restraints and sedative medications should be avoided if possible, as they can worsen delirium. If absolutely necessary for safety, use the lowest effective dose and reassess frequently.
6. **Enhance Communication and Orientation:** Frequent reorientation to time, place, and person helps. Speak calmly and clearly, and provide reassurance. Family members and familiar caregivers should be involved in the care process.
7. **Manage Sleep Disturbances:** Promote a regular sleep-wake cycle. Encourage physical activity during the day if possible, and create a quiet, dark environment at night. Avoid sleep-inducing medications if possible.
8. **Address Behavioral and Psychological Symptoms:** Non-pharmacological interventions should be the first line. This includes reassurance, redirection, and the presence of familiar people. Pharmacological interventions may be necessary for severe agitation or psychosis but should be used judiciously.
9. **Involve Multidisciplinary Teams:** The management of delirium often requires a team approach, including doctors, nurses, pharmacists, physical and occupational therapists, and social workers.
10. **Monitor and Reassess Regularly:** Delirium can fluctuate, and patients' conditions can change rapidly. Regular monitoring and reassessment are essential to ensure that management strategies are effective and to make adjustments as needed.
11. **Preventive Measures:** In at-risk populations (like older adults in hospitals), proactive measures such as early mobilization, proper hydration and nutrition, regular orientation, adequate pain control, and avoiding high-risk medications can help prevent delirium.
12. **Education and Support for Caregivers and Family:** Educating caregivers and family members about delirium, its implications, and ways to assist can be beneficial.

Effective management of delirium can significantly impact the patient's recovery and overall outcome. It is important to approach it as a medical emergency and seek a comprehensive, timely intervention.

What is the prognosis of delirium?

The prognosis of delirium varies widely and depends on several factors, including the underlying cause, the patient's age, their overall health status, and the promptness and effectiveness of treatment. Here are some general points regarding the prognosis of delirium:

1. **Reversibility:** Delirium is often reversible if the underlying cause is promptly identified and treated. In many cases, patients can fully recover with appropriate management.
2. **Duration:** The duration of delirium can vary. It may last for only a few hours or days in some cases, but in other situations, particularly when the underlying cause is complex or severe, it can persist for weeks or even months.

3. **Elderly and Frail Patients:** Older adults, especially those with pre-existing cognitive impairments like dementia, often have a poorer prognosis. Delirium in these patients can lead to a rapid decline in both cognitive and physical functioning.

4. **Hospitalization and Complications:** Delirium is associated with longer hospital stays, increased risk of complications, and a higher likelihood of being discharged to a rehabilitation facility or nursing home rather than returning home.

5. **Increased Mortality Risk:** Delirium, especially when not promptly addressed, is associated with an increased risk of death. This risk is higher in older adults and those with more severe underlying health issues.

6. **Long-Term Cognitive Impact:** Some patients, particularly older individuals, may experience long-term cognitive decline following an episode of delirium. This decline can be part of a gradual deterioration or a more abrupt change.

7. **Psychological and Emotional Impact:** Patients who have experienced delirium may suffer from anxiety, depression, or post-traumatic stress disorder (PTSD) after the episode, especially if it was prolonged or severe.

8. **Functional Decline:** Prolonged delirium can lead to a decline in a patient's ability to perform daily activities independently.

9. **Importance of Preventive Measures:** In high-risk populations, such as hospitalized older adults, preventive measures can significantly improve prognosis by reducing the incidence and severity of delirium.

10. **Early Intervention:** Early recognition and treatment of delirium are crucial for improving outcomes. This includes both addressing the cause and providing supportive care to manage symptoms.

In summary, while many patients with delirium recover fully, especially with timely and appropriate treatment, some may experience lasting effects, particularly if they are older or have underlying health conditions. The prognosis of delirium underscores the importance of early intervention, comprehensive management, and preventive strategies in at-risk populations.

What is dementia, and its types?

Dementia is a broad term used to describe a decline in cognitive function severe enough to interfere with daily life. It is not a specific disease but rather a general term that encompasses a wide range of specific medical conditions, including Alzheimer's disease and others. Dementia is characterized by impairment in memory, communication, and thinking.

Here are some of the most common types of dementia:

1. **Alzheimer's Disease:** This is the most common type of dementia, accounting for an estimated 60-80% of cases. Alzheimer's is characterized by the formation of amyloid plaques and tau tangles in the brain, leading to the death of brain cells.

2. **Vascular Dementia:** This type occurs due to microscopic bleeding and blood vessel blockage in the brain. It is often triggered by a stroke or other conditions that damage blood vessels, leading to changes in thinking skills.

3. **Lewy Body Dementia:** Characterized by the presence of Lewy bodies (abnormal aggregates of protein) in brain cells. Symptoms include changes in alertness and attention, recurrent visual hallucinations, and Parkinsonian movement features.

4. **Frontotemporal Dementia (FTD):** This type includes several disorders that primarily affect the frontal and temporal lobes of the brain. It is often associated with personality changes, difficulty with language, and behavior changes.

5. **Mixed Dementia:** In some cases, a person may have more than one type of dementia. Alzheimer's disease and vascular dementia frequently occur together.

6. **Parkinson's Disease Dementia:** This form of dementia occurs in the later stages of Parkinson's disease, a progressive neurological disorder. It shares some characteristics with Alzheimer's and Lewy body dementia.

7. **Creutzfeldt-Jakob Disease:** A rare, rapidly fatal disorder that causes dementia symptoms that worsen significantly over time. It is caused by an abnormal version of a protein called a prion.

8. **Normal Pressure Hydrocephalus:** Caused by the build-up of fluid in the brain. Symptoms include difficulty walking, memory loss, and inability to control urine.

9. **Huntington's Disease:** A progressive brain disorder caused by a defective gene. It affects the brain, causing changes in mood, mental abilities, and coordination.
10. **Wernicke-Korsakoff Syndrome:** A chronic memory disorder caused by severe deficiency of thiamine (vitamin B1), most commonly caused by alcohol misuse.

Each type of dementia may have a different underlying cause and can vary in how quickly symptoms progress and in the pattern of cognitive decline. Early diagnosis and intervention are important for managing the symptoms of dementia, although most types are progressive and have no cure currently. The management usually focuses on improving quality of life, managing symptoms, and providing support to the patient and their caregivers.

What are the symptoms of dementia?

Dementia is characterized by a decline in cognitive function and usually involves multiple cognitive and behavioral symptoms. These symptoms vary depending on the type and stage of dementia, but some common ones include:

1. **Memory Loss:** One of the most common early signs, particularly short-term memory issues. This may include forgetting recently learned information, repeating questions, forgetting important dates or events, or increasingly needing memory aids.
2. **Difficulty with Complex Tasks:** Trouble with planning, organizing, problem-solving, and multitasking. Tasks that were once easy may become challenging and time-consuming.
3. **Disorientation and Confusion:** People with dementia may become lost in familiar places, confused about the time or date, or have difficulty understanding information.
4. **Language Problems:** Difficulty finding the right words, following or joining a conversation, or calling things by the wrong name.
5. **Impaired Visual and Spatial Abilities:** Difficulty judging distance or seeing objects in three dimensions; navigating stairs or parking may become hard.
6. **Poor Judgment and Decision Making:** This might include poor understanding of safety risks, making unusual or inappropriate choices in social interactions, or mishandling finances.
7. **Mood and Personality Changes:** Increased irritability, anxiety, or depression; shifts in personality; reduced interest in social activities; withdrawal from work or social engagements.
8. **Apathy:** Loss of motivation, initiative, or interest in hobbies and activities.
9. **Behavioral Changes:** Uncharacteristic behaviors such as agitation, aggression, wandering, or repeating the same actions or words.
10. **Difficulty Performing Familiar Tasks:** Struggling with daily tasks like dressing, cooking, or grooming.
11. **Physical Symptoms:** In later stages, physical abilities may decline, including walking, balance, and coordination.
12. **Changes in Sleep Patterns:** Insomnia, waking up during the night, or sleeping more during the day.
13. **Hallucinations or Delusions:** In some types of dementia, individuals may experience hallucinations, delusions, or paranoia.

It is important to note that having one or more of these symptoms does not necessarily mean a person has dementia. Other health conditions or normal aging can cause many of these symptoms. However, if someone is experiencing multiple symptoms that are worsening over time and affecting daily life, it is important to consult a healthcare professional for a thorough evaluation. Early diagnosis and intervention can help manage symptoms, improve quality of life, and plan for the future.

What happens in early stage of dementia?

In the early stage of dementia, also known as mild dementia or the initial stage, changes in cognitive abilities and behavior may be subtle and often go unnoticed by others. During this stage, individuals may still be able to function independently in many aspects of their daily life, but they may start experiencing difficulties that hint at the onset of dementia. Key characteristics of the early stage of dementia include:

1. **Memory Lapses:** Forgetfulness becomes more noticeable. This might include forgetting names, appointments, or recent events, misplacing items, or having difficulty recalling information they just read.
2. **Difficulty with Complex Tasks:** Challenges in planning, organizing, or following through with

more complex tasks, like managing finances or planning a dinner party, may arise.

3. **Word-Finding Difficulties:** Trouble finding the right words during conversations, or taking longer to articulate thoughts.
4. **Mood Changes:** Increased feelings of anxiety, irritability, or depression. These mood changes may be a reaction to noticing their own difficulties.
5. **Subtle Changes in Personality:** Slight shifts in personality traits, such as becoming more withdrawn, less interested in socializing, or more rigid in thinking.
6. **Difficulty in Work Performance:** Those who are still working may start to have trouble with tasks that were previously manageable.
7. **Disorientation:** Occasional confusion about the date or time of day.
8. **Difficulty with Directions:** Getting lost in familiar places or trouble following a series of directions.
9. **Decreased Initiative:** Less motivation to initiate activities or engage in hobbies they once enjoyed.
10. **Repeating Stories or Questions:** Unintentionally repeating stories, anecdotes, or questions in conversation.

During the early stages of dementia, it is not uncommon for individuals and their families to attribute these changes to normal aging or stress. However, these early signs can impact daily life and may signal the need for a medical evaluation.

Early diagnosis is important as it allows for early intervention, planning for the future, and potentially slowing the progression of symptoms. Management in the early stages often focuses on lifestyle modifications, cognitive stimulation, and support for the individual and their family. Medications may also be prescribed in some cases to address symptoms such as memory decline or mood changes.

What happens in intermediate stage of dementia?

The intermediate stage of dementia, also known as moderate dementia, is characterized by more pronounced symptoms than the early stage. In this phase, individuals generally require greater assistance with daily activities and may experience significant changes in cognitive abilities and behavior. Here are some key aspects of the intermediate stage of dementia:

1. **Increased Memory Loss:** Memory impairment becomes more obvious, including forgetting significant aspects of personal history and having difficulty remembering familiar people, such as close friends or family members.
2. **Greater Difficulty with Communication:** Problems with language increase, such as struggling to follow or join a conversation, frequently pausing to find the right word, or using the wrong words.
3. **Confusion and Disorientation:** Individuals may become more disoriented regarding time and place. They may not know where they are, even in familiar settings, or have difficulty understanding events happening around them.
4. **Impaired Judgment and Reasoning:** Difficulty with complex mental tasks becomes more apparent. This includes trouble handling finances, understanding safety risks, or making sound decisions.
5. **Behavioral and Mood Changes:** Symptoms such as agitation, irritability, apathy, withdrawal, and sometimes depression or anxiety become more common. Sleep disturbances and sundowning (increased confusion and agitation in the late afternoon and evening) may occur.
6. **Difficulty with Daily Activities:** Increasing dependence on others for activities of daily living, such as dressing, bathing, and grooming. They may wear the same clothes repeatedly or forget to bathe.
7. **Physical Changes:** Decreased coordination and motor skills can lead to problems with walking or a higher risk of falls. There may also be changes in appetite and eating habits.
8. **Incontinence:** As the disease progresses, bladder and bowel control may become a problem.
9. **Personality Changes:** More noticeable changes in personality may occur, such as becoming suspicious, paranoid, or fearful, or exhibiting inappropriate behaviors.
10. **Wandering:** Some individuals may wander or become lost, even in familiar surroundings.
11. **Recognition Difficulties:** Difficulty recognizing family members and close friends.

During the intermediate stage of dementia, safety becomes a major concern due to increased confusion and physical decline. Caregiver support is crucial, as individuals with moderate dementia typically require substantial assistance with their daily activities. This stage can be challenging for both the individual and their caregivers, often necessitating adjustments in living arrangements and increased caregiving support.

Management typically includes continued medical care, behavioral strategies to address mood and behavior changes, modification of the living environment to ensure safety, and support for caregivers in handling the increasing care needs. Community resources, support groups, and respite care can also be valuable for caregivers during this stage.

What happens in late stage of dementia?

In the late stage of dementia, also known as advanced or severe dementia, individuals experience significant impairment in their cognitive and physical abilities. This stage requires intensive care and support. The symptoms are more pronounced and often include:

1. **Severe Memory Loss:** Individuals may not recognize close family members or loved ones and may have little to no verbal communication. Long-term memory, as well as short-term memory, is significantly impaired.
2. **Near-Total Dependence:** Individuals in this stage typically require full-time assistance with all aspects of daily living, including eating, dressing, bathing, and toileting.
3. **Loss of Physical Abilities:** There is often a significant decline in physical capabilities. Individuals may become bedridden or unable to sit without support. Loss of mobility increases the risk of complications like bedsores and infections.
4. **Difficulty with Communication:** Verbal communication may be minimal or absent. Understanding language and expressing thoughts become extremely difficult.
5. **Changes in Eating and Swallowing:** Difficulty in swallowing (dysphagia) can lead to choking hazards and nutritional deficiencies. Many individuals require modified diets or feeding assistance.
6. **Incontinence:** Bladder and bowel control are typically lost, necessitating the use of incontinence products and assistance with toileting.
7. **Susceptibility to Infections:** Increased vulnerability to infections, such as pneumonia, urinary tract infections, and skin infections.
8. **Behavioral Symptoms:** While some individuals become quieter and more withdrawn, others may experience increased agitation, restlessness, or verbal outbursts.
9. **Loss of Weight and Muscle Mass:** Decreased food intake and the body's declining ability to process nutrients often lead to significant weight loss and muscle wasting.
10. **Sensory Processing:** Individuals may experience changes in their response to pain or temperature. They might not be able to communicate discomfort or pain effectively.
11. **Emotional Responses:** Even if cognitive skills are significantly diminished, some individuals may still respond to emotional stimuli or the presence of loved ones through non-verbal communication or expressions.

During the late stage of dementia, the focus of care is primarily on providing comfort and quality of life. Palliative care, which includes managing physical symptoms, ensuring a peaceful environment, and supporting emotional well-being, becomes central. Families and caregivers often face emotional and practical challenges during this stage, and support from healthcare professionals, community resources, and support groups is crucial.

Decisions regarding medical interventions, hospitalizations, and end-of-life care need to be made, often guided by advance directives or discussions with the individual's healthcare proxy or family members. The goal is to ensure dignity and comfort for the individual while providing support and guidance for their caregivers and loved ones.

What is the differential diagnosis of dementia?

Differential diagnosis is the process of distinguishing a particular disease or condition from others that present similar clinical features. For dementia, this is especially important because various conditions can mimic dementia or cause cognitive impairment. The differential diagnosis for dementia includes:

1. **Delirium:** Unlike dementia, delirium develops quickly and often fluctuates throughout the day. Patients with delirium might experience hallucinations, severe disorientation, and fluctuating levels of consciousness.
2. **Depression:** Especially in older adults, depression can cause symptoms similar to dementia, such

as forgetfulness and concentration problems. This is sometimes referred to as "pseudodementia."

3. **Vitamin Deficiencies:** Deficiencies in certain vitamins, particularly B12 and folate, can lead to cognitive impairment.
4. **Thyroid Disorders:** Both hyperthyroidism and hypothyroidism can cause symptoms that resemble dementia.
5. **Chronic Alcoholism:** Chronic alcohol abuse can lead to a condition known as Wernicke-Korsakoff syndrome, which is characterized by severe memory impairment and confabulation.
6. **Normal Pressure Hydrocephalus:** This condition, caused by an accumulation of cerebrospinal fluid in the brain, can lead to dementia-like symptoms, including gait disturbances and incontinence, in addition to cognitive deficits.
7. **Brain Tumors:** Tumors in certain parts of the brain can cause symptoms that mimic dementia.
8. **Medication Side Effects:** Certain medications, especially those with anticholinergic properties, can impair cognitive function.
9. **Infectious Diseases:** Conditions such as HIV/AIDS, syphilis, and Lyme disease can affect cognitive function.
10. **Metabolic Disorders:** Conditions like Hypoglycaemia or hypercalcemia can cause cognitive changes.
11. **Autoimmune Disorders:** Diseases such as lupus and multiple sclerosis can affect cognitive function.
12. **Sleep Disorders:** Poor sleep quality, including conditions like sleep apnea, can lead to cognitive impairment.
13. **Psychiatric Disorders:** Other mental health conditions, including schizophrenia and bipolar disorder, can have symptoms that overlap with dementia.
14. **Structural Brain Changes:** Traumatic brain injury, subdural hematomas, and other structural changes to the brain can cause symptoms similar to dementia.
15. **Seizure Disorders:** In some cases, seizure activity can result in cognitive impairment.

A thorough assessment, including medical history, physical examination, laboratory tests, and often neuroimaging (like MRI or CT scans), is essential for making an accurate diagnosis. Since many of the conditions that mimic dementia are treatable, correct diagnosis is crucial for effective management and potentially reversing cognitive impairment.

What tests must be employed to screen dementia?

Screening for dementia typically involves a combination of clinical evaluation, cognitive testing, and sometimes additional diagnostic procedures. The goal is to assess cognitive functions thoroughly, identify any deficits, and determine their impact on daily life. Here is an overview of the typical screening process:

1. **Clinical Evaluation:** A comprehensive medical history and physical examination are essential. The evaluation should include a thorough review of the patient's medical history, current medications, past and present medical conditions, family history, and lifestyle factors.
2. **Neurological Examination:** To assess neurological health, including reflexes, muscle strength, muscle tone, sense of touch and sight, coordination, and balance.
3. **Cognitive and Neuropsychological Tests:** These tests assess memory, problem-solving skills, attention, language, and other intellectual functions. Common tests include:
   - **Mini-Mental State Examination (MMSE):** A widely used test for assessing cognitive function.
   - **Montreal Cognitive Assessment (MoCA):** A screening assessment for detecting mild cognitive dysfunction.
   - **Clock Drawing Test:** Used to assess visual-spatial skills and executive function.
   - **Memory Assessment Scales:** To evaluate different types of memory functions.
4. **Laboratory Tests:** Blood tests to rule out other causes of cognitive impairment, such as thyroid disorders, vitamin deficiencies (particularly B12), infections, or metabolic abnormalities.
5. **Psychiatric Evaluation:** To assess for depression or other mental health conditions that can cause symptoms similar to dementia.

6. **Functional Assessment:** Evaluation of the ability to perform daily activities (like paying bills, taking medication, driving, and personal care).
7. **Neuroimaging:** Brain imaging studies, such as Magnetic Resonance Imaging (MRI) or Computed Tomography (CT) scans, can be used to identify strokes, tumors, or other problems that could cause cognitive changes.
8. **Electroencephalogram (EEG):** In some cases, to assess for seizure activity or other neurological disorders.
9. **Genetic Testing:** May be considered, especially if there is a family history of dementia, particularly in cases of early-onset Alzheimer's disease.
10. **Lumbar Puncture (Spinal Tap):** Occasionally, to analyze cerebrospinal fluid for infections, inflammatory diseases, and markers of neuro-degeneration.

The specific combination of tests will depend on the individual's symptoms, medical history, and the clinical judgment of the healthcare provider. Early and accurate diagnosis is crucial for managing dementia effectively, including initiating appropriate treatments, planning for future care needs, and providing education and support for both patients and caregivers.

What measures must the caregivers take in cases of dementia?

Caring for someone with dementia is challenging and requires a combination of practical strategies, emotional support, and often, changes to the living environment. Here are key measures caregivers should consider:

1. **Educate Yourself About Dementia:** Understanding the condition helps in managing expectations and preparing for future challenges. It is also important to know the progression of the disease and what to expect in each stage.
2. **Create a Safe and Structured Environment:** Modify the home to make it safer and more comfortable. This can include installing grab bars, removing trip hazards, and using locks on cabinets that contain harmful substances.
3. **Establish a Routine:** People with dementia often benefit from a predictable routine. Try to keep daily activities, mealtimes, and bedtime consistent.
4. **Encourage Independence:** Allow the person with dementia to do as much for themselves as possible. This helps maintain their skills and promotes a sense of accomplishment.
5. **Effective Communication:** Use simple words and sentences. Speak clearly and calmly. Maintain eye contact and use nonverbal cues and touch to help convey your message.
6. **Manage Behavioral Changes:** Learn strategies to address common behavioral symptoms such as agitation, aggression, wandering, and sleep disturbances.
7. **Nutrition and Hydration:** Ensure a balanced diet and encourage regular fluid intake to prevent dehydration.
8. **Physical Activity and Social Interaction:** Encourage regular physical activity suited to their abilities and promote social interaction to enhance their quality of life.
9. **Regular Medical Check-ups:** Ensure that the person with dementia receives regular medical care and that their health needs are being met.
10. **Manage Medications:** Keep track of medications, including dosages and schedules, and watch for potential side effects.
11. **Plan for the Future:** Discuss and make legal and financial plans for the future while the person with dementia can still participate and express their wishes.
12. **Support for the Caregiver:** Caregiving can be emotionally and physically draining. Caregivers should seek support from family, friends, and community resources. Joining a caregiver support group can provide emotional support and practical advice.
13. **Respite Care:** Utilize respite care services to take breaks and prevent caregiver burnout.
14. **Be Flexible and Patient:** As dementia progresses, the abilities of the person will change. Caregivers need to be adaptable and patient as they navigate these changes.
15. **End-of-Life Care:** In advanced stages, consider palliative care services to manage symptoms and provide comfort.
16. **Emotional Support:** Provide emotional support through companionship, conversation, and engagement in activities that the person enjoys and can participate in.

Caring for someone with dementia is a significant responsibility and can be challenging. It is crucial for caregivers to also take care of their own health and well-being. Seeking support from healthcare professionals, social services, and support networks can make a substantial difference in managing the demands of caregiving.

What is the treatment of dementia?

Treatment for dementia focuses on managing symptoms, improving quality of life, and supporting both the patient and their caregivers. There is currently no cure for most types of dementia, including Alzheimer's disease, but various strategies can help manage the condition. Treatment typically involves a combination of medication, lifestyle changes, and supportive care:

1. **Medications:**
   - **Cholinesterase Inhibitors:** Drugs like donepezil, rivastigmine, and galantamine are often prescribed for Alzheimer's disease. They work by increasing levels of a chemical messenger involved in memory and judgment.
   - **Memantine:** This medication works differently from cholinesterase inhibitors, regulating the activity of glutamate, another chemical messenger in the brain, and is used in moderate to severe Alzheimer's.
   - **Medications for Behavioral Symptoms:** Antidepressants, antipsychotics, or anxiolytics can be used to treat symptoms such as depression, aggression, agitation, or sleep disturbances.
   - **Medications for Cognitive Symptoms:** Some drugs might help manage memory loss or other cognitive symptoms.
2. **Managing Underlying Health Conditions:** Treatment of coexisting medical conditions, such as heart disease, diabetes, or high blood pressure, is important in managing dementia.
3. **Lifestyle Changes and Home Remedies:**
   - **Regular Physical Activity:** Exercise can help improve mood, cardiovascular health, and maintain muscle strength.
   - **Healthy Diet:** A balanced diet can support overall health and may reduce the risk of some types of dementia.
   - **Cognitive Stimulation:** Activities like puzzles, memory games, and reading can help keep the mind engaged.
   - Social Interaction: Regular social interaction can help improve mood and maintain function.
4. **Supportive Therapies:**
   - **Occupational Therapy:** Can help people with dementia maintain their skills and independence for as long as possible.
   - **Music or Art Therapy:** Can enhance quality of life and improve mood.
   - **Behavioral Therapy:** To help manage challenging behaviors without medications.
5. **Caregiver Education and Support:** Teaching caregivers how to respond to behavioral changes and communicate effectively is crucial. Support groups and respite care services can also be beneficial.
6. **Environment and Routine:** Creating a safe, structured environment can help reduce confusion and agitation. Keeping a consistent routine is also helpful.
7. **Safety Considerations:** Measures like removing trip hazards, installing safety locks, and ensuring adequate supervision can prevent accidents.
8. **Legal and Financial Planning:** Early in the disease course, discussing and arranging legal and financial matters is advisable.
9. **Advanced Care Planning:** Discussing and documenting care preferences for the later stages of the disease is important.
10. **Palliative Care:** In advanced stages, the focus may shift to palliative care, emphasizing comfort and quality of life.

Each person with dementia is unique, and their treatment plan should be tailored to their specific needs and circumstances. It is important to work closely with healthcare professionals to develop a comprehensive care plan.

How must be the caregivers in family be assisted in dementia?

Assisting family caregivers of individuals with dementia is crucial, as caring for a loved one with dementia can be physically and emotionally demanding. Here are several ways to support family caregivers:

1. **Education and Information:** Provide caregivers with information about dementia, its progression, and what to expect. Understanding the disease can help them manage their loved one's symptoms better and prepare for future challenges.

2. **Training:** Offer training on specific skills needed for dementia care, such as communication techniques, behavior management strategies, safety measures, and personal care tasks.
3. **Support Groups:** Encourage participation in support groups where caregivers can share experiences, tips, and emotional support with others in similar situations.
4. **Respite Care:** Arrange for respite care services to give caregivers regular breaks. This can include adult day care services, in-home respite, or short-term residential care facilities.
5. **Health and Wellness:** Remind caregivers to take care of their own health. This includes regular medical check-ups, stress management, exercise, and proper nutrition.
6. **Counseling Services:** Provide access to counseling or therapy to help caregivers deal with the emotional and psychological challenges of caregiving.
7. **Community Resources:** Connect caregivers with community resources, such as local Alzheimer's Association chapters, senior centers, or social services, which may offer practical assistance, educational programs, and support.
8. **Financial and Legal Guidance:** Help caregivers understand and access financial resources, legal services, and benefits that can assist with the costs of care. This can include information about Medicare, Medicaid, veteran's benefits, and long-term care insurance.
9. **Home Safety Evaluations:** Offer guidance on making the home environment safer for someone with dementia, which can include installing grab bars, removing trip hazards, and ensuring adequate lighting.
10. **Emergency Preparedness:** Assist in developing a plan for emergencies, including medical crises or wandering incidents.
11. **Regular Check-ins:** Regularly check in with caregivers to see how they're doing and what support they might need.
12. **Technology Aids:** Introduce caregivers to technologies that can help in care, such as reminder systems, safety devices, and GPS trackers for wandering.
13. **Care Coordination and Planning:** Help caregivers coordinate care among various healthcare providers and understand future care options, including home care services, memory care facilities, and hospice care.
14. **Validation and Recognition:** Acknowledge the hard work and dedication of caregivers. Validation can be a significant source of emotional support.
15. **Peer Support:** Facilitate connections with other caregivers who have gone through similar experiences, for shared advice and emotional support.

Supporting family caregivers is not just about providing resources; it is also about acknowledging their role and helping them maintain their well-being while they care for their loved ones. This holistic approach is crucial for the sustained health and effectiveness of the caregiver.

What are the legal issues in dementia?

Legal issues are a significant concern in dementia care, both for individuals with dementia and their caregivers. Addressing these issues early in the disease process is crucial for ensuring that the person's wishes are respected and that legal and financial matters are handled appropriately as the disease progresses. Key legal issues include:

1. **Advance Directives:** These are legal documents that specify an individual's preferences for medical care if they become unable to make decisions for themselves. This includes a living will and healthcare proxy or durable power of attorney for health care.
2. **Power of Attorney:** Establishing a power of attorney allows a person with dementia to appoint someone to make legal and financial decisions on their behalf when they are no longer capable of doing so. This can include decisions about property, finances, and other legal matters.
3. **Guardianship or Conservatorship:** If no power of attorney is in place and the individual's decision-making ability has significantly declined, it may be necessary to seek legal guardianship or conservatorship. This gives a designated person the legal authority to make decisions on behalf of the individual with dementia.
4. **Estate Planning:** Individuals should be encouraged to make arrangements regarding their estate while they still have the capacity to do so. This includes creating or updating their will,

establishing trusts, and making plans for the distribution of their assets.

5. **Financial Planning:** Managing finances can become challenging as dementia progresses. It is important to organize financial documents, understand the individual's financial situation, and plan for future costs of care.
6. **Long-term Care Planning:** Discussing and planning for long-term care needs, including potential residential care, home care, and end-of-life care. Understanding insurance coverage, Medicaid eligibility, and other potential sources of funding for long-term care is crucial.
7. **Capacity and Consent:** Legal issues around the capacity to make decisions and consent to treatment or research participation. As dementia progresses, individuals may lose the capacity to give informed consent.
8. **Protection Against Abuse and Fraud:** People with dementia are vulnerable to abuse, neglect, and financial scams. Legal measures may be needed to protect them from exploitation.
9. **Employment Issues:** If the individual with dementia is still employed, there may be legal considerations related to their employment, such as when to retire, how to access disability benefits, and workplace accommodations.
10. **Driving and Dementia:** Addressing when it is no longer safe to drive and taking legal steps to ensure the person with dementia stops driving when necessary.
11. **End-of-Life Decisions:** Discussing and documenting wishes regarding end-of-life care, including Do Not Resuscitate (DNR) orders and hospice care preferences.

It is advisable for individuals with dementia and their families to consult with legal professionals who specialize in elder law or estate planning to navigate these issues effectively. These professionals can provide guidance tailored to the individual's specific circumstances and ensure that all legal documents are properly prepared and executed.

What is Alzheimer's Disease?

Alzheimer's disease is a progressive neurodegenerative disorder and the most common cause of dementia in older adults. It is characterized by a decline in cognitive function and memory, affecting the ability to perform everyday activities. Key features and aspects of Alzheimer's disease include:

1. **Amyloid Plaques and Tau Tangles:** Alzheimer's disease is pathologically characterized by the accumulation of amyloid-beta plaques and tau protein tangles in the brain. These abnormal protein deposits disrupt communication between nerve cells and eventually lead to cell death.
2. **Memory Loss:** One of the earliest and most noticeable symptoms is memory loss, particularly difficulty remembering recent events or conversations. As the disease progresses, memory impairments worsen.
3. **Cognitive Decline:** This includes problems with reasoning, judgment, and complex task management. Decision-making ability deteriorates, and understanding or developing new concepts becomes challenging.
4. **Language Problems:** Difficulty with language and communication, such as struggling to find the right words, repeating phrases, or difficulty following conversations.
5. **Disorientation:** Individuals may become disoriented to time and place, getting lost in familiar environments and losing track of dates and seasons.
6. **Changes in Behavior and Personality:** Depression, anxiety, social withdrawal, mood swings, distrust in others, increased aggressiveness, or changes in sleeping habits.
7. **Difficulty with Daily Activities:** As the disease progresses, there is an increased dependence on others for basic tasks like dressing, bathing, and eating.
8. **Motor Function and Coordination:** In later stages, coordination and motor functions may be affected, leading to difficulty walking or increased risk of falls.
9. **Progressive Nature:** Alzheimer's disease is progressive, meaning symptoms gradually worsen over time. It typically develops slowly and intensifies over a period of years, eventually leading to severe impairment.
10. **Risk Factors:** Age is the greatest known risk factor, although genetics (family history) also plays a role. Other potential risk factors include cardiovascular disease, head injury, and lifestyle factors.

11. **Diagnosis:** There is no single test for Alzheimer's. Diagnosis is based on medical history, physical and neurological examinations, cognitive tests, and sometimes brain imaging and other tests to rule out other causes of dementia.

12. **Treatment:** Currently, there is no cure for Alzheimer's. Treatment focuses on managing symptoms, slowing the progression of the disease, and improving quality of life. Medications can help with memory symptoms and other cognitive changes. Supportive care, including structured environments, routines, and emotional support, is also important.

13. **Research and Hope:** Ongoing research is focused on finding new ways to treat and prevent Alzheimer's, including exploring the role of genetics, lifestyle factors, and the development of new medications.

Alzheimer's disease has a profound impact not only on the individuals who suffer from it but also on their families and caregivers. Early diagnosis and intervention can be beneficial in managing the disease and planning for the future.

What is the pathology of Alzheimer's dementia?

The pathology of Alzheimer's dementia is characterized by distinctive changes in the brain, involving both structural and chemical alterations. These changes are believed to contribute to the progressive cognitive decline seen in Alzheimer's disease. Key pathological features include:

1. **Amyloid Plaques:** One of the hallmarks of Alzheimer's pathology is the accumulation of beta-amyloid plaques outside neurons. These plaques are dense deposits of protein and cellular material that build up in the spaces between nerve cells. The beta-amyloid protein is derived from a larger precursor protein and is thought to play a crucial role in disrupting cell function.

2. **Neurofibrillary Tangles:** Inside the brain cells, abnormal tau proteins twist into tangles, leading to the breakdown of the neuron's transport system. Tau is a protein that, when functioning normally, helps stabilize microtubules in neurons. In Alzheimer's, tau proteins undergo abnormal chemical changes and form paired helical filaments, disrupting the neuron's internal transport system.

3. **Neuronal and Synaptic Loss:** The presence of plaques and tangles leads to the loss of neurons (nerve cells) and synapses (connections between neurons) throughout the brain. This loss is associated with a decline in neurotransmitters, chemicals that transmit signals between neurons, which is essential for normal brain function.

4. **Brain Atrophy:** Progressive atrophy (shrinking) of brain tissue occurs in Alzheimer's disease, particularly in regions important for memory and cognitive functions, such as the hippocampus and cerebral cortex. This atrophy can be observed in brain imaging studies, like MRI scans.

5. **Inflammation:** The brain's response to the accumulation of plaques and tangles includes inflammation, which may exacerbate neuronal damage.

6. **Vascular Changes:** Reduced blood flow and vascular changes are also commonly observed in Alzheimer's, contributing to brain cell damage.

7. **Genetic Factors:** Certain genetic mutations have been linked to Alzheimer's, particularly in early-onset forms of the disease. The most well-known genetic risk factor for late-onset Alzheimer's is the APOE-e4 allele, although having this gene variant does not mean an individual will definitely develop the disease.

The exact cause of Alzheimer's disease is still not fully understood, and it is likely that a combination of genetic, environmental, and lifestyle factors play a role. Understanding the pathology of Alzheimer's is crucial for developing effective treatments and interventions. Current research continues to explore these pathological processes in the hopes of finding ways to prevent, slow, or reverse the progression of the disease.

What are the Symptoms and Signs of Alzheimer's dementia?

Alzheimer's dementia manifests through a variety of symptoms and signs, which typically develop slowly and worsen over time. The progression can be divided into mild (early-stage), moderate (middle-stage), and severe (late-stage) Alzheimer's disease. Key symptoms and signs include:

1. **Memory Loss:** One of the earliest and most prominent symptoms. Initially, this involves difficulty remembering recent events or conversations. As the disease progresses, memory loss becomes more severe, affecting long-term memory.

2. **Difficulty with Planning and Solving Problems:** Challenges in developing and following plans,

working with numbers, and dealing with complex tasks. Individuals may have trouble following recipes, managing bills, or making decisions.

3. **Difficulty Completing Familiar Tasks:** Struggling with daily tasks, both at home and at work, that were previously routine and easy to complete.
4. **Confusion with Time or Place:** Losing track of dates, seasons, and the passage of time. Individuals may become disoriented about where they are or how they got there.
5. **Trouble Understanding Visual Images and Spatial Relationships:** Vision problems leading to difficulty with balance or reading. They may also have problems judging distance and determining color or contrast, contributing to driving challenges.
6. **New Problems with Words in Speaking or Writing:** Trouble following or joining a conversation. Stopping in the middle of a conversation and having no idea how to continue, or repeating themselves. They may struggle with vocabulary, have problems finding the right word, or call things by the wrong name.
7. **Misplacing Things and Losing the Ability to Retrace Steps:** Placing items in unusual places. They may lose things and be unable to go back over their steps to find them. In some cases, they may accuse others of stealing.
8. **Decreased or Poor Judgment:** This can include confusion about what is safe or socially appropriate. There might be decreased attention to grooming and hygiene, or unwise decisions with money.
9. **Withdrawal from Work or Social Activities:** Pulling away from social activities, work projects, or hobbies. They may have trouble keeping up with a favorite sports team or completing a favorite hobby.
10. **Changes in Mood and Personality:** The development of depression, fearfulness, anxiety, or being easily upset at home, at work, with friends, or in places where they are out of their comfort zone.
11. **Behavioral and Psychological Symptoms:** Agitation, aggression, wandering, restlessness, and sleep disturbances are more common in the middle to late stages.
12. **Physical Decline:** In the later stages, physical abilities decline, including walking, balance, and eventually swallowing.

It is important to note that experiencing one or more of these symptoms does not necessarily mean a person has Alzheimer's. Other medical conditions can cause similar symptoms, so it is important to seek a thorough medical evaluation for an accurate diagnosis. Early diagnosis and intervention can help manage the symptoms of Alzheimer's disease and improve quality of life.

What is the difference between Alzheimer's Disease and Lewy Body Dementia?

Alzheimer's disease and Lewy Body Dementia (LBD) are both common types of dementia but have distinct characteristics and differences in their symptoms, progression, and underlying pathology. Understanding these differences is important for diagnosis and management. Here is a comparison of the two:

Alzheimer's Disease (AD)

1. **Pathology:** Characterized by the build-up of beta-amyloid plaques and tau tangles in the brain.
2. **Memory Loss:** Early and prominent symptom; particularly short-term memory is affected.
3. **Cognitive Decline:** Gradual and steady progression of cognitive decline, particularly in memory, problem-solving, and planning.
4. **Language and Communication:** Difficulty finding words and following conversations appears relatively early.
5. **Behavioral Changes:** Occur, but usually later in the disease progression.
6. **Motor Symptoms:** Not typically present in early stages.
7. **Diagnosis:** Primarily based on clinical evaluation of symptoms, medical history, and cognitive testing. Brain imaging and other tests can provide supporting information.

Lewy Body Dementia (LBD)

1. **Pathology:** Characterized by the presence of Lewy bodies, abnormal deposits of the protein alpha-synuclein, in the brain's nerve cells.
2. **Memory Loss:** Can occur, but is typically not the most prominent symptom in the early stages.
3. **Cognitive Decline:** Fluctuating cognition with varying levels of alertness and attention is a

hallmark. Executive function is often more affected than memory in early stages.

4. **Language and Communication:** Less affected in the early stages compared to Alzheimer's.
5. **Behavioral Changes:** Hallucinations (especially visual) and delusions are common early in the disease. Fluctuations in attention and alertness are also significant.
6. **Motor Symptoms:** Parkinsonian symptoms (such as rigidity, bradykinesia, tremor, and shuffling gait) are commonly seen and often occur early in the disease process.
7. **Diagnosis:** In addition to cognitive testing and medical history, diagnosis is supported by the presence of key symptoms like parkinsonism and visual hallucinations. Brain imaging can help in differentiating it from other types of dementia.

General Comparison

- **Progression:** Alzheimer's typically has a more gradual onset and steady progression, while LBD often presents with a rapid onset and more fluctuating course.
- **Treatment Response:** People with LBD may have a different response to dementia medications compared to those with Alzheimer's and are often more sensitive to antipsychotic medications, which can worsen their symptoms.
- **Sleep Disturbances:** LBD is often associated with significant sleep disturbances, including REM sleep behavior disorder, which can precede other symptoms.

In summary, while there are overlapping features in Alzheimer's disease and Lewy Body Dementia, key differences in their clinical presentations, progression, and responses to treatment are crucial for accurate diagnosis and appropriate management. Proper diagnosis is essential since the treatment strategies and management of symptoms can vary significantly between the two conditions.

What is Vascular Dementia?

Vascular dementia is the second most common type of dementia after Alzheimer's disease and is caused by reduced blood flow to the brain. This reduced blood flow, often due to strokes or other conditions affecting the blood vessels, leads to brain damage and associated cognitive decline. Here are key aspects of vascular dementia:

1. **Causes and Risk Factors:**
   - **Stroke-Related:** Can occur after a stroke interrupts blood flow to the brain, causing brain cells to die.
   - **Small Vessel Disease:** Caused by changes in smaller blood vessels, leading to more widespread brain damage over time.
   - Risk factors include high blood pressure, high cholesterol, diabetes, heart disease, smoking, and atrial fibrillation.
2. **Symptoms:**
   - **Cognitive Impairment:** Memory, thinking, and reasoning skills are affected, though the pattern of impairment can vary.
   - **Executive Functioning Problems:** Difficulty with planning, organizing, and following through with tasks.
   - **Personality Changes:** May include depression, apathy, and social withdrawal.
   - **Physical Symptoms:** Problems with walking and balance, weakness or numbness in limbs, depending on the area of the brain affected.
   - **Rapid Onset and Stepwise Progression:** Symptoms often appear suddenly and worsen in a 'stepwise' manner, where each stroke or vascular event causes a further decline.
3. **Diagnosis:**
   - **Medical History and Physical Examination:** Including assessment of cardiovascular risk factors and neurological function.
   - **Neuropsychological Testing:** To assess cognitive functions more thoroughly.
   - **Brain Imaging:** MRI or CT scans can reveal evidence of strokes or other vascular changes.
4. **Treatment and Management:**
   - **Managing Risk Factors:** Controlling blood pressure, cholesterol, diabetes, and stopping smoking are crucial.
   - **Medications:** To prevent further strokes or vascular events (like antiplatelets or anticoagulants) and to manage specific symptoms.
   - **Rehabilitation Therapies:** Physical therapy, occupational therapy, and speech therapy can help maximize function and independence.

- **Cognitive and Behavioral Interventions:** To address cognitive symptoms and provide behavioral support.
- **Support for Daily Activities:** Assisting with activities of daily living and providing adaptive devices or modifications to the living environment.

5. **Prognosis:**
   - Vascular dementia can progress over time, especially if the underlying vascular issues are not adequately managed. However, with good control of risk factors, further progression can sometimes be slowed.
6. **Prevention:**
   - The best way to prevent vascular dementia is by controlling risk factors for stroke and heart disease, such as maintaining a healthy diet, regular exercise, not smoking, and managing health conditions like hypertension and diabetes.

Vascular dementia highlights the strong connection between overall cardiovascular health and brain health. Effective management of vascular risk factors can play a significant role in preventing or slowing the progression of this form of dementia.

What are the types of vascular dementia?

Vascular dementia is a broad term that encompasses several types, each resulting from different vascular problems in the brain. The type of vascular dementia a person has depends on the part of the brain where blood flow is impaired and the cause of the impairment. Here are the primary types:

1. **Multi-Infarct Dementia (MID):** This is the most common type of vascular dementia. It occurs due to multiple strokes causing infarcts (areas of dead tissue) in the brain. These strokes may be noticeable or may be so small that they don't cause any noticeable symptoms. MID typically presents with a stepwise decline in cognitive function – each stroke causes the brain function to suddenly worsen.
2. **Strategic Infarct Dementia:** Caused by a stroke in a specific area of the brain that is critical for cognitive functioning, such as the thalamus, angular gyrus, or the frontal lobes.
3. **Subcortical Vascular Dementia (also known as Binswanger's Disease):** This type involves changes to the small blood vessels in the subcortical white matter of the brain. It leads to widespread damage and a slow, progressive decline in cognitive function. Symptoms can include difficulty with memory, mood changes, and problems with walking.
4. **Single-Infarct Dementia:** Occurs when a single stroke in a critical area of the brain leads to cognitive impairment.
5. **Hemorrhagic Dementia:** Caused by bleeding in the brain due to a cerebral hemorrhage, which can result from conditions like high blood pressure or cerebral amyloid angiopathy.
6. **Mixed Dementia:** A combination of vascular dementia and another type of dementia, such as Alzheimer's disease. Mixed dementia is increasingly recognized as a common occurrence in older adults.

Each type of vascular dementia can present differently depending on the areas of the brain affected, the severity of the damage, and the individual's overall health. The progression of symptoms can also vary, with some types showing a gradual decline and others a more abrupt change following each vascular event.

Diagnosis of the specific type of vascular dementia usually involves a combination of medical history assessment, neurological exams, and brain imaging studies like MRI or CT scans. Managing underlying cardiovascular risk factors is a key part of treatment and prevention strategies for all types of vascular dementia.

What are the Symptoms and Signs of vascular dementia?

Vascular dementia, resulting from reduced blood flow to the brain, presents with a range of symptoms that can vary greatly depending on the specific areas of the brain affected and the severity of the vascular damage. Common symptoms and signs include:

1. **Cognitive Impairment:**
   - **Memory Loss:** Difficulties with short-term memory.
   - **Executive Dysfunction:** Problems with planning, organizing, problem-solving, and following through with tasks.
2. **Neurological Symptoms:**
   - **Physical Weakness or Paralysis:** Usually on one side of the body, similar to stroke symptoms.

- **Problems with Coordination and Balance:** Difficulty walking or a tendency to fall.

3. **Language and Communication:**
   - **Aphasia:** Difficulty in understanding or producing speech.
   - **Slowed Thinking:** Taking longer to process information and respond.
4. **Personality and Behavioral Changes:**
   - **Apathy:** Lack of interest in usual activities.
   - **Mood Swings or Depression:** Rapid changes in mood, episodes of irritability, or depressive symptoms.
   - **Social Withdrawal:** Avoiding social interactions and activities.
5. **Confusion and Disorientation:**
   - Difficulty in understanding time and place.
   - Becoming easily confused, especially in unfamiliar environments.
6. **Impaired Judgment:**
   - Difficulty in making decisions or behaving appropriately in social situations.
7. **Urinary Symptoms:**
   - Incontinence or urgency, which may be due to brain signals not properly controlling bladder functions.
8. **Gait Disturbances:**
   - A shuffling walk or 'magnetic' gait, where the feet seem to stick to the floor.
9. **Stepwise Progression:**
   - Unlike Alzheimer's disease, which typically has a gradual, continuous decline, vascular dementia often shows a 'stepwise' progression. This means symptoms may suddenly worsen following a stroke or mini-stroke, then stabilize for a time before worsening again with further vascular events.
10. **Fluctuating Symptoms:**
    - The symptoms may vary or fluctuate over time, depending on the state of blood flow in the brain.
11. **Night-time Confusion:**
    - Increased confusion or agitation during the night.

It is important to recognize that vascular dementia can coexist with other forms of dementia, like Alzheimer's disease, leading to a mixed dementia picture. This can make the exact symptomatology more complex. The presence and severity of these symptoms can fluctuate based on the progression of the disease, treatment of underlying conditions, and overall health status of the individual. Early diagnosis and management can help in slowing the progression and improving the quality of life for individuals with vascular dementia.

How do you diagnose vascular dementia?

Diagnosing vascular dementia involves a combination of clinical assessment, medical history, neurological examination, and diagnostic tests. The goal is to identify the symptoms consistent with dementia, establish the vascular cause, and rule out other possible causes. Here is an overview of the diagnostic process:

1. **Medical and Personal History:** Understanding the patient's medical history, including prior strokes, heart attacks, or risk factors for vascular disease (like high blood pressure, high cholesterol, diabetes, smoking history) is crucial. A detailed personal history that includes changes in behavior, cognitive function, and daily activities is also gathered, often with input from family members or caregivers.
2. **Neurological Examination:** This assesses brain and nerve function and may include tests of memory, problem-solving, attention, language skills, visual-spatial skills, reflexes, muscle strength, movement, coordination, balance, and sensory function.
3. **Cognitive and Neuropsychological Testing:** Detailed tests to assess cognitive function more thoroughly, focusing on areas like memory, executive function (planning, organizing, problem-solving), language, and visuospatial skills.
4. **Laboratory Tests:** Blood tests to check for vitamin deficiencies (like B12), thyroid function, and other conditions that can cause symptoms similar to dementia.
5. **Brain Imaging:**
   - **MRI or CT Scans:** These are critical for diagnosing vascular dementia. They can reveal evidence of strokes, brain atrophy, and other changes in brain structure. MRI is more sensitive than CT in detecting smaller lesions and damage in the brain.

- **Doppler Ultrasound:** To assess blood flow in the carotid arteries, which supply blood to the brain.

6. **Cardiac Evaluation:** Since vascular dementia can be related to heart problems, tests like an electrocardiogram (EKG) or echocardiogram might be performed.

7. **Ruling Out Other Causes:** It is important to differentiate vascular dementia from other types of dementia like Alzheimer's. This can sometimes be challenging as some individuals may have mixed dementia, which includes features of both Alzheimer's and vascular dementia.

8. **Review of Medications:** Evaluating current medications to rule out side effects that might mimic symptoms of dementia.

The diagnosis of vascular dementia is made based on the presence of cognitive decline, evidence of cerebrovascular disease (as shown in brain imaging), and a clear relationship between the two. Since there is no single definitive test for vascular dementia, it is diagnosed based on the overall clinical picture. Early and accurate diagnosis is important for managing the condition and potentially slowing its progression.

What is the prognosis of vascular dementia?

The prognosis of vascular dementia varies depending on several factors, including the extent and location of brain damage, the underlying vascular conditions, the individual's overall health, and how well risk factors are managed. Key aspects of the prognosis for vascular dementia include:

1. **Progression:** Vascular dementia typically progresses in a stepwise manner, where symptoms may suddenly worsen due to stroke or mini-stroke and then stabilize for a time. The rate of progression can vary widely among individuals.

2. **Variable Rate of Decline:** Unlike Alzheimer's disease, which generally has a gradual, steady decline, the course of vascular dementia can be more unpredictable due to its dependence on cardiovascular health and new vascular events.

3. **Impact of Stroke Prevention:** Active management of risk factors like high blood pressure, high cholesterol, diabetes, smoking cessation, and a healthy lifestyle can significantly impact the progression of the disease. Preventing further strokes or mini-strokes is crucial in slowing the progression of vascular dementia.

4. **Mixed Dementia:** Many people with vascular dementia also have Alzheimer's disease pathology, which can influence the progression and prognosis.

5. **Comorbid Conditions:** The presence of other medical conditions, especially those related to heart and vascular health, can affect the prognosis. Coexisting conditions can complicate management and may accelerate cognitive decline.

6. **Quality of Life:** With appropriate support, individuals with vascular dementia can maintain a good quality of life, especially in the earlier stages of the disease. As the condition progresses, increased care and support may be required.

7. **Life Expectancy:** Vascular dementia can potentially shorten life expectancy, particularly if the underlying cardiovascular issues are not well-managed. However, life expectancy can vary greatly depending on individual health factors and the severity of vascular brain damage.

8. **Symptom Management:** While there is no cure for vascular dementia, treatment to manage symptoms, rehabilitative therapies, and supportive care can improve quality of life.

9. **Importance of Early Detection:** Early diagnosis and intervention to manage vascular risk factors can slow the progression of dementia and improve outcomes.

The prognosis for vascular dementia is highly individual and depends on a variety of factors. Regular medical care, management of cardiovascular risk factors, and supportive interventions are key to managing the disease and maintaining the best possible quality of life.

What is the treatment of vascular dementia?

The treatment of vascular dementia focuses on managing the underlying vascular conditions, controlling symptoms, and maximizing the individual's quality of life. Since there is no cure for vascular dementia, the goal is to slow the progression of the disease and address the symptoms that affect daily living. Treatment typically involves a combination of medical management, lifestyle modifications, and supportive care:

1. **Managing Underlying Vascular Conditions:**
   - **Blood Pressure Control:** High blood pressure is a major risk factor for vascular dementia. Controlling blood pressure through medications and lifestyle changes is crucial.

- **Cholesterol Management:** Statins or other cholesterol-lowering drugs may be prescribed.
- **Diabetes Management:** Keeping blood sugar levels under control is important.
- **Heart Disease Management:** Treating underlying heart conditions and maintaining heart health.
- **Stroke Prevention:** Antiplatelet agents (like aspirin) or anticoagulants may be used to prevent strokes.

2. **Lifestyle Modifications:**
   - **Diet and Nutrition:** A heart-healthy diet, such as the Mediterranean diet, can be beneficial.
   - **Physical Activity:** Regular exercise improves cardiovascular health and can help maintain muscle tone and balance.
   - **Smoking Cessation and Limiting Alcohol Intake:** These lifestyle changes are important for reducing the risk of further vascular damage.
3. **Cognitive and Behavioral Interventions:**
   - **Cognitive Stimulation:** Activities like puzzles, memory games, and social interactions can help stimulate the brain.
   - **Behavioral Management:** Non-pharmacological approaches are often first-line for addressing behavioral issues like agitation or aggression.
4. **Medications for Cognitive Symptoms:**
   - Though primarily used in Alzheimer's disease, medications like cholinesterase inhibitors (e.g., donepezil) and memantine may sometimes be prescribed to manage cognitive symptoms in vascular dementia.
5. **Support for Activities of Daily Living:**
   - Occupational therapy can provide strategies for coping with daily tasks.
   - Speech therapy may be beneficial if there are language or swallowing difficulties.
6. **Psychological Support:**
   - Counseling or therapy for the patient and family to manage the emotional challenges of the diagnosis.
   - Support groups can provide shared experiences and strategies.
7. **Safety Considerations:**
   - Modifications in the living environment to prevent falls and ensure safety.
   - In later stages, assistance with mobility, feeding, and personal care may be necessary.
8. **Monitoring and Regular Follow-up:**
   - Regular check-ups to monitor the progression of dementia and adjust treatments as necessary.
9. **Legal and Financial Planning:**
   - Early planning for future healthcare, living arrangements, and financial management is advised.
10. **Caregiver Support:**
    - Education and resources for caregivers, respite care options, and support groups.

Vascular dementia treatment requires a multidisciplinary approach, involving doctors, nurses, therapists, and caregivers. While treatment cannot reverse the damage to the brain, it can help slow down the progression of dementia and improve the quality of life for both the person with dementia and their caregivers.

What is Lewy Body Dementia (LBD)?

Lewy Body Dementia (LBD) is a type of progressive dementia that leads to a decline in thinking, reasoning, and independent function due to abnormal microscopic deposits that damage brain cells over time. These deposits are made of a protein called alpha-synuclein, and the clumps are referred to as Lewy bodies, named after the neurologist who discovered them. LBD is one of the most common causes of dementia, alongside Alzheimer's disease and vascular dementia.

LBD is characterized by two related clinical disorders:

1. **Dementia with Lewy Bodies (DLB):** In DLB, cognitive symptoms severe enough to interfere with daily living appear before or concurrently with Parkinson's-like movement symptoms.
2. **Parkinson's Disease Dementia (PDD):** In PDD, the movement symptoms of Parkinson's disease appear first, followed by the development of dementia symptoms more than a year later.

Key Features of Lewy Body Dementia:

1. **Cognitive Decline:** Fluctuating cognition with pronounced variations in attention and alertness;

problems with executive function, planning, handling complex tasks, and visual-spatial abilities.

2. **Visual Hallucinations:** Detailed and recurrent visual hallucinations are common and one of the hallmark symptoms.
3. **Movement Disorders:** Symptoms similar to Parkinson's disease, such as slowness of movement, stiffness, tremors, and walking difficulty.
4. **REM Sleep Behavior Disorder:** Acting out dreams, sometimes violently, which can precede other LBD symptoms.
5. **Fluctuating Alertness:** Fluctuations in alertness and attention, including periods of drowsiness, long periods of staring into space, or disorganized speech.
6. **Other Symptoms:** May include depression, apathy, anxiety, paranoia, and delusions.

Diagnosis:

Diagnosing LBD can be challenging, as its early symptoms are often similar to those of Alzheimer's and Parkinson 's disease. There is no single test for LBD, so doctors diagnose it based on the range of symptoms. This process usually involves:

- A thorough medical history.
- Neurological and physical exams.
- Cognitive tests.
- Brain imaging to rule out other conditions.

Treatment:

Treatment for LBD is focused on managing symptoms, as there is no cure for the disease currently. The approach may include:

- **Medications:** Cholinesterase inhibitors for cognitive symptoms, and in some cases, Parkinson's disease medications for movement symptoms.
- Non-pharmacological interventions for behavior and mood symptoms, like structured environments and routines.
- Management of sleep and mood disorders.
- Physical therapy for movement problems.
- Occupational and speech therapy.

Challenges in Management:

People with LBD may react differently or be more sensitive to certain medications compared to people with Alzheimer's, particularly those used to treat hallucinations. Therefore, treatment requires careful monitoring and adjustment.

LBD is a complex condition that significantly impacts both the person with the disease and their caregivers. Providing comprehensive care and support for both is essential.

What is pathology of LB dementia?

Lewy Body Dementia (LBD) is characterized by distinctive pathological changes in the brain, which are key to understanding the disease. The primary pathological feature of LBD is the presence of Lewy bodies and Lewy neurites, which are abnormal aggregates of protein that develop inside nerve cells. These protein deposits primarily consist of a protein called alpha-synuclein. Here is an overview of the pathology of LBD:

1. **Lewy Bodies and Lewy Neurites:**
   - Lewy bodies are spherical, intracellular aggregates found in the neurons, predominantly in the cortex (outer layer of the brain).
   - Lewy neurites are abnormal neuritic processes filled with alpha-synuclein and are often found in the hippocampus and amygdala, regions involved in memory and emotion.
   - The accumulation of Lewy bodies and neurites disrupts normal neuronal function and communication, leading to the symptoms of LBD.
2. **Alpha-Synuclein Protein:**
   - Alpha-synuclein is a protein found abundantly in the brain, but its normal function is not well understood.
   - In LBD (and Parkinson's disease), alpha-synuclein forms clumps, which are thought to be toxic to brain cells.
3. **Neurodegeneration:**
   - Over time, the accumulation of Lewy bodies leads to progressive degeneration of brain tissue, especially in areas that control cognition, movement, and behavior.
   - This neurodegeneration causes a decline in mental abilities, motor skills, and affects autonomic body functions.
4. **Dopaminergic Neuron Loss:**
   - Similar to Parkinson's disease, LBD involves the loss of dopamine-producing neurons in the

substantia nigra, part of the midbrain. This loss contributes to the Parkinsonian motor symptoms observed in LBD.

5. **Cortical Involvement:**
   - In dementia with Lewy bodies (DLB), the cerebral cortex is more extensively involved than in Parkinson's disease dementia (PDD), which explains the more pronounced cognitive symptoms seen in DLB.
6. **Other Pathological Changes:**
   - LBD pathology often coexists with other types of brain pathology, including Alzheimer's disease pathology (amyloid plaques and tau tangles).
   - Vascular changes and brain atrophy are also commonly observed in LBD.
7. **Neurotransmitter Changes:**
   - Apart from dopamine, there are changes in other neurotransmitters, including acetylcholine (involved in memory and learning), contributing to cognitive and behavioral symptoms.

The pathology of LBD is complex, and its overlap with other neurodegenerative disorders like Parkinson's disease and Alzheimer's disease can make diagnosis and treatment challenging. Research continues to evolve in understanding the exact mechanisms by which Lewy bodies cause brain cell damage and how these processes can be halted or reversed.

What are the clinical features of LB dementia?

Lewy Body Dementia (LBD) encompasses a spectrum of clinical features that can vary significantly from person to person. It is characterized by a combination of cognitive, behavioral, motor, and sleep-related symptoms. The clinical features of LBD can be divided into core symptoms, supportive features, and indicative biomarkers:

Core Symptoms

1. **Fluctuating Cognition:** This includes pronounced variations in attention and alertness. Individuals may have periods of clear thinking and awareness, followed by times of confusion and clouded attention.
2. **Recurrent Visual Hallucinations:** Well-formed and detailed hallucinations, typically visual, are a common feature. These hallucinations are often recurrent and can be one of the earliest symptoms.
3. **Parkinsonism:** Motor symptoms similar to Parkinson's disease, such as rigidity, bradykinesia (slowness of movement), tremors, and gait disturbances.

Supportive Features

1. **REM Sleep Behavior Disorder:** Acting out dreams, sometimes violently, is a significant feature often preceding cognitive decline.
2. **Severe Neuroleptic Sensitivity:** Extreme sensitivity to antipsychotic medications, with a tendency to worsen symptoms.
3. **Non-Visual Hallucinations:** Auditory or other non-visual hallucinations can occur.
4. **Cognitive Symptoms:** Impairment in executive function (planning, decision-making), memory, and visuospatial abilities.
5. **Behavioral and Mood Symptoms:** Depression, apathy, anxiety, agitation, and delusions.
6. **Autonomic Dysfunction:** This can include blood pressure fluctuations, urinary incontinence, constipation, and erectile dysfunction.

Indicative Biomarkers

1. **Brain Imaging:** Showing reduced dopamine transporter uptake in basal ganglia, revealed through SPECT or PET imaging.
2. **Polysomnographic Confirmation:** Confirmation of REM sleep without atonia.
3. **Other Biomarkers:** These are still under research but include abnormalities in alpha-synuclein, PET imaging of amyloid, and tau in the brain.

Other Clinical Features

1. **Sensitivity to Medications:** People with LBD may have adverse reactions to certain medications used to treat hallucinations or Parkinsonism, which can exacerbate symptoms.
2. **Overlap with Other Dementias:** LBD may coexist with Alzheimer's disease or Parkinson's disease, complicating the clinical picture.
3. **Progression:** The symptoms of LBD progressively worsen over time, although the rate of progression can vary between individuals.

The clinical presentation of LBD can be complex, and symptoms can overlap with other neurodegenerative diseases, making diagnosis challenging. Early and accurate diagnosis is essential for managing symptoms and improving the quality of life for individuals with LBD and their caregivers.

How do you diagnose LB dementia?

Diagnosing Lewy Body Dementia (LBD) can be challenging due to its overlap with other dementia types like Alzheimer's disease and Parkinson's disease dementia. There is no single test to diagnose LBD, so it typically involves a combination of clinical assessment, patient history, neurological examination, cognitive testing, and sometimes additional diagnostic tools. Here is an overview of the process:

1. **Clinical Assessment:**
   - Detailed evaluation of symptoms, including cognitive, behavioral, and motor symptoms.
   - Assessment of core features of LBD such as fluctuating cognition, visual hallucinations, and Parkinsonian motor symptoms.
2. **Medical and Family History:**
   - Gathering information about the patient's medical history, family history of dementia or Parkinson's disease, and any history of similar symptoms.
3. **Neurological Examination:**
   - Assessing motor function to check for signs of Parkinsonism (rigidity, tremors, bradykinesia).
   - Evaluating reflexes, muscle strength, movement, coordination, and balance.
4. **Cognitive Testing:**
   - Neuropsychological tests to assess memory, executive function, attention, language, and visuospatial abilities.
   - Monitoring for fluctuations in attention and alertness.
5. **Sleep Evaluation:**
   - Inquiry about sleep disturbances, particularly REM Sleep Behavior Disorder (RBD), which involves acting out dreams.
   - A polysomnogram (sleep study) may be recommended to document RBD.
6. **Psychiatric Evaluation:**
   - Assessing for hallucinations, delusions, and other psychiatric symptoms.
   - Differentiating these symptoms from other causes, such as delirium or psychiatric disorders.
7. **Brain Imaging:**
   - MRI or CT scans to rule out other conditions that could cause similar symptoms, like strokes or brain tumors.
   - SPECT or PET scans to assess brain function and dopamine transporter activity, which can support a diagnosis of LBD.
8. **Response to Medication:**
   - Observing how symptoms respond to medications can provide diagnostic clues, though this approach must be used cautiously due to potential medication sensitivities in LBD.
9. **Exclusion of Other Conditions:**
   - Ruling out other possible causes of symptoms, such as Alzheimer's disease, vascular dementia, or frontotemporal dementia.
10. **Biomarkers Research:**
    - While not yet routinely used in clinical practice, research into biomarkers, including alpha-synuclein levels in the cerebrospinal fluid, is ongoing.

Diagnosis of LBD is often based on the consensus criteria developed by experts in the field and requires careful consideration of the patient's symptoms, history, and test results. Since LBD can significantly impact medication choices and management strategies, an accurate diagnosis is crucial for optimal patient care.

What is the treatment of LB dementia?

The treatment of Lewy Body Dementia (LBD) is primarily focused on managing symptoms, as there is currently no cure for the disease. Treatment strategies are tailored to the individual's specific symptoms and may change as the disease progresses. Key components of LBD treatment include:

1. **Medication Management:**
   - **Cognitive Symptoms:** Cholinesterase inhibitors, such as donepezil, rivastigmine, or galantamine, are often used to improve cognition and alertness.
   - **Parkinsonism:** Medications used for Parkinson's disease, like levodopa, can help with movement symptoms, but must be used cautiously as they can exacerbate hallucinations and confusion.

- **Psychiatric Symptoms:** Atypical antipsychotics may be prescribed for severe hallucinations or delusions, but they carry risks and must be used carefully due to increased sensitivity in LBD patients.

2. **Non-Pharmacological Interventions:**
   - **Cognitive Stimulation:** Activities that engage the brain, such as puzzles, memory games, and social interaction, can help maintain cognitive function.
   - **Physical Therapy:** To address movement issues and prevent falls.
   - **Occupational Therapy:** To help maintain independence in daily activities.
   - **Speech Therapy:** For any issues with speech or swallowing.
3. **Management of Sleep Disorders:**
   - Treatment for REM Sleep Behavior Disorder might include medications like melatonin or clonazepam.
   - Maintaining good sleep hygiene is also important.
4. **Behavioral Strategies:**
   - Techniques to manage behavioral issues like agitation or aggression, including environmental modifications, structured routines, and minimizing triggers that cause distress.
5. **Support and Education for Caregivers:**
   - Providing education about LBD to caregivers.
   - Support groups and counseling can be beneficial for caregivers.
6. **Safety Considerations:**
   - Ensuring a safe environment, especially for patients experiencing hallucinations, confusion, or mobility issues.
7. **Regular Medical Check-ups:**
   - Ongoing monitoring of the patient's overall health and adjustment of treatments as necessary.
8. **End-of-Life Planning:**
   - Discussing and preparing for end-of-life care, including advance directives and palliative care options.
9. **Psychological Support:**
   - Counseling or therapy for both the patient and their caregivers to address the emotional and psychological impact of the disease.

It is crucial to approach LBD treatment with a multidisciplinary perspective, involving neurologists, psychiatrists, physical therapists, occupational therapists, speech therapists, and primary care providers. Due to the complexity of LBD and its varied symptoms, treatment plans are highly individualized and require careful monitoring and adjustments over time.

What is the prognosis of LB dementia?

Lewy Body Dementia (LBD) is a progressive brain disorder characterized by the accumulation of Lewy bodies, abnormal aggregates of protein, in the brain. The prognosis for LBD can vary significantly among individuals, but it is generally considered a progressive and incurable disease. Here are some key points regarding the prognosis of LBD:

1. **Progression Rate:** LBD typically progresses at a variable rate. Some individuals experience a rapid decline, while others may have a more gradual progression of symptoms.
2. **Symptoms:** Symptoms can include cognitive impairment, visual hallucinations, sleep disturbances, and Parkinsonian motor symptoms. As the disease progresses, these symptoms typically worsen.
3. **Life Expectancy:** On average, individuals with LBD live 5 to 8 years after the onset of symptoms. However, this can vary widely, and some people may live longer.
4. **Management:** There is no cure for LBD, but symptoms can sometimes be managed with medication and non-pharmacological interventions. Management focuses on improving quality of life and may involve a multidisciplinary team.
5. **Complications:** In later stages, complications such as severe motor dysfunction, communication difficulties, and poor response to medications can arise. There is also an increased risk of pneumonia and other infections due to immobility and swallowing difficulties.
6. **Supportive Care:** As LBD progresses, supportive care becomes increasingly important. This may include assistance with daily activities, physical therapy, occupational therapy, and palliative care.

It is important to note that every individual's experience with LBD is unique, and the course of the disease can be unpredictable. Ongoing medical care and support from healthcare providers, caregivers, and support groups are crucial in managing LBD.

What is HIV-Associated Dementia?

HIV-Associated Dementia (HAD), also known as AIDS Dementia Complex (ADC), is a neurological disorder associated with HIV infection and AIDS. It occurs when the HIV virus directly affects the brain and nervous system. Here are key aspects of HIV-Associated Dementia:

1. **Causes and Pathophysiology:** HAD results from the direct effects of HIV on the central nervous system. The virus can infect brain cells, leading to inflammation and damage to neurons. The exact mechanisms are complex and involve a combination of direct viral effects, immune activation, and neuronal injury.

2. **Symptoms:** Symptoms of HAD can range from mild to severe and typically involve cognitive, motor, and behavioral changes. Cognitive symptoms may include memory loss, difficulty concentrating, and confusion. Motor symptoms can include clumsiness, poor coordination, and weakness. Behavioral changes might include apathy, social withdrawal, and changes in mood.

3. **Progression:** The progression of HAD can vary. In some individuals, symptoms develop slowly and progressively worsen over time. In others, the onset may be more abrupt.

4. **Diagnosis:** Diagnosing HAD involves a combination of neurological exams, neuropsychological testing, brain imaging, and ruling out other causes of dementia. It is important to differentiate HAD from other conditions that can occur in people with HIV, such as opportunistic infections and medication side effects.

5. **Treatment and Management:** Antiretroviral therapy (ART), which controls HIV replication, is the cornerstone of HAD treatment. Effective ART can often prevent or alleviate symptoms of HAD by suppressing HIV in the brain. Additional treatments may address specific symptoms, such as cognitive therapies, physical therapy, and psychiatric medications for mood or behavioral issues.

6. **Prevention:** The best prevention for HAD is early and effective treatment of HIV infection with ART. Keeping the virus under control can significantly reduce the risk of developing HAD.

7. **Prognosis:** With the advent of effective ART, the incidence of HAD has significantly decreased, and the prognosis has improved. However, in cases where HAD develops, the severity and progression can vary. Some individuals may experience a stabilization or improvement of symptoms with treatment, while others may continue to experience a decline in function.

It is important for individuals with HIV to receive regular medical care, including neurological assessments, to monitor for signs of HAD and other neurological complications associated with HIV.

What is pathology of HIV-Associated Dementia?

The pathology of HIV-Associated Dementia (HAD), also known as AIDS Dementia Complex (ADC), is complex and involves multiple factors related to HIV infection and its impact on the brain. Understanding the pathology requires examining several key areas:

1. **HIV Infection of the Brain:** HIV can enter the brain early after initial infection. The virus crosses the blood-brain barrier, often carried by infected monocytes (a type of white blood cell). Once inside the brain, these cells can infect microglia (the resident immune cells of the brain) and possibly astrocytes (cells that support and protect neurons).

2. **Neuroinflammation:** A significant aspect of HAD pathology is chronic neuroinflammation. Infected microglial cells and activated astrocytes release inflammatory cytokines and chemokines, leading to an inflammatory response that can be damaging to brain tissue.

3. **Neuronal Damage:** While HIV does not usually infect neurons directly, the virus-induced inflammatory environment in the brain can lead to neuronal injury and death. Neurotoxins released by infected and activated glial cells, including cytokines and viral proteins (like gp120 and Tat), can cause direct neuronal damage. This process is often referred to as indirect neurotoxicity.

4. **Synaptic and Dendritic Damage:** There is evidence of synaptic and dendritic damage in HAD, which contributes to the cognitive and motor symptoms observed in the disease. This damage is likely a result of the neuroinflammatory milieu and neurotoxic effects of viral proteins.

5. **Amyloid Deposition:** Some research has indicated that HIV infection may accelerate the process of amyloid deposition in the brain, a hallmark of Alzheimer's disease, suggesting some overlap in the pathology of these conditions.

6. **Brain Atrophy and White Matter Changes:** Neuroimaging studies often reveal brain atrophy (shrinkage) and white matter changes in individuals with HAD. These changes are associated with the severity of cognitive and motor impairments.

7. **Blood-Brain Barrier Disruption:** HIV infection can disrupt the integrity of the blood-brain barrier, making it more permeable and allowing more immune cells and potentially harmful substances into the brain.

8. **Role of Antiretroviral Therapy (ART):** While ART has significantly reduced the incidence and severity of HAD, its role in the pathology is complex. Effective ART reduces viral load in the brain, which can prevent or mitigate HAD. However, some antiretroviral drugs have limited penetration into the brain, and certain drugs might contribute to neurotoxicity.

9. **Viral Escape:** There is a concept of "viral escape" in the central nervous system, where the virus in the brain may become genetically distinct from the virus in the rest of the body. This can happen because the brain is somewhat isolated from the immune system, allowing different viral strains to evolve.

10. **Genetic and Host Factors:** Individual genetic factors and the overall health of the person's immune system can influence the severity and progression of HAD. This includes genetic variants that affect immune responses and brain cell functions.

In summary, the pathology of HIV-Associated Dementia is characterized by HIV infection of brain cells, chronic neuroinflammation, indirect neuronal damage, and changes in brain structure and function. The interaction between the virus, the immune system, and various neural cell types plays a crucial role in the development and progression of HAD. Continuous research is essential for better understanding and treating this complex condition.

What are Symptoms and Signs of HIV-Associated Dementia?

HIV-Associated Dementia (HAD), also known as AIDS Dementia Complex, is a neurological condition that can occur in advanced stages of HIV infection. The symptoms and signs of HAD can be quite varied, affecting cognitive, motor, and behavioral functions. Here are some of the key symptoms and signs:

1. **Cognitive Impairment:**
   - **Memory Loss:** Difficulty in recalling recent events or learning new information.
   - **Concentration and Attention Deficits:** Trouble focusing on tasks or maintaining attention.
   - **Slowed Processing Speed:** Slower thought processes and difficulty understanding complex information.
   - **Executive Dysfunction:** Problems with planning, organizing, problem-solving, and multitasking.
2. **Motor Symptoms:**
   - **Poor Coordination:** Clumsiness or difficulty in coordinating movements.
   - **Weakness:** Generalized weakness, sometimes more pronounced in specific limbs.
   - **Bradykinesia:** Slowness of movement.
   - **Tremors or Shaking:** Unintentional trembling or shaking, which may be subtle.
   - **Gait Abnormalities:** Changes in walking, such as a shuffling gait.
3. **Behavioral and Mood Changes:**
   - **Apathy:** Lack of interest or motivation in daily activities.
   - **Irritability:** Increased irritability or short temper.
   - **Depression:** Symptoms of depression, including persistent sadness, loss of interest in pleasurable activities, and changes in sleep and appetite.
   - **Social Withdrawal:** Tendency to withdraw from social interactions and activities.
4. **Speech and Language Difficulties:**
   - **Difficulty in Articulation:** Trouble in clearly articulating words.
   - **Slowed Speech:** Slowing down of speech or taking longer to respond in conversations.
5. **Other Neurological Signs:**
   - **Seizures:** In some cases, seizures can occur.

- **Psychosis:** Rarely, symptoms such as hallucinations or delusions might manifest.

6. **Advanced Symptoms:**
   - In later stages, HAD can lead to more severe cognitive and motor deterioration, significantly impairing a person's ability to carry out daily activities.

7. **Variability of Symptoms:**
   - The onset of symptoms can be gradual or rapid, and the severity can range from mild to severe. Not all individuals with HIV will develop HAD, and the symptoms can vary significantly from person to person.

It is important to note that these symptoms can also be caused by other conditions, including other neurological disorders, infections, and side effects of medication. Therefore, a thorough medical evaluation is necessary to distinguish HAD from other possible causes. With the widespread use of effective antiretroviral therapy (ART), the incidence and severity of HAD have significantly decreased. Regular medical care and effective HIV treatment can help manage or prevent the development of HAD.

How do you Diagnose HIV-Associated Dementia?

Diagnosing HIV-Associated Dementia (HAD) involves a comprehensive assessment to rule out other potential causes of symptoms and to confirm that the cognitive, motor, and behavioral changes are indeed due to HIV infection of the brain. The process typically includes the following steps:

1. **Clinical Assessment:**
   - **Medical History:** Detailed medical history, including the history of HIV infection, antiretroviral therapy (ART) adherence, and any other medical conditions or medications that could affect cognitive function.
   - **Symptom Evaluation:** Assessment of cognitive, motor, and behavioral symptoms reported by the patient or observed by others.

2. **Neuropsychological Testing:**
   - Tests to assess various cognitive functions such as memory, attention, language, problem-solving, and executive functions. These tests help quantify the degree of cognitive impairment.

3. **Neurological Examination:**
   - A thorough neurological exam to evaluate motor function, coordination, reflexes, and other neurological functions.

4. **Laboratory Tests:**
   - Blood tests to check for other causes of dementia-like symptoms, such as vitamin deficiencies, thyroid dysfunction, syphilis, or other infections.
   - HIV viral load and CD4 count to assess the current status of HIV infection.

5. **Brain Imaging:**
   - MRI or CT scans of the brain to rule out other causes of dementia (such as stroke, brain tumors, or other neurodegenerative diseases) and to look for patterns of brain atrophy or other changes that might be consistent with HAD.

6. **Lumbar Puncture:**
   - Sometimes, a lumbar puncture (spinal tap) is performed to analyze cerebrospinal fluid (CSF) for HIV viral load, signs of inflammation, and other infections that can affect the brain.

7. **Exclusion of Other Causes:**
   - It is crucial to rule out other potential causes of dementia, especially in individuals with HIV, as they may be prone to various neurological complications, including opportunistic infections and side effects of medications.

8. **Monitoring and Follow-Up:**
   - Regular monitoring of cognitive function and HIV disease status, as changes over time can provide important diagnostic clues.

It is important to note that HAD is a diagnosis of exclusion, meaning it is considered after other potential causes have been ruled out. The involvement of a multidisciplinary team, including neurologists, psychiatrists, and infectious disease specialists, is often beneficial in the diagnostic process. With the advancement in HIV treatment, the incidence of HAD has decreased significantly, and early initiation of ART can help prevent or mitigate its development.

What is the prognosis of HIV-Associated Dementia?

The prognosis of HIV-Associated Dementia (HAD) has significantly improved with the advent of effective antiretroviral therapy (ART), but it still varies based on several factors. Here are key points regarding the prognosis:

1. **Impact of Antiretroviral Therapy:** ART has dramatically changed the outlook for HAD. Effective ART can not only prevent its onset in people living with HIV but can also halt or reverse the progression of cognitive decline in those who develop HAD. Early and consistent treatment of HIV is crucial.
2. **Severity at Diagnosis:** The severity of dementia at the time of diagnosis can impact prognosis. Individuals with milder forms of cognitive impairment may respond better to ART and have a more favorable outcome.
3. **Adherence to Treatment:** Adherence to ART is a critical factor in prognosis. Inconsistent adherence can lead to less effective control of HIV, potentially worsening the neurological impact.
4. **Comorbid Conditions:** The presence of other comorbid conditions, such as other infections, substance abuse, or other neurological disorders, can complicate the treatment of HAD and affect the overall prognosis.
5. **Cognitive and Functional Status:** The degree of cognitive and functional impairment can influence the outcome. Individuals with significant impairment may experience a decline in their ability to perform daily activities, impacting their quality of life.
6. **Immune System Health:** The overall health of the immune system, as indicated by CD4 counts and HIV viral load, plays a role in the progression of HAD. A stronger immune system typically correlates with a better prognosis.
7. **Age and General Health:** Older age and poorer general health can negatively impact the prognosis. Younger individuals and those in good general health may have a more favorable outcome.
8. **Neurological and Psychiatric Complications:** The development of other neurological or psychiatric complications associated with HIV can also influence the prognosis.

In summary, while HAD was once considered a severely debilitating condition with a poor prognosis, advances in HIV treatment have significantly improved outcomes. Early diagnosis, effective and consistent use of ART, management of comorbid conditions, and regular medical follow-up are key to optimizing the prognosis for individuals with HAD. However, the variability in individual responses and the complexity of HIV management mean that each case needs to be considered on an individual basis.

What is the Treatment of HIV-Associated Dementia?

The treatment of HIV-Associated Dementia (HAD) primarily focuses on optimizing antiretroviral therapy (ART) and addressing specific symptoms. Here are the main components of HAD treatment:

1. **Optimizing Antiretroviral Therapy (ART):**
   - The cornerstone of HAD treatment is effective ART. This therapy reduces the viral load in the body, including the brain, and can stabilize or improve cognitive function.
   - Some antiretroviral drugs have better penetration into the central nervous system (CNS) and might be more effective for HAD. The choice of ART should be guided by a specialist in HIV treatment.
2. **Management of Symptoms:**
   - **Cognitive Symptoms:** Cognitive rehabilitation therapies may help. In some cases, medications used for other forms of dementia, like Alzheimer's disease (e.g., cholinesterase inhibitors), might be considered, although their efficacy in HAD is not well-established.
   - **Motor Symptoms:** Physical therapy and exercise can help manage motor symptoms. Medications might be used for specific symptoms, such as tremors or spasticity.
   - **Behavioral and Psychiatric Symptoms:** Antidepressants, anxiolytics, or antipsychotics can be used to treat associated depression, anxiety, or psychotic symptoms, under careful supervision due to potential interactions with ART.
3. **Addressing Comorbid Conditions:**
   - Managing other medical conditions, including opportunistic infections, is essential for overall health and can positively influence HAD treatment outcomes.
4. **Supportive Care:**
   - Supportive care includes nutritional support, managing daily living activities, and ensuring a safe environment, especially for those with advanced cognitive impairment.

- Counseling and support for both the patient and caregivers are important, as HAD can be challenging to manage on both an emotional and practical level.

5. **Regular Monitoring and Follow-Up:**
   - Regular neurological assessments and monitoring of HIV status (CD4 count and viral load) are important to assess the effectiveness of treatment and make any necessary adjustments.

6. **Research and Experimental Treatments:**
   - Ongoing research may provide new treatment options in the future. Participation in clinical trials could be considered, where appropriate.

It is important to note that while ART can significantly improve the prognosis and symptoms of HAD, it may not completely reverse the condition, especially if diagnosed at a later stage. Multidisciplinary care involving neurologists, psychiatrists, infectious disease specialists, and other healthcare professionals is essential for optimal management of HAD.

What is Frontotemporal (FTD) Dementia?

Frontotemporal Dementia (FTD) is a group of brain disorders caused by degeneration of the frontal and temporal lobes of the brain. It is one of the less common types of dementia and tends to occur at a younger age than Alzheimer's disease, often between the ages of 45 and 65. FTD is characterized by progressive changes in behavior, personality, language, and movement. The symptoms of FTD can vary significantly depending on the specific areas of the brain that are affected.

FTD is broadly categorized into several types:

1. **Behavioral Variant Frontotemporal Dementia (bvFTD):**
   - This is the most common form of FTD. It primarily affects behavior and personality. Individuals may exhibit disinhibition, apathy, loss of empathy, compulsive behavior, and neglect of personal hygiene.
   - There are often changes in eating habits, such as overeating or developing a preference for sweets.
   - Cognitive skills such as memory and spatial awareness may remain relatively intact, especially in the early stages.

2. **Primary Progressive Aphasia (PPA):**
   - PPA is characterized by the gradual impairment of language skills. It is subdivided into several types, including:
     - o **Semantic Variant PPA:** Difficulty understanding or finding words and a gradual loss of the ability to understand language.
     - o **Nonfluent/Agrammatic Variant PPA:** Difficulty producing speech, making grammatical errors, and speaking in short, halting sentences.
   - The ability to plan, reason, and concentrate may initially be preserved.

3. **Movement Disorders:**
   - Some forms of FTD are associated with movement disorders similar to Parkinson's disease or motor neuron disease. Symptoms might include tremor, rigidity, muscle weakness, and coordination problems.

The exact cause of FTD is unknown, but it involves the progressive loss of nerve cells in the frontal and/or temporal lobes. There is a genetic component in some cases, with mutations in specific genes such as C9orf72, MAPT, and GRN being linked to the disorder.

Diagnosis of FTD involves a thorough medical history, neurological examination, brain imaging (such as MRI or PET scans), and neuropsychological testing to assess cognitive functions. It is important to differentiate FTD from other types of dementia, as the treatment and management strategies can vary.

Treatment of FTD focuses on managing symptoms and providing support. There are currently no treatments available to slow or stop the progression of the disease. Medications may be used to manage specific symptoms such as depression, agitation, or behavioral problems. Supportive care, including speech therapy, occupational therapy, and physical therapy, can be beneficial in managing the symptoms and improving quality of life.

Caregiver support is also crucial, as FTD can be particularly challenging for families and caregivers due to the early age of onset and the profound changes in behavior and personality. Support groups, counseling, and respite care can be valuable resources for caregivers.

Ongoing research is focused on understanding the underlying causes of FTD and developing more effective treatments.

What is the pathology of FTD?

Frontotemporal Dementia (FTD) is characterized by progressive degeneration of the frontal and temporal lobes of the brain. The pathology of FTD is complex and involves several key aspects:

1. **Neuronal Loss and Atrophy:** The most striking feature of FTD is the significant shrinkage (atrophy) of the frontal and temporal lobes. This atrophy is due to the loss of neurons in these areas.

2. **Tau Protein Abnormalities:** In many cases of FTD, there are abnormal accumulations of the tau protein in neurons and glial cells. Tau is a protein that stabilizes microtubules in neurons, and its abnormal accumulation, known as tauopathy, disrupts neuronal function and leads to cell death. This is seen in some subtypes of FTD, such as Pick's disease.

3. **TDP-43 Proteinopathies:** In other cases of FTD, there is abnormal accumulation of the TDP-43 protein (Transactive response DNA-binding protein 43). Abnormal TDP-43 is found in the majority of cases of FTD, particularly those with behavioral variant FTD and some forms of primary progressive aphasia.

4. **FUS Protein Inclusions:** Another protein, FUS (Fused in Sarcoma), can abnormally accumulate in some variants of FTD. FUS is involved in DNA repair and RNA metabolism, and its pathology is less common than tau or TDP-43 pathologies.

5. **Genetic Mutations:** There are known genetic mutations associated with FTD. The most common include mutations in the C9orf72, GRN (progranulin), and MAPT (microtubule-associated protein tau) genes. These mutations can lead to the production of abnormal proteins or a reduction in necessary proteins, contributing to the disease process.

6. **Neuroinflammation:** There is evidence of neuroinflammation in FTD, with activated microglia and astrocytes observed in the brains of affected individuals. This inflammation may contribute to neuronal damage and loss.

7. **Synaptic Changes:** Changes and loss of synapses, the connections between neurons, are also a feature of FTD, contributing to the disruption of neural networks and cognitive deficits.

8. **Neurochemical Changes:** There are alterations in neurotransmitter systems, including serotonin, dopamine, and acetylcholine, which may contribute to some of the behavioral and cognitive symptoms of FTD.

The pathology of FTD varies somewhat between indivi- duals and particularly between the different subtypes of the disease. This variability can influence the clinical presentation and progression of the disease. Understanding the underlying pathology of FTD is crucial for developing targeted treatments, which currently remain limited.

How to Diagnose FTD?

Diagnosing Frontotemporal Dementia (FTD) can be challenging, particularly in the early stages, as its symptoms often overlap with those of psychiatric disorders and other types of dementia. However, a systematic approach involving several key steps can help in accurately diagnosing FTD:

1. **Detailed Medical and Family History:**
   - Collecting a comprehensive history of the patient's symptoms, including when they started, how they have progressed, and any family history of similar symptoms or neurological diseases.

2. **Neurological Examination:**
   - A thorough neurological examination to assess motor function, reflexes, muscle strength, coordination, and other aspects of the nervous system.

3. **Neuropsychological Testing:**
   - Detailed cognitive testing to evaluate memory, executive functions (such as problem-solving and organizing), language skills, and behavior. This helps in identifying patterns of cognitive strengths and weaknesses typical of FTD.

4. **Psychiatric Evaluation:**
   - Since FTD symptoms can mimic psychiatric conditions, a psychiatric evaluation is important to rule out primary psychiatric disorders like depression, bipolar disorder, or schizophrenia.

5. **Brain Imaging:**
   - Structural imaging (MRI or CT scans) to identify atrophy (shrinkage) in the frontal and temporal lobes, characteristic of FTD.
   - Functional imaging (such as PET or SPECT scans) may also be used to assess brain activity patterns that can support a diagnosis of FTD.

6. **Blood Tests and Other Investigations:**
   - To rule out other causes of dementia, such as vitamin deficiencies, thyroid dysfunction, or infectious diseases.

7. **Genetic Testing:**
   - If there is a family history suggesting a genetic cause, genetic counseling and testing for known FTD-related mutations (e.g., C9orf72, MAPT, GRN) may be recommended.
8. **Specialist Consultations:**
   - Referrals to specialists, such as neurologists, psychiatrists, or geriatricians, who have experience with dementia and related disorders.
9. **Observation of Disease Progression:**
   - Monitoring the progression of symptoms over time, as this can provide valuable diagnostic information. FTD typically shows a gradual, progressive decline in behavior and/or language skills.
10. **Exclusion of Other Conditions:**
    - It is crucial to systematically rule out other neurological disorders and conditions that might mimic FTD, such as Alzheimer's disease, vascular dementia, Lewy body dementia, and chronic subdural hematomas.

Diagnosis of FTD is often a process of elimination and may require a combination of the above approaches. It is important for the diagnosis to be revisited and updated as new symptoms emerge or as the condition progresses. Early diagnosis is beneficial for planning future care, considering treatment options, and making important decisions while the individual can still participate actively.

What is the Prognosis of FTD?

The prognosis of Frontotemporal Dementia (FTD) varies among individuals, but it is a progressive condition for which there is currently no cure. The progression and impact of the disease can differ significantly based on the subtype of FTD and individual factors. Here are key points regarding the prognosis:

1. **Life Expectancy:**
   - On average, individuals with FTD live approximately 7 to 13 years after the onset of symptoms, but this can vary widely.
   - FTD often begins at a younger age than other types of dementia, typically between 45 and 65 years.
2. **Rate of Progression:**
   - The progression of FTD can be variable. Some individuals experience a rapid decline, while others may have a slower progression.
   - The specific subtype of FTD (behavioral variant, primary progressive aphasia, etc.) can also influence the rate of progression.
3. **Behavioral and Cognitive Decline:**
   - In the behavioral variant of FTD, early symptoms often involve changes in personality and behavior. As the disease progresses, cognitive impairment becomes more pronounced.
   - In primary progressive aphasia, language abilities decline progressively, often with relative preservation of other cognitive functions in the early stages.
4. **Motor Symptoms:**
   - Some individuals with FTD develop motor symptoms, such as parkinsonism or motor neuron disease-like symptoms, which can affect mobility and physical function.
5. **Dependency:**
   - Over time, individuals with FTD will require increasing levels of care and support for daily activities.
6. **Complications:**
   - In later stages, complications such as difficulty swallowing, mobility issues, and increased susceptibility to infections (like pneumonia) can occur.
7. **Quality of Life:**
   - The impact on quality of life can be significant, both for the individual and for caregivers. Behavioral changes, in particular, can be challenging for families.
8. **No Disease-Modifying Treatments:**
   - Currently, there are no treatments available to slow or stop the progression of FTD. Treatment focuses on managing symptoms and providing supportive care.
9. **Genetic Factors:**
   - In cases where FTD is genetic, the specific mutation may influence the disease course.

It is important for individuals with FTD and their families to have access to support services, including counseling, support groups, and palliative care resources. Planning for the future, considering legal and financial matters, and establishing a care team are important steps following a diagnosis of FTD.

What is the treatment of FTD?

The treatment of Frontotemporal Dementia (FTD) is primarily supportive and symptomatic, as there is currently no cure or treatment to slow the progression of the disease. The management strategies are tailored to the individual's symptoms and needs, and often involve a multidisciplinary approach. Here are the main components of FTD treatment:

1. **Medication Management:**
   - While no medications can cure FTD, certain drugs may help manage symptoms.
   - Antidepressants can be used to treat behavioral symptoms like depression or obsessive-compulsive behaviors.
   - Antipsychotics may be prescribed cautiously for severe behavioral disturbances, although they must be used carefully due to potential side effects.
   - There is limited evidence for the effectiveness of cholinesterase inhibitors (commonly used in Alzheimer's disease) in FTD, and they may actually worsen symptoms in some individuals.
2. **Behavioral and Psychiatric Support:**
   - Behavioral interventions to manage challenging behaviors. This might include modifying the environment, establishing routines, and using non-drug based behavioral strategies.
   - Psychological support and psychiatric care for mood disturbances, depression, or other mental health issues.
3. **Speech and Language Therapy:**
   - For those with language variants of FTD, speech and language therapy can be helpful in managing communication difficulties.
4. **Occupational and Physical Therapy:**
   - These therapies can assist in maintaining mobility, function, and independence for as long as possible.
   - Occupational therapy can also help in adapting the living environment to the individual's needs.
5. **Nutritional Support:**
   - Managing dietary needs, especially if there are changes in eating behaviors or difficulties with swallowing.
6. **Support for Caregivers:**
   - Education and support for family members and caregivers, as caring for someone with FTD can be particularly challenging.
   - Access to support groups, respite care, and counseling services.
7. **Legal and Financial Planning:**
   - Early planning for the future, including legal and financial affairs, as decision-making capacity may decline over time.
8. **Safety and Supervision:**
   - Ensuring a safe living environment, as individuals with FTD may have poor judgment or engage in risky behaviors.
9. **Research and Clinical Trials:**
   - Participation in clinical trials for new treatments may be considered.
10. **Palliative Care:**
    - In advanced stages, palliative care focuses on comfort and quality of life, managing symptoms, and providing support to the individual and family.

It is important for treatment and care plans to be regularly reviewed and adapted as the disease progresses and needs change. Interdisciplinary care involving neurologists, psychiatrists, speech therapists, occupational therapists, and social workers, along with strong support for caregivers, is essential in managing FTD effectively.

What is Normal–Pressure Hydrocephalus (NPH)?

Normal-Pressure Hydrocephalus (NPH) is a neurological disorder characterized by the accumulation of cerebrospinal fluid (CSF) in the brain's ventricles, leading to increased pressure within the skull. Despite its name, the pressure within the ventricles is often not significantly higher than normal. NPH can occur in adults of any age but is most common in the elderly. It is characterized by a classic triad of symptoms:

1. **Gait Disturbance:** This is often the earliest and most prominent symptom. It starts as a mild difficulty in walking and progresses to a more pronounced unsteadiness. The gait is typically described as a slow, shuffling walk with difficulty turning and a tendency to fall.
2. **Urinary Incontinence:** This symptom usually appears after the onset of gait disturbance. It

begins with mild urgency and progresses to more severe incontinence.

3. **Cognitive Impairment:** This includes memory loss, difficulty in concentrating, and a general slowing of mental processes. The cognitive changes are often subtle initially but can progress to more pronounced dementia-like symptoms.

The pathophysiology of NPH is not fully understood. It is thought to involve a disruption in the production, flow, or absorption of cerebrospinal fluid, leading to an accumulation of fluid in the ventricles. This expansion of the ventricles can then lead to pressure on and damage to brain tissues, particularly those affecting gait and bladder control.

Diagnosis of NPH can be challenging, as its symptoms overlap with other conditions such as Alzheimer's disease, Parkinson's disease, and other forms of dementia. The diagnosis typically involves a clinical evaluation, brain imaging (such as MRI or CT scans) to assess ventricular enlargement, and sometimes a lumbar puncture to test CSF pressure and composition.

Treatment for NPH often involves surgical intervention, usually the placement of a shunt in the brain to drain excess cerebrospinal fluid into another part of the body, typically the abdomen, where it can be absorbed. This can lead to significant improvement in symptoms, especially if the condition is diagnosed and treated early. However, the degree of improvement can vary, and not all patients respond to shunt surgery. Regular follow-up and monitoring are necessary to manage the shunt and assess for any complications or the need for adjustments.

What are the Symptoms and Signs of NPH?

Normal Pressure Hydrocephalus (NPH) is characterized by a classic triad of symptoms, often described as "wet, wobbly, and wacky," referring to urinary incontinence, gait disturbance, and cognitive impairment, respectively. Here are the details of these symptoms and signs:

1. **Gait Disturbance:**
   - The most common and often the first symptom to appear.
   - Typically presents as a shuffling, magnetic gait. Individuals may have difficulty lifting their feet off the ground, as if their feet are "stuck" to the floor.
   - There may be a loss of balance and coordination, leading to a higher risk of falls.
   - Gait disturbance in NPH is more pronounced than the typical unsteadiness seen in the elderly.
2. **Urinary Incontinence:**
   - Usually appears after the onset of gait disturbance.
   - Initially presents as urinary urgency and frequency, progressing to frank incontinence in later stages.
   - Incontinence in NPH is often not related to urinary tract infections or other urological conditions.
3. **Cognitive Impairment:**
   - Changes in cognition include memory loss, difficulty concentrating, and a general slowing of mental processes.
   - There can be changes in personality, such as increased apathy or decreased interest in usual activities.
   - Some individuals may experience confusion, disorientation, or difficulty in understanding complex tasks.
   - Unlike Alzheimer's disease, in which memory loss is an early and prominent feature, memory problems in NPH may be less pronounced initially.
4. **Additional Neurological Symptoms:**
   - Some patients may also exhibit mild weakness in the legs, changes in speech, or other neurological signs.

It is important to note that the symptoms of NPH can be similar to those of other conditions, such as Parkinson's disease, Alzheimer's disease, and other types of dementia. This overlap can make diagnosis challenging. A thorough medical evaluation, including neurological examination, brain imaging, and sometimes a lumbar puncture, is necessary to distinguish NPH from other conditions.

Early diagnosis and treatment are crucial, as the symptoms of NPH can sometimes be reversible with appropriate intervention, such as the surgical placement of a shunt to drain excess cerebrospinal fluid. However, the degree of improvement varies among individuals, and not all patients respond to treatment. Regular follow-up with healthcare providers is essential for managing NPH effectively.

How to diagnose NPH?

Diagnosing Normal Pressure Hydrocephalus (NPH) involves a combination of clinical evaluation, imaging studies, and sometimes diagnostic tests to assess the response to cerebrospinal fluid (CSF) removal. Here is a step-by-step approach:

1. **Clinical Assessment:**
   - A thorough medical history and physical examination, focusing on the classic triad of NPH symptoms: gait disturbance, urinary incontinence, and cognitive impairment.
   - Evaluation of other medical conditions that could explain the symptoms, such as Parkinson's disease, stroke, or other forms of dementia.
2. **Neurological Examination:**
   - Detailed examination to assess gait, balance, muscle strength, reflexes, and cognitive function.
3. **Brain Imaging:**
   - MRI or CT scan of the brain to look for enlarged ventricles, which are a hallmark of NPH. Imaging can also help rule out other causes of symptoms, like tumors or stroke.
   - Sometimes, additional imaging tests such as a CSF flow study may be performed.
4. **Lumbar Puncture (Spinal Tap):**
   - A lumbar puncture can be done to remove a small amount of CSF. This can sometimes lead to a temporary improvement in symptoms, which supports the diagnosis of NPH.
   - The procedure also measures CSF pressure, which is typically normal or slightly elevated in NPH.
5. **Gait Assessment:**
   - Detailed assessment of walking before and after a lumbar puncture can provide valuable diagnostic information, as improvement in gait following CSF removal is suggestive of NPH.
6. **Neuropsychological Testing:**
   - Cognitive testing may be conducted to assess the degree of cognitive impairment and monitor changes over time.
7. **Continuous CSF Drainage Test:**
   - In some cases, an extended CSF drainage test, such as via a lumbar drain over several days, may be conducted. Improvement in symptoms with continuous drainage further supports the diagnosis of NPH.
8. **Ruling Out Other Conditions:**
   - It is crucial to differentiate NPH from other neurodegenerative disorders, as the treatment and prognosis differ significantly.

NPH is often under-diagnosed or misdiagnosed because its symptoms overlap with those of other, more common conditions in the elderly. Accurate diagnosis is essential, as NPH is one of the few reversible causes of dementia if treated appropriately, typically with surgical intervention to drain excess CSF. A multidisciplinary approach involving neurologists, neurosurgeons, and other specialists is often beneficial in diagnosing and managing NPH.

What is the Treatment of NPH?

The primary treatment for Normal Pressure Hydrocephalus (NPH) is surgical, aimed at reducing the accumulation of cerebrospinal fluid (CSF) in the brain. The specific treatments include:

1. **Ventriculoperitoneal (VP) Shunt:**
   - The most common treatment for NPH.
   - A VP shunt is a device implanted surgically that drains excess CSF from the ventricles in the brain to the peritoneal cavity (in the abdomen), where the fluid can be absorbed.
   - The shunt usually has a valve to regulate the flow of CSF and prevent over-drainage.
2. **Ventriculoatrial (VA) Shunt:**
   - Similar to a VP shunt, but the CSF drains into the right atrium of the heart.
   - Used less commonly than VP shunts due to a higher risk of complications.
3. **Endoscopic Third Ventriculostomy (ETV):**
   - A minimally invasive surgical procedure where a small hole is made in the floor of the third ventricle, allowing CSF to bypass the obstruction and flow directly to the site of absorption around the brain and spinal cord.
   - ETV is less commonly used in NPH compared to shunting but can be an option in certain cases.
4. **Adjustable Shunts:**
   - Some shunts have adjustable valves that can be modified non-invasively after surgery to optimize CSF drainage without additional surgery.

5. **Monitoring and Follow-up:**
   - Regular follow-up is essential to monitor shunt function and to check for complications like infection, blockage, or over-drainage.
   - Neuroimaging studies may be done periodically to assess ventricle size and shunt function.
6. **Management of Symptoms:**
   - Physical therapy is often recommended to improve gait and balance.
   - Occupational therapy can assist with daily living activities and cognitive function.
   - Medication may be prescribed for associated symptoms like urinary incontinence or depression.
7. **Complication Management:**
   - Complications from shunt placement, such as infection, shunt malfunction, or abdominal issues (for VP shunts), need prompt medical attention.

The success of treatment varies among individuals. Some patients experience significant improvement in their symptoms following shunt placement, particularly in gait. Cognitive symptoms and urinary incontinence may also improve but are generally less responsive than gait disturbances. Early diagnosis and treatment generally lead to a better outcome. The decision to proceed with surgery is based on a careful consideration of potential benefits and risks, and it often involves a multidisciplinary team including neurologists, neurosurgeons, and other healthcare professionals.

What is Behavioral variant Frontotemporal Dementia (bvFTD) and how to manage it?

Behavioral variant Frontotemporal Dementia (bvFTD) is a subtype of Frontotemporal Dementia primarily characterized by significant changes in personality, behavior, and social interaction, often preceding or being more prominent than cognitive deficits. It results from degeneration in the frontal and anterior temporal lobes of the brain, areas associated with behavior, emotion, and personality.

Key Features of bvFTD include:

1. **Behavioral Changes:** Disinhibition, inappropriate social behavior, lack of empathy, impulsivity, and apathy.
2. **Personality Alterations:** Drastic changes from the person's previous character; becoming either apathetic or excessively driven.
3. **Emotional Blunting:** Reduced ability to empathize with others, leading to apparent insensitivity to the feelings of others.
4. **Poor Judgment and Impulse Control:** Inability to plan or organize activities, and acting impulsively without considering consequences.
5. **Compulsive or Ritualistic Behavior:** Repetitive or ritualistic behaviors, such as hand-washing, counting, or hoarding.
6. **Eating Habits Changes:** Overeating, change in dietary preferences (like a newfound preference for sweets), or other changes in eating behaviors.
7. **Cognitive Impairment:** Executive function deficits, such as difficulties in planning, organizing, or problem-solving, often appear as the disease progresses.

Management of bvFTD:

1. **Medication:**
   - While no medication can stop the progression of bvFTD, some can help manage symptoms. SSRIs or other antidepressants may alleviate behavioral symptoms or depression.
   - Antipsychotics should be used cautiously, as patients with bvFTD can be particularly sensitive to side effects.
2. **Behavioral Strategies:**
   - Behavioral management strategies tailored to the individual's symptoms, such as setting routines, simplifying tasks, and creating a safe and structured environment.
   - Minimizing triggers that lead to agitation or inappropriate behaviors.
3. **Support for Caregivers:**
   - Education and support for caregivers are vital, as managing a loved one with bvFTD can be very challenging.
   - Support groups, respite care, and counseling can provide much-needed support and information.
4. **Occupational and Physical Therapy:**
   - These therapies can help maintain function and independence for as long as possible.
   - Physical activity and structured exercises can also be beneficial.

5. **Speech and Language Therapy:**
   - Though language may not be initially affected, speech therapy can be beneficial as the disease progresses.
6. **Legal and Financial Planning:**
   - Early planning for the future, considering legal and financial affairs, is important as decision-making capacity may decline.
7. **Safety Measures:**
   - Implementing safety measures at home to prevent accidents due to poor judgment or impulsive behaviors.
8. **Nutritional Support:**
   - Addressing changes in eating habits to ensure a balanced diet and prevent weight gain or nutritional deficiencies.
9. **Regular Medical Follow-up:**
   - Regular follow-ups with healthcare professionals to monitor the progression and manage the symptoms effectively.
10. **Palliative Care:**
    - In advanced stages, focus on comfort and quality of life, managing symptoms, and providing support to the individual and family.

Each patient with bvFTD is unique, and management strategies should be individualized. It is also important to recognize that the needs of a person with bvFTD will change over time as the disease progresses, requiring adjustments in care strategies. Collaboration with a multidisciplinary team, including neurologists, psychiatrists, social workers, and other healthcare professionals, is essential for comprehensive care. Additionally, educating and preparing family members about the nature of the disease and its expected progression is crucial for effective and compassionate care.

What is Sundowning and how to manage it?

Sundowning, also known as "sundown syndrome," is a phenomenon often observed in people with dementia, Alzheimer's disease, or other cognitive impairments. It refers to the increase in confusion, agitation, anxiety, and restlessness that typically occurs in the late afternoon and evening, or as the sun goes down. This can be distressing both for the individual experiencing it and for their caregivers.

Causes of Sundowning: The exact cause of sundowning is not well understood, but it is believed to be related to disruptions in the body's internal clock (circadian rhythm) caused by dementia and Alzheimer's disease. Other contributing factors may include fatigue, low lighting, increased shadows, disruption of the sleep-wake cycle, and an inability to distinguish dreams from reality.

Symptoms of Sundowning:

- Increased confusion and agitation in the evening.
- Restlessness and pacing.
- Irritability or aggression.
- Anxiety and fear.
- Yelling or mood swings.
- Hallucinations or delusions.

Management Strategies for Sundowning:

1. **Maintain a Consistent Routine:** Keep a regular schedule for waking, meals, activities, and bedtime to help regulate the internal clock.
2. **Increase Light Exposure:** Exposure to natural light during the day can help reset the person's circadian rhythms. Bright light therapy in the morning may also be beneficial.
3. **Create a Calm Environment in the Evening:** Reduce noise, clutter, and the number of people around to minimize stimulation. Soft music, calming activities, and a quiet environment can be soothing.
4. **Ensure Physical Activity and Engagement During the Day:** Regular physical activity and engagement in activities during the day can help reduce restlessness in the evening.
5. **Monitor Diet:** Limit caffeine and sugar intake in the afternoon and evening to avoid interfering with sleep.
6. **Address Medical Issues:** Check for any physical discomfort, pain, hunger, thirst, or need to use the toilet that may be contributing to agitation.
7. **Use of Medications:** Medication may be used as a last resort if behavioral strategies are not effective. This should be done under strict medical supervision due to potential side effects and interactions with other medications.
8. **Ensure Safety:** As sundowning may increase the risk of wandering or accidents, ensure that the environment is safe and secure. Use safety measures such as door alarms or locks and remove any hazards.

9. **Comfort and Reassurance:** Provide comfort and reassurance to the person. They may become more anxious or agitated if they sense frustration or anger from their caregivers.

10. **Caregiver Support:** Caring for someone experiencing sundowning can be challenging. Caregivers should seek support when needed and consider respite care to prevent burnout.

11. **Sleep Hygiene:** Promote good sleep hygiene by creating a comfortable sleeping environment and establishing a calming bedtime routine.

12. **Consult Healthcare Professionals:** Regularly review the person's health and medications with healthcare professionals, as changes in health status can affect behavior.

Understanding and being prepared for sundowning can help caregivers manage these symptoms more effectively. It is also important to remember that every individual is different, and what works for one person may not work for another, so it may take some trial and error to find the most effective strategies.

How about the problem of treatment of opioid addiction in Punjab with buprenorphine?

The problem of opioid addiction in Punjab, India, has been a significant public health concern, and the use of buprenorphine as a treatment option is one of the strategies employed to combat this issue. Buprenorphine is a medication used in the treatment of opioid dependence and is part of a broader approach known as Medication-Assisted Treatment (MAT).

Key Aspects of Buprenorphine Treatment in Punjab:

1. **Buprenorphine as a MAT Option:** Buprenorphine is a partial opioid agonist, which means it activates the same brain receptors as other opioids but produces a lesser effect. It helps in reducing cravings and withdrawal symptoms, making it easier for individuals to stop using harmful opioids.

2. **Implementation and Accessibility:** The Punjab government has taken steps to make buprenorphine more accessible to those struggling with opioid addiction. This includes establishing de-addiction centers and outpatient opioid-assisted treatment programs where buprenorphine is dispensed.

3. **Combating Stigma:** There is an ongoing effort to reduce the stigma associated with addiction and its treatment. Encouraging people to seek help without fear of social repercussions is a critical component of the treatment strategy.

4. **Regulation and Monitoring:** To prevent misuse and diversion of buprenorphine, strict regulatory mechanisms are in place. This includes monitoring prescriptions and ensuring that the medication is only available through authorized centers.

5. **Integrated Treatment Approach:** Effective treatment often involves a combination of medication, counseling, and support groups. Addressing not just the physical aspect of addiction but also psychological, social, and behavioral factors is crucial.

6. **Challenges and Barriers:** Despite these efforts, there are challenges such as the availability of illegal opioids, social stigma, and the need for more widespread and consistent implementation of treatment programs.

7. **Research and Evaluation:** Ongoing research and evaluation of treatment programs are necessary to understand their effectiveness and to make necessary adjustments in strategies.

8. **Education and Awareness:** Public awareness campaigns about the dangers of opioid abuse and the availability of treatment options are vital components of the strategy to combat opioid addiction.

9. **Support for Families:** Providing support and resources to families affected by opioid addiction is also an important aspect of the overall treatment and recovery process.

The approach to treating opioid addiction with buprenorphine in Punjab is a multifaceted one, involving medical treatment, regulatory measures, public awareness, and social support. It is a part of a broader effort to address the complex issue of opioid addiction, which requires ongoing commitment from government authorities, healthcare providers, and the community.

What about management of dystonia?

Dystonia is a neurological movement disorder characterized by involuntary muscle contractions, leading to repetitive movements or abnormal postures. Management of dystonia is aimed at reducing symptoms and improving quality of life, as there is currently no cure. Treatment approaches are often tailored to the individual's specific type of dystonia, its severity, and the body areas affected. Here are key strategies in the management of dystonia:

1. **Medications:**
   - Oral medications, such as anticholinergics (e.g., trihexyphenidyl), benzodiazepines (e.g., diazepam), and baclofen, can be used to reduce muscle spasms and improve function.
   - Dopaminergic agents are sometimes used, especially if dystonia is associated with Parkinson's disease or other conditions affecting dopamine pathways.
2. **Botulinum Toxin Injections:**
   - Botulinum toxin (Botox) injections are a common treatment for focal dystonia, such as cervical dystonia or blepharospasm. They work by temporarily weakening the overactive muscles.
   - The effects typically last for about three months, so repeated injections are often necessary.
3. **Physical Therapy and Rehabilitation:**
   - Tailored exercises, stretches, and other physical therapy techniques can help manage symptoms, improve mobility, and prevent complications like contractures.
   - Occupational therapy can assist with adaptations to daily activities and the use of assistive devices.
4. **Deep Brain Stimulation (DBS):**
   - DBS is a surgical treatment option for certain types of severe dystonia that don't respond well to other treatments. It involves implanting electrodes in specific brain areas to modulate abnormal brain activity.
5. **Selective Denervation Surgery:**
   - In some cases, particularly for cervical dystonia, selective denervation surgery (cutting the nerves responsible for the overactive muscles) can provide long-term relief.
6. **Stress Management and Counseling:**
   - Stress and emotional factors can exacerbate dystonia. Techniques for stress reduction, counseling, and support groups can be beneficial.
7. **Complementary Therapies:**
   - Some individuals find relief with complementary therapies like acupuncture, yoga, or meditation, although their effectiveness is less well-documented in scientific literature.
8. **Lifestyle Modifications:**
   - Adjustments in daily activities and ergonomic changes can help reduce the impact of dystonia on quality of life.
9. **Regular Monitoring and Follow-Up:**
   - Dystonia can change over time, so regular follow-up with healthcare providers is important to adjust treatment plans as needed.

The management of dystonia is typically overseen by a neurologist, possibly in collaboration with other specialists such as physical therapists, occupational therapists, and pain management experts. Since dystonia can affect individuals differently, a personalized approach to treatment is often necessary.

What are the causes of dystonia?

Dystonia is a complex movement disorder, and its exact causes can vary depending on the type of dystonia. The condition is characterized by involuntary muscle contractions leading to abnormal movements and postures. Here are the primary known causes and risk factors associated with dystonia:

1. **Genetic Factors:**
   - Many forms of dystonia are linked to specific genetic mutations. For example, DYT1 dystonia, a common form of early-onset generalized dystonia, is often associated with a mutation in the TOR1A gene.
   - Genetic dystonia can be inherited or occur due to new mutations.
2. **Neurochemical Imbalance:**
   - Dystonia may result from imbalances in certain neurotransmitters (chemical messengers in the brain), particularly those involved in motor control, such as dopamine.
3. **Brain Injury or Trauma:**
   - Brain injuries, including those from trauma, stroke, tumors, hypoxia (lack of oxygen), or infections, can lead to secondary dystonia.
   - Perinatal injuries (injuries occurring around the time of birth) are also a known risk factor.
4. **Infections and Autoimmune Disorders:**
   - Certain infections or autoimmune conditions that affect the brain or nervous system can trigger dystonia.

5. **Reaction to Certain Medications:**
   - Drug-induced dystonia can occur as a side effect of certain medications, particularly those that affect dopamine, such as antipsychotics and some nausea medications.
6. **Other Neurological Disorders:**
   - Dystonia can be a feature of other neurological conditions like Parkinson's disease, Huntington's disease, and Wilson's disease.
7. **Environmental Factors:**
   - Some research suggests that environmental exposures, possibly in combination with genetic susceptibility, might play a role in the development of dystonia.
8. **Idiopathic Dystonia:**
   - In many cases, the cause of dystonia is unknown (idiopathic). This is particularly true for adult-onset focal dystonias like cervical dystonia (affecting the neck) and blepharospasm (affecting the eyelids).

Understanding the underlying cause of dystonia is important for determining the appropriate treatment and management strategy. For some individuals, a specific cause may not be identifiable, which can make treatment more challenging. In these cases, management focuses on alleviating symptoms and improving quality of life.

How to diagnose dystonia?

Diagnosing dystonia can be challenging due to its variable presentation and the fact that it shares symptoms with several other neurological conditions. The diagnostic process typically involves a combination of medical history evaluation, physical and neurological examinations, and various diagnostic tests. Here is a step-by-step approach to diagnosing dystonia:

1. **Medical History:**
   - Detailed assessment of the patient's medical history, including the onset, duration, and progression of symptoms.
   - Family history to identify any genetic patterns, as some forms of dystonia are inherited.
2. **Neurological Examination:**
   - Comprehensive evaluation of the patient's motor and sensory skills, muscle strength, reflexes, coordination, balance, and gait.
   - Observation of involuntary movements or abnormal postures.
3. **Laboratory Tests:**
   - Blood tests to rule out metabolic or systemic disorders that can cause secondary dystonia, such as Wilson's disease, thyroid disorders, or certain infections.
4. **Genetic Testing:**
   - If there is a family history or if the symptoms suggest a specific type of genetic dystonia, genetic testing can be conducted to identify mutations associated with dystonia.
5. **Imaging Studies:**
   - Brain imaging with MRI (Magnetic Resonance Imaging) or CT (Computed Tomography) scans to look for structural abnormalities, stroke, tumors, or other conditions that might cause secondary dystonia.
6. **Electrophysiological Studies:**
   - Tests like electromyography (EMG) to assess muscle activity and nerve function.
7. **Response to Medication:**
   - Sometimes, response to medications (like anticholinergics or botulinum toxin) is part of the diagnostic process, particularly in cases where the cause is unclear.
8. **Exclusion of Other Conditions:**
   - It is important to rule out other conditions that mimic dystonia, including Parkinson's disease, Huntington's disease, and certain psychiatric disorders.
9. **Specialist Referral:**
   - Referral to a neurologist or movement disorder specialist, particularly those with expertise in dystonia, can be crucial for an accurate diagnosis.
10. **Observation Over Time:**
    - In some cases, the diagnosis may become clearer over time as symptoms develop or change.

Since dystonia can vary greatly in its presentation and may coexist with other neurological disorders, a thorough and comprehensive approach is essential for an accurate diagnosis. This process not only helps in understanding the type and cause of dystonia but also guides the subsequent treatment and management strategies.

What is the Treatment of dystonia?

The treatment of dystonia focuses on relieving symptoms, improving quality of life, and maximizing the patient's ability to function. Since dystonia can vary widely in its forms and severity, treatment is highly individualized. Here are the main components of dystonia treatment:

1. **Medications:**
   - Anticholinergics (e.g., trihexyphenidyl) can reduce tremors and muscle rigidity.
   - Baclofen may help alleviate muscle spasms.
   - Dopaminergic Agents are used, especially if the dystonia is associated with Parkinson's disease or dopaminergic response dystonia.
   - Benzodiazepines (e.g., diazepam) can be effective for some types of dystonia, particularly those involving spasms or anxiety.
   - **Note:** Medication efficacy varies among individuals, and some trial and error may be necessary to find the most effective regimen with the fewest side effects.
2. **Botulinum Toxin Injections:**
   - Botulinum toxin (e.g., Botox) injections into affected muscles are a common treatment for focal dystonia (such as cervical dystonia and blepharospasm).
   - These injections temporarily paralyze the overactive muscles, providing relief from involuntary movements and postures.
3. **Physical Therapy and Rehabilitation:**
   - Exercises, stretches, and massage can help manage symptoms and maintain range of motion.
   - Physical therapy can also help with pain management and functional improvement.
4. **Occupational Therapy:**
   - Occupational therapy assists patients in adapting their daily activities and work environment to their abilities, which can improve independence and quality of life.
5. **Speech Therapy:**
   - For those with dystonia affecting speech and swallowing (like laryngeal dystonia), speech therapy can be very helpful.
6. **Surgical Options:**
   - In severe cases, especially when dystonia is not responsive to other treatments, surgical options such as Deep Brain Stimulation (DBS) might be considered.
   - DBS involves implanting electrodes in specific areas of the brain, which are then connected to a pacemaker-like device that sends electrical impulses to the brain.
7. **Stress Management:**
   - Techniques for managing stress, such as relaxation techniques, yoga, and meditation, can be beneficial since stress can exacerbate symptoms.
8. **Complementary Therapies:**
   - Some patients find relief with acupuncture, biofeedback, or other complementary therapies, though their effectiveness is less well-documented in scientific literature.
9. **Treatment of Secondary Effects:**
   - Addressing secondary effects of dystonia, such as pain, depression, or sleep disturbances, is an important part of overall care.
10. **Regular Monitoring and Adjustments:**
    - Regular follow-up with healthcare providers is necessary to monitor the effectiveness of treatments and make adjustments as needed.

Each individual's response to treatment can vary, and what works for one person may not work for another. Hence, a multidisciplinary approach involving neurologists, physical therapists, occupational therapists, and other healthcare professionals is often the most effective strategy in managing dystonia.

What is Erectile dysfunction (ED) and its management?

Erectile Dysfunction (ED) is a common medical condition where a man has difficulty achieving or maintaining an erection sufficient for sexual intercourse. It can have physical, psychological, or a combination of causes. The management of ED involves addressing these underlying causes, lifestyle modifications, and various treatment options.

Causes of ED:

1. **Physical Causes:** These include cardiovascular disease, diabetes, hypertension, high cholesterol, obesity, hormonal imbalances (like low testosterone), neurological disorders, and certain medications.

2. **Psychological Causes:** Stress, anxiety, depression, and relationship problems can contribute to or cause ED.

3. **Lifestyle Factors:** Smoking, excessive alcohol consumption, lack of physical activity, and poor diet can contribute to the development of ED.

Management of ED:

1. **Medical Evaluation:** It is important to consult a healthcare provider for a thorough medical evaluation to identify any underlying health issues contributing to ED. This may include blood tests, physical examination, and sometimes, specialized tests.

2. **Lifestyle Modifications:**

   - Regular exercise, a healthy diet, maintaining a healthy weight, quitting smoking, and limiting alcohol consumption can improve ED.
   - Managing stress and getting adequate sleep are also important.

3. **Medications:**

   - Oral medications such as sildenafil (Viagra), tadalafil (Cialis), and vardenafil (Levitra) are commonly prescribed and work by enhancing the effects of nitric oxide, a natural chemical the body produces that relaxes muscles in the penis.
   - It is important to use these medications under medical supervision, as they can have interactions with other drugs, especially nitrates used for heart disease.

4. **Psychological Counseling:**

   - If psychological factors such as stress, anxiety, or depression are contributing to ED, counseling or therapy can be beneficial.
   - Couples counseling can also be helpful when relationship problems are affecting sexual function.

5. **Vacuum Erection Devices:**

   - A mechanical vacuum pump can be used to induce an erection by increasing blood flow to the penis.

6. **Intraurethral Suppositories and Intracavernosal Injections:**

   - Medications can be administered directly into the penis to achieve an erection.

7. **Surgical Treatment:**

   - In cases where other treatments are not effective or suitable, surgical options like penile implants may be considered.

8. **Management of Chronic Health Conditions:**

   - Effective management of conditions like diabetes, high blood pressure, and heart disease can improve ED.

9. **Hormonal Therapy:**

   - If hormonal imbalances are identified (like low testosterone), hormone replacement therapy may be considered.

10. **Alternative Therapies:**

    - Some men explore alternative treatments like herbal supplements; however, their effectiveness is not widely supported by scientific evidence, and they should be used cautiously.

11. **Regular Follow-Up:**

    - Ongoing communication with a healthcare provider is important for adjusting treatment plans, discussing side effects, and monitoring overall health.

Managing ED often requires a holistic approach that includes medical treatment, lifestyle changes, and, in some cases, psychological support. It is important for individuals with ED to openly discuss their condition and treatment options with their healthcare provider to determine the most effective and safe approach for their specific situation.

What are types of ED?

Erectile Dysfunction (ED) can be categorized into different types based on its underlying causes. Understanding these types is important for effective treatment and management. The main types of ED are:

1. **Organic ED:**

   - This type is due to physical health problems, which can be further subdivided into:
   - **Vascular ED:** Related to problems with blood flow to the penis, often due to conditions like atherosclerosis, heart disease, or high blood pressure.
   - **Neurogenic ED:** Caused by nerve damage or dysfunction, which can occur in conditions like diabetes, spinal cord injury, multiple sclerosis, or after certain types of surgery.

- **Hormonal ED:** Linked to hormonal imbalances, such as low testosterone levels or thyroid disorders.
- **Anatomical ED:** Due to structural abnormalities of the penis, such as Peyronie's disease.

2. **Psychogenic ED:**
   - This type is primarily caused by psychological factors, including:
     - **Performance Anxiety:** Anxiety specifically related to sexual performance.
     - **Stress and Mental Health Issues:** General stress, depression, and other mental health conditions can affect sexual function.
     - **Relationship Problems:** Issues in a relationship can contribute to ED.
3. **Mixed ED:**
   - A combination of both organic and psychogenic factors. This is quite common, as physical health issues can lead to psychological distress that further exacerbates ED.
4. **Medication-Induced ED:**
   - Caused by certain medications that affect sexual function. These can include antidepressants, antihypertensives, and some medications used to treat prostate conditions.
5. **Age-Related ED:**
   - While not a distinct category, the likelihood of developing ED increases with age, often due to a combination of physical and psychological changes.

Identifying the type of ED is crucial for effective treatment. For example, vascular ED might be managed with medications that improve blood flow, lifestyle changes, and treating underlying cardiovascular conditions. Psychogenic ED, on the other hand, may benefit more from therapy, stress management techniques, or changes in the patient's relationship dynamics.

In practice, many men with ED have a combination of these factors, and a comprehensive approach to treatment is often required. A healthcare provider can help determine the underlying cause of ED through a detailed medical history, physical examination, and appropriate tests.

What are causes of ED?

Erectile Dysfunction (ED) can be caused by a variety of factors that can be broadly classified into physical (organic), psychological, and lifestyle-related categories. It is important to note that these factors can sometimes overlap, and more than one factor can contribute to ED. Here are the primary causes:

1. **Physical Causes:**
   - **Cardiovascular Diseases:** Conditions like hypertension, atherosclerosis, and heart disease can impair blood flow to the penis, leading to ED.
   - **Diabetes:** Often causes neuropathy and vascular problems, which can affect erectile function.
   - **Neurological Disorders:** Conditions like Parkinson's disease, multiple sclerosis, stroke, and spinal cord injuries can disrupt the nerve signals involved in achieving an erection.
   - **Hormonal Imbalances:** Low testosterone levels, thyroid conditions, and other hormonal disorders can contribute to ED.
   - **Medications:** Certain medications, including antihypertensives, antidepressants, and medications for prostate conditions, can have ED as a side effect.
   - **Kidney Disease:** Chronic kidney disease can cause chemical changes in the body that affect hormones, circulation, nerve function, and energy levels.
   - **Peyronie's Disease:** A condition that causes fibrous scar tissue to develop in the penis, leading to curved, painful erections.
2. **Psychological Causes:**
   - **Stress and Anxiety:** Including stress from work, financial burdens, or family issues.
   - **Depression:** Can affect a person's overall desire for sex as well as erectile function.
   - **Relationship Problems:** Communication issues, trust issues, or other relationship dynamics.
   - **Performance Anxiety:** Worrying about sexual performance can create a negative feedback loop leading to ED.
3. **Lifestyle Factors:**
   - **Smoking:** Can damage blood vessels and restrict blood flow to the penis.

- **Alcohol and Substance Abuse:** Excessive alcohol intake and certain recreational drugs can affect sexual function.
- **Obesity and Poor Diet:** Can contribute to cardiovascular problems and diabetes, which in turn can cause ED.
- **Lack of Physical Activity:** A sedentary lifestyle can lead to health conditions that cause ED.
- **Poor Sleep Patterns:** Disorders like sleep apnea can lead to reduced testosterone levels and ED.

In many cases, ED is multifactorial, meaning that multiple factors contribute to its development. Identifying the underlying cause or causes is crucial for effective treatment. This often involves a comprehensive evaluation by a healthcare provider, including a detailed medical and sexual history, physical examination, and sometimes, diagnostic tests.

What are drugs causing ED?

Several medications can cause or contribute to erectile dysfunction (ED) as a side effect. It is important to note that while these drugs may contribute to ED, they are often necessary for managing other health conditions. Patients should not stop taking any prescribed medication without consulting their healthcare provider. Some of the common categories of medications that can lead to ED include:

1. **Antihypertensives:**
   - **Beta-Blockers (e.g., propranolol, atenolol):** Commonly used for high blood pressure and heart conditions. They can decrease nerve impulses to blood vessels and the heart, potentially affecting erectile function.
   - **Diuretics (e.g., hydrochlorothiazide, furosemide):** Often called "water pills," they can decrease blood flow to the penis.
2. **Antidepressants and Antipsychotics:**
   - **Selective Serotonin Reuptake Inhibitors (SSRIs) (e.g., fluoxetine, sertraline):** Used for depression and anxiety, can affect sexual desire and function.
   - **Tricyclic Antidepressants (e.g., amitriptyline):** Can also interfere with sexual function.
   - **Antipsychotics (e.g., risperidone, haloperidol):** Used for schizophrenia and certain mood disorders, can impact hormone levels and erectile function.
3. **Antiandrogens:**
   - Used to treat prostate cancer and other conditions, these drugs can lower testosterone levels, affecting sexual desire and function.
4. **Drugs for Benign Prostatic Hyperplasia (BPH):**
   - **Alpha-Blockers (e.g., tamsulosin, doxazosin):** While used to treat urinary symptoms due to BPH, they can cause ejaculation problems or ED in some men.
   - **5-Alpha Reductase Inhibitors (e.g., finasteride, dutasteride):** Can also impact sexual function.
5. **Opioids:**
   - Long-term use of opioid painkillers can affect testosterone production and sexual function.
6. **Central Nervous System Depressants:**
   - Including some sedatives and hypnotics used for sleep disorders or anxiety, these can interfere with sexual response and libido.
7. **H2 Blockers (e.g., cimetidine):**
   - Used for gastrointestinal disorders like peptic ulcer disease, can have antiandrogenic effects and impact libido and erectile function.

It is essential for patients experiencing ED to review their medication list with their healthcare provider. Often, alternative medications or adjustments in dosages can mitigate the side effects while effectively managing the primary health condition. Additionally, lifestyle modifications, psychological support, and other interventions can be beneficial in managing ED.

How to do a Clinical evaluation of ED?

A clinical evaluation of Erectile Dysfunction (ED) is a comprehensive process that aims to identify the underlying causes of the condition and to determine the most appropriate treatment. This evaluation typically includes the following steps:

1. **Medical and Sexual History:**
   - **Duration and Severity of Symptoms:** Understanding when the ED started and how it has progressed over time.
   - **Specific Symptoms:** Details about erection quality, libido (sexual desire), orgasm, and ejaculation.
   - **Medical History:** Information about chronic diseases, surgeries, medications, and lifestyle factors that might contribute to ED.

- **Sexual History:** Questions about sexual relationships, experiences, and any recent changes in sexual activity or performance.

2. **Psychological Assessment:**
   - Screening for psychological factors like stress, anxiety, depression, or relationship issues that might be contributing to ED.
3. **Physical Examination:**
   - A general physical exam to assess overall health.
   - A focused genital examination to check for penile abnormalities, hormonal problems (like gynecomastia or decreased body hair), or circulatory issues.
4. **Laboratory Tests:**
   - **Blood Tests:** To check for diabetes, high cholesterol, thyroid problems, testosterone levels, and other possible underlying conditions.
   - **Urine Tests:** To screen for diabetes and other health conditions.
5. **Other Diagnostic Tests:**
   - **Nocturnal Penile Tumescence (NPT) Test:** Measures erectile function during sleep.
   - **Penile Doppler Ultrasound:** Assesses blood flow in the penis and can detect vascular abnormalities.
   - **Penile Biothesiometry:** Tests nerve function in the penis.
   - **Dynamic Infusion Cavernosometry and Cavernosography (DICC):** Invasive tests used in specific cases to evaluate the venous leak.
6. **Questionnaires:**
   - Self-administered questionnaires like the International Index of Erectile Function (IIEF) can be useful for assessing the severity of ED and its impact on quality of life.
7. **Referral to Specialists:**
   - If needed, referrals to a urologist, endocrinologist, cardiologist, or psychologist/psychiatrist for further evaluation and management.
8. **Lifestyle Evaluation:**
   - Discussion about lifestyle factors such as smoking, alcohol use, exercise habits, and diet that can influence ED.
9. **Review of Current Medications:**
   - Some medications may contribute to ED, and a review can help identify any potential drug-related causes.
10. **Partner Involvement:**
    - In some cases, involving the patient's partner in discussions can provide additional insights and support.
11. **Follow-Up Assessments:**
    - Ongoing monitoring and follow-up assessments may be necessary to evaluate the effectiveness of any treatment and to make adjustments as needed.

The clinical evaluation of ED is a sensitive issue and requires a respectful and non-judgmental approach by the healthcare provider. Open communication and a thorough understanding of the patient's overall health, lifestyle, and psychological state are key to determining the most effective treatment strategy.

How is ED investigated?

Investigating Erectile Dysfunction (ED) involves a series of steps to determine the underlying causes and to guide appropriate treatment. The investigation usually starts with a comprehensive clinical evaluation and may include various diagnostic tests:

1. **Medical and Sexual History:**
   - Detailed questioning about sexual function, onset and duration of ED, and any associated factors like changes in libido, ejaculation, or orgasm.
   - Review of medical history for conditions linked to ED, such as diabetes, hypertension, cardiovascular disease, neurological disorders, and hormonal imbalances.
   - Assessment of psychological factors including stress, anxiety, depression, and relationship issues.
   - Evaluation of lifestyle factors such as smoking, alcohol consumption, drug use, and exercise habits.
2. **Physical Examination:**
   - General physical exam to assess overall health.
   - Focused genitourinary examination to look for physical abnormalities of the penis, testes, and prostate.

- Assessment of secondary sexual characteristics like hair distribution, breast size (to detect gynecomastia), and body composition.

3. **Laboratory Tests:**
   - Blood tests to check glucose levels, lipid profile, kidney function, liver function, thyroid function, and testosterone levels.
   - Urinalysis to identify signs of diabetes or other underlying conditions.
4. **Psychological Assessment:**
   - If psychological factors are suspected, referral to a psychologist or psychiatrist may be beneficial for further evaluation.
5. **Specialized Tests:**
   - **Nocturnal Penile Tumescence (NPT) and Rigidity Testing:** Monitors erections during sleep to differentiate between physical and psychological causes of ED.
   - **Penile Doppler Ultrasound:** Assesses blood flow in the penis, useful in identifying vascular issues.
   - **Penile Biothesiometry:** Evaluates nerve sensitivity in the penis.
   - **Dynamic Infusion Cavernosometry and Cavernosography (DICC):** Invasive tests used in certain cases to evaluate venous leak.
   - **Neurological Testing:** Such as bulbocavernosus reflex or sensory testing, especially if a neurological cause is suspected.
6. **Questionnaires and Inventories:**
   - Tools like the International Index of Erectile Function (IIEF) help quantify the severity of ED and its impact on quality of life.
7. **Review of Current Medications:**
   - Some medications can contribute to ED, so a thorough review of all medications, including over-the-counter drugs and supplements, is essential.
8. **Lifestyle Assessment:**
   - Discussion of lifestyle factors that can impact ED, including diet, physical activity, alcohol consumption, and tobacco use.

These investigations not only aid in diagnosing the cause of ED but also help in formulating a comprehensive and individualized treatment plan. It is important for individuals experiencing ED to consult a healthcare professional for a thorough evaluation. Additionally, ongoing follow-up may be necessary to monitor the effectiveness of treatment strategies and make adjustments as needed.

What is the Treatment of ED?

The treatment of Erectile Dysfunction (ED) involves a variety of approaches tailored to the individual's needs and the underlying cause of the condition. A comprehensive treatment plan often includes lifestyle changes, psychological support, medical therapies, and sometimes surgical interventions. Here are the primary treatments for ED:

1. **Lifestyle Modifications:**
   - **Healthy Diet and Exercise:** A balanced diet and regular exercise can improve cardiovascular health and blood flow, potentially improving ED.
   - **Weight Loss:** If overweight, losing weight can have a significant positive impact on ED.
   - **Quit Smoking:** Smoking cessation is important as smoking can impair blood flow.
   - **Limit Alcohol:** Excessive alcohol can worsen ED.
   - **Stress Management:** Techniques like meditation, yoga, and counseling can help reduce stress.
2. **Oral Medications:**
   - **Phosphodiesterase type 5 inhibitors (PDE5 inhibitors):** These are the first-line treatment for many men and include sildenafil (Viagra), tadalafil (Cialis), and vardenafil (Levitra). They work by enhancing the effects of nitric oxide, which relaxes muscles in the penis and increases blood flow.
   - **Hormone Replacement Therapy:** If tests show low testosterone levels, testosterone replacement therapy may be recommended.
3. **Psychological Counseling:**
   - For men whose ED is caused by stress, anxiety, depression, or relationship issues, counseling or therapy can be beneficial.
4. **Vacuum Erection Devices (Penis Pumps):**
   - These devices create a vacuum around the penis, drawing blood into it and causing an erection. A tension ring is then applied at the base of the penis to maintain the erection.

5. **Intracavernosal Injections:**
   - Medications such as alprostadil can be injected directly into the penis, causing an erection.
6. **Intraurethral Medication:**
   - Alprostadil can also be placed into the urethra in pellet form.
7. **Penile Implants (Prostheses):**
   - Surgical insertion of devices into both sides of the penis. These implants can be inflatable or semirigid rods.
8. **Vascular Surgery:**
   - In rare cases, particularly in younger men with ED due to pelvic trauma, vascular surgery to repair blood vessel blockages can restore erectile function.
9. **Management of Underlying Conditions:**
   - Addressing underlying medical conditions such as diabetes, high blood pressure, or heart disease is crucial.
10. **Alternative Therapies:**
    - Some men explore herbal supplements and alternative treatments. Caution is advised as the efficacy and safety of these treatments are not always well-established.

It is essential for individuals with ED to discuss their condition openly with a healthcare provider to determine the most appropriate and safe treatment options. The effectiveness of treatments can vary, and what works for one person may not work for another. Regular follow-up is also important to assess the efficacy and adjust the treatment plan as needed.

What is drug dependence?

Drug dependence, also known as substance dependence, is a medical condition characterized by an adaptive state that develops from repeated drug administration, and which results in withdrawal upon cessation of drug use. This condition encompasses both psychological and physical elements. Here are key aspects to understand about drug dependence:

1. **Physical Dependence:**
   - Occurs when the body adapts to the drug, leading to tolerance (needing more of the drug to achieve the same effect) and withdrawal symptoms when the drug use is reduced or stopped.
   - Withdrawal symptoms can vary depending on the substance but often include physical and mental health symptoms that are uncomfortable and, in some cases, life-threatening.
2. **Psychological Dependence:**
   - Refers to the emotional and mental preoccupation with the drug. This can include cravings for the drug and using it despite understanding the harmful consequences.
   - Psychological dependence often drives the compulsion to use the drug to feel 'normal' or to avoid negative emotions or states of mind.
3. **Substances Commonly Associated with Dependence:**
   - A wide range of substances can lead to dependence, including alcohol, opioids (like heroin and prescription painkillers), benzodiazepines, stimulants (like cocaine and methamphetamine), cannabis, tobacco, and certain prescription medications.
4. **Development of Dependence:**
   - Not everyone who uses drugs becomes dependent. The risk depends on multiple factors including the type of substance, the dose and frequency of use, genetic factors, environmental influences, and individual psychological factors.
5. **Impact on Health and Functioning:**
   - Drug dependence can have serious consequences for physical and mental health, relationships, occupational and social functioning, and legal status.
   - Long-term dependence can lead to chronic health problems, mental health disorders, difficulties in personal and professional relationships, financial problems, and legal issues.
6. **Treatment:**
   - Treatment can include detoxification (managing withdrawal), inpatient and outpatient rehabilitation programs, counseling, support groups, and sometimes medications to manage cravings and withdrawal symptoms.
   - Treatment plans are often tailored to the individual's specific needs and may involve a combination of therapy, social support, and sometimes medication.

7. **Recovery and Relapse:**
   - Recovery is a long-term process and may involve multiple attempts. Relapse, or a return to drug use after an attempt to stop, is common and considered a part of the recovery process.

Understanding drug dependence as a complex and multifaceted condition is crucial. It requires a comprehensive approach for treatment and support, often involving healthcare professionals, mental health specialists, family, and peer support networks.

What is addiction?

Addiction, also known as substance use disorder, is a complex and chronic brain disease characterized by compulsive drug seeking and use despite harmful consequences. It involves a set of behaviors and psychological changes that are more extensive than drug dependence. Here are the key aspects of addiction:

1. **Compulsive Behavior:**
   - Individuals with addiction feel an overwhelming, often uncontrollable urge to use substances, regardless of the negative impact on their health, social life, or other areas of functioning.
2. **Changes in the Brain:**
   - Addiction leads to changes in the brain's reward system. The repeated use of substances alters the way the brain experiences pleasure and can lead to craving the substance.
   - These changes in the brain can persist long after the substance is stopped, which contributes to the risk of relapse.
3. **Tolerance and Dependence:**
   - Tolerance develops as the body becomes accustomed to the substance, requiring higher doses to achieve the same effect.
   - Dependence is a physical state where the body adapts to the presence of the substance, leading to withdrawal symptoms when use is reduced or stopped.
4. **Withdrawal Symptoms:**
   - When not using the substance, individuals may experience withdrawal symptoms, which can be physical (like nausea, shaking, or sweating) or psychological (like irritability, anxiety, or depression).
5. **Continued Use Despite Negative Consequences:**
   - A hallmark of addiction is the continued use of the substance despite clear evidence of harm to oneself or others.
6. **Impact on Daily Life:**
   - Addiction can lead to difficulties in maintaining employment, relationships, and meeting daily responsibilities. It can also have legal and financial consequences.
7. **Psychological Factors:**
   - Psychological factors, including stress, trauma, and other mental health disorders, can contribute to the development and continuation of addiction.
8. **Treatment:**
   - Treatment for addiction is often multifaceted and can include detoxification, rehabilitation programs, counseling, behavioral therapy, support groups, and sometimes medication.
   - Treatment focuses on more than just abstaining from the substance; it also addresses related health and psychological issues, social relationships, and lifestyle changes.
9. **Chronic Nature and Relapse:**
   - Addiction is considered a chronic disease, similar to diabetes or heart disease, meaning it can be managed but not cured. Relapse, or returning to substance use, is common and considered part of the recovery process.

Understanding addiction as a comprehensive and long-term condition is essential. It requires ongoing management and a supportive environment for recovery. Additionally, overcoming stigma and viewing addiction as a medical condition, not a moral failing, is crucial in providing effective care and support to those affected.

What is drug abuse?

Drug abuse, also known as substance abuse, is the use of a drug in ways or amounts that are harmful to the user or others. It differs from addiction in that it does not always include the compulsive use, tolerance, or withdrawal that characterize addiction. However, drug abuse can lead to addiction over time. Here are key aspects to understand about drug abuse:

1. **Pattern of Use:**
   - Drug abuse involves using substances inappropriately, such as taking more than the

recommended dose of prescription medications, using someone else's prescription, or using illegal substances.

2. **Impact on Functioning:**
   - Drug abuse can negatively impact daily functioning, including performance at work or school and in personal relationships.
3. **Risky Behavior:**
   - Engaging in risky or harmful behavior while under the influence of drugs, such as driving while intoxicated or engaging in unsafe sexual practices.
4. **Health Consequences:**
   - Abuse of drugs can lead to serious health issues, including physical and mental health disorders. The type and severity of these health problems vary depending on the substance used.
5. **Legal and Social Consequences:**
   - Drug abuse can lead to legal issues, such as arrest for possession of illegal substances or for behaviors conducted under the influence. Social consequences might include strained or broken relationships with family and friends.
6. **Continued Use Despite Problems:**
   - Continued use of the substance despite having persistent or recurrent social, occupational, health, or legal problems caused or exacerbated by drug use indicates a problem of abuse.
7. **Denial of Problem:**
   - Individuals abusing drugs often do not recognize the extent of their problematic behavior and its impact on themselves and others.
8. **Psychological Factors:**
   - Various psychological factors, including stress, trauma, peer pressure, or other mental health disorders, can contribute to or exacerbate drug abuse.
9. **Prevention and Education:**
   - Efforts to prevent drug abuse often include education about the risks and consequences of drug use, developing life skills to resist peer pressure, and creating awareness of the signs and dangers of abuse.
10. **Treatment and Support:**
    - Treatment for drug abuse may involve counseling, behavioral therapy, participation in support groups, and sometimes medication, depending on the substance being abused.
    - Early intervention is crucial to prevent the progression from abuse to addiction.

Recognizing and addressing drug abuse early is important for preventing more serious problems, including addiction and long-term health issues. Support from healthcare professionals, family, friends, and community resources can be vital in helping individuals who struggle with substance abuse.

What is illicit drug use?

Illicit drug use refers to the use of illegal drugs or the misuse of prescription medications. This typically includes drugs that are forbidden by law or drugs that are legally available but used in ways other than prescribed. The term "illicit" highlights the illegality or unauthorized nature of the activity.

Key aspects of illicit drug use include:

1. **Legality:** The drugs are illegal to possess, distribute, or use. This can include drugs like heroin, cocaine, methamphetamine, and certain hallucinogens, which are prohibited under law.
2. **Misuse of Prescription Drugs:** This involves using prescription drugs in a way not intended by the prescribing doctor. This can include taking higher doses than prescribed, using someone else's prescription, or taking the medication for reasons other than medical need, such as for recreational purposes.
3. **Health Risks:** Illicit drug use is often associated with various health risks, including addiction, overdose, and the transmission of infectious diseases through shared needles. It can also lead to various mental and physical health problems.
4. **Societal Impact:** Beyond individual health risks, illicit drug use can have broader societal implications, including crime, economic costs, and social welfare issues.

It is important to note that the classification of drugs as illicit can vary between different countries and over time within the same country, depending on changes in law and societal attitudes.

What is recreational drug use?

Recreational drug use refers to the use of psychoactive substances primarily for pleasure, leisure, or enjoyment, rather than for medical reasons. This practice contrasts with medicinal drug use, which is intended for treating or preventing specific health conditions. Recreational drugs are often used to alter one's mental state, providing effects such as relaxation, euphoria, increased sociability, or altered perception.

These substances can be legal, such as alcohol and tobacco, or illegal, like cannabis, cocaine, ecstasy, and heroin. The legality and social acceptance of these substances vary widely between different cultures and countries.

What are narcotics?

"Narcotics" is a term that can have different meanings based on the context in which it is used. Traditionally, the term referred to a class of substances that dull the senses and relieve pain, often inducing sleep. Originally, it was primarily associated with opium, opium derivatives, and their synthetic substitutes.

In a medical context, narcotics are more accurately known as opioids. This group includes both natural and synthetic substances that act on opioid receptors in the brain to produce pain-relieving effects. Examples of opioids include morphine, heroin, fentanyl, oxycodone, and methadone. These substances are used medically for pain relief but have a high potential for abuse and addiction.

In a legal and law enforcement context, the term "narcotics" is often used more broadly to refer to a range of illicit drugs, not all of which are opioids. In this sense, the term can include drugs like cocaine, methamphetamine, and cannabis, in addition to opioids. This usage is less precise from a pharmacological standpoint, as many of these substances do not have the pain-relieving properties of traditional narcotics.

It is important to note that the term "narcotics" can sometimes carry a negative connotation and may be used in a stigmatizing way. In recent years, there has been a shift towards more specific and clinically accurate terminology, like "opioids," to describe these substances, especially in medical and health-related contexts.

What is schedule of drugs?

The "schedule of drugs" refers to a classification system used by various governments to categorize drugs and other substances based on their potential for abuse, medical value, and safety. This system is a key element in regulating the manufacture, possession, and use of pharmaceuticals and psychoactive substances. Different countries have their own scheduling systems, but one of the most well-known is the scheduling system used by the United States under the Controlled Substances Act (CSA).

In the U.S., the Drug Enforcement Administration (DEA) and the Food and Drug Administration (FDA) classify substances into one of five "schedules" based on the following criteria:

1. **Schedule I:** These substances have a high potential for abuse, no currently accepted medical use in the U.S., and a lack of accepted safety for use under medical supervision. Examples include heroin, LSD, ecstasy (MDMA), and cannabis (although the classification of cannabis is a subject of ongoing debate and varies by state).
2. **Schedule II:** These drugs have a high potential for abuse, with use potentially leading to severe psychological or physical dependence. However, they have some accepted medical uses with severe restrictions. Examples include cocaine, methamphetamine, methadone, oxycodone, and fentanyl.
3. **Schedule III:** Substances in this category have a potential for abuse less than substances in Schedules I or II and have currently accepted medical uses in the U.S. Abuse may lead to moderate or low physical dependence or high psychological dependence. An example is anabolic steroids.
4. **Schedule IV:** Drugs in this schedule have a lower potential for abuse than Schedule III drugs, are currently accepted for medical use in the U.S., and may lead to limited physical or psychological dependence relative to Schedule III substances. Examples include Xanax (alprazolam), Valium (diazepam), and Ambien (zolpidem).
5. **Schedule V:** These substances have a lower potential for abuse than Schedule IV drugs, have currently accepted medical uses in the U.S., and have limited potential for causing dependence. Many cough preparations with small amounts of codeine are classified under this schedule.

This scheduling system helps to guide legal and regulatory measures, influencing everything from criminal penalties to medical prescriptions. It is important to note that these schedules are subject to change as new substances emerge and as more is understood about existing ones. Also, while the U.S. scheduling system is influential, drug scheduling can vary significantly from country to country.

What are the principals of treatments of Addiction in general?

The treatment of addiction, a complex and often chronic condition, involves multiple principles that address the diverse aspects of the disorder. These principles are designed to treat not only the addiction itself but also its underlying causes and the various physical, psychol-ogical, and social issues associated with it. The key principles of addiction treatment include:

1. **Individualized Treatment:** Addiction treatment should be tailored to the unique needs of the individual. This includes considering factors like the type of substance used, the severity of the addiction, personal health history, and any co-occurring mental health conditions.
2. **Comprehensive Approach:** Effective treatment usually requires a combination of approaches. This can include behavioral therapy, medication, counseling, and support groups. Addressing related medical, psychological, social, vocational, and legal problems is also crucial in achieving the best outcomes.
3. **Access to Treatment:** Early and easy access to treatment is crucial. Prompt treatment can prevent the addiction from worsening and reduce the impact on an individual's life.
4. **Long-Term Perspective:** Addiction is typically a chronic disease, and like other chronic diseases, it often requires long-term management. Treatment duration should be adequate, and ongoing support or maintenance therapy may be necessary.
5. **Behavioral Therapies and Counseling:** These are the most common forms of addiction treatment and can help individuals engage in the treatment process, modify their attitudes and behaviors related to substance abuse, and increase their life skills to handle stressful circumstances and environmental cues that may trigger intense craving for substances.
6. **Medication Management:** When applicable, medication can play a critical role in recovery, particularly in the treatment of opioid, alcohol, and nicotine addiction. Medications can be used to manage withdrawal symptoms, prevent relapse, and treat co-occurring conditions.
7. **Monitoring:** Continuous monitoring of an individual's drug and alcohol use during treatment can help the treatment providers make necessary adjustments and can be a means to prevent relapse.
8. **Integration of Mental Health Services:** Many individuals with addiction also suffer from other mental health disorders (dual diagnosis). Treating both the addiction and the mental health condition simultaneously can be crucial for effective management.
9. **Supportive Services:** Services that support the treatment process, such as vocational training, legal assistance, and housing support, can be important elements of a comprehensive treatment program.
10. **Continuous Evaluation and Modification of Treatment:** As individuals change and grow during recovery, their treatment plans should be re-evaluated and modified as needed to ensure that it continues to meet their needs.
11. **Relapse Prevention:** Education and therapy to recognize and manage triggers and cravings play a crucial role in preventing relapse.
12. **Involvement of Family and Community:** Support from family and community can enhance the effectiveness of treatment. Involving them in the treatment process can provide additional support and help rebuild damaged relationships.

It is important to remember that recovery from addiction is a personal journey and can vary significantly from person to person. What works for one individual might not be as effective for another, which is why the principles of addic-tion treatment emphasize personalized and flexible approaches.

What are usual symptoms of drug withdrawal?

Drug withdrawal symptoms vary widely depending on the type of substance used, the duration of use, the dose, and the individual's physical and mental health. However, there are some common symptoms associated with withdrawal from various substances. These symptoms can be physi-cal, psychological, or a combination of both, and their severity can range from mild to life-threatening. Here are some typical withdrawal symptoms for various classes of drugs:

1. **Opioids (Heroin, Morphine, Prescription Pain Relievers):**
   - **Physical Symptoms:** Muscle aches, restless-ness, abdominal cramping, diarrhea, nausea, vomiting, sweating, tremors, rapid heartbeat.

- **Psychological Symptoms:** Anxiety, insomnia, agitation, depression.

2. **Benzodiazepines (Valium, Xanax, Ativan):**
   - **Physical Symptoms:** Sweating, palpitations, muscle stiffness or pain, tremors, seizures.
   - **Psychological Symptoms:** Anxiety, panic attacks, irritability, insomnia, poor concentration, nightmares.
3. **Alcohol:**
   - **Physical Symptoms:** Tremors, sweating, nausea, vomiting, headache, increased heart rate, high blood pressure, fever, seizures, hallucinations.
   - **Psychological Symptoms:** Anxiety, depression, irritability, confusion, insomnia, nightmares.
4. **Stimulants (Cocaine, Amphetamines, Methamphetamine):**
   - **Physical Symptoms:** Fatigue, increased appetite, sleep disturbances.
   - **Psychological Symptoms:** Depression, anxiety, irritability, restlessness, poor concentration, cravings.
5. **Cannabis (Marijuana):**
   - **Physical Symptoms:** Mild and less common, but can include headaches, sweating, chills, fever.
   - **Psychological Symptoms:** Irritability, restlessness, anxiety, cravings, disturbed sleep, decreased appetite.
6. **Nicotine (Cigarettes, Vaping):**
   - **Physical Symptoms:** Increased appetite, weight gain, restlessness, trouble sleeping.
   - **Psychological Symptoms:** Irritability, frustration, anger, anxiety, depression, difficulty concentrating, cravings.

It is important to note that withdrawal can be dangerous and even life-threatening in some cases, particularly with substances like alcohol and benzodiazepines. Medical supervision is often recommended, especially for individuals who have been using heavily or for an extended period. In a medically supervised setting, withdrawal can be managed more safely, and medications can be used to alleviate symptoms and reduce the risk of complications.

How to treat cocaine addiction?

Treating cocaine addiction involves a combination of therapeutic approaches, as there is currently no FDA-approved medication specifically for treating cocaine addiction. The treatment plan is usually tailored to the individual's needs, taking into account the severity of the addiction, any co-occurring mental health disorders, and the individual's social and family circumstances. Key components of cocaine addiction treatment typically include:

1. **Behavioral Therapies:** These are the most effective treatments for cocaine addiction.
   - **Cognitive-Behavioral Therapy (CBT):** Helps patients recognize, avoid, and cope with situations in which they are most likely to use cocaine.
   - **Contingency Management (CM):** Uses a voucher-based system where patients earn "points" based on negative drug tests, which they can exchange for items that encourage healthy living.
   - **Therapeutic Communities (TCs):** Drug-free residences where people in recovery from substance use disorders help each other to understand and change their behaviors.
2. **Group Therapy and Support Groups:** Support groups like Narcotics Anonymous (NA) or other community-based groups provide peer support for individuals quitting or reducing cocaine use.
3. **Individual Counseling:** This can help address the root causes of addiction, improve personal skills for resisting drug use, and support other treatments.
4. **Dual Diagnosis Treatment:** If there are co-occurring mental health disorders such as depression or anxiety, it is important to treat these concurrently with the addiction.
5. **Family Therapy:** Involving family members can improve the support network for the person in recovery and help resolve issues within family dynamics that may contribute to drug use.
6. **Medication-Assisted Treatment (MAT):** While there are no specific medications for cocaine addiction, medications may be used to treat withdrawal symptoms or co-occurring mental health issues.
7. **Inpatient Rehabilitation Programs:** These programs provide an environment away from usual triggers and stresses, offering intensive care and support.

8. **Aftercare and Relapse Prevention:** Ongoing support is crucial for maintaining sobriety. This can include continued therapy, support groups, and lifestyle changes to avoid relapse.
9. **Lifestyle Changes and Holistic Therapies:** Regular exercise, a healthy diet, sufficient sleep, stress management practices, and activities like yoga or meditation can support overall well-being and recovery.

It is important to remember that recovery from cocaine addiction is an ongoing process, and relapse can be part of this journey. Continuous support, patience, and adapting treatment strategies as needed are essential components of effective treatment. Seeking professional help from a healthcare provider or addiction specialist is the first step in this process.

How to treat alcohol addiction?

Treating alcohol addiction, also known as alcohol use disorder (AUD), typically involves a combination of medical, psychological, and support interventions. The approach depends on the individual's specific needs and the severity of their addiction. Here are the key components of alcohol addiction treatment:

1. **Medical Detoxification:** The first step in treatment is often detoxification, which is best done under medical supervision, especially for individuals with severe dependence. This process helps manage the acute and potentially dangerous physiological effects of stopping alcohol consumption, including withdrawal symptoms.
2. **Behavioral Therapies:** These are the most common treatments for AUD and help patients modify their attitudes and behaviors related to alcohol use, enhance healthy life skills, and persist with other forms of treatment.
   - **Cognitive-Behavioral Therapy (CBT):** Helps individuals develop strategies to cope with cravings and avoid situations that might trigger relapse.
   - **Motivational Enhancement Therapy:** Focuses on building motivation and creating a plan for change.
   - **Family Therapy:** Involves family members in the treatment process, which can improve family relationships and support systems.
3. **Medication-Assisted Treatment (MAT):** Certain medications can help reduce the desire to drink, manage withdrawal symptoms, or create adverse reactions if alcohol is consumed. Examples include Naltrexone, Acamprosate, and Disulfiram.
4. **Support Groups and Peer Support:** Groups like Alcoholics Anonymous (AA) and other community or online support groups offer a network of individuals facing similar challenges, providing a platform for sharing experiences and strategies for maintaining sobriety.
5. **Dual Diagnosis Treatment:** If the individual has co-occurring mental health disorders, such as depression or anxiety, it is important to treat these conditions alongside the AUD.
6. **Lifestyle Changes and Holistic Therapies:** Adopting a healthy lifestyle with regular exercise, a balanced diet, adequate sleep, and stress-reducing activities (like yoga, meditation, or hobbies) can support overall well-being and recovery.
7. **Inpatient or Outpatient Rehabilitation Programs:** Inpatient programs provide intensive treatment in a residential setting, while outpatient programs allow individuals to live at home while receiving treatment.
8. **Aftercare and Relapse Prevention:** Continuing care, including ongoing therapy, support groups, and check-ins with healthcare providers, helps prevent relapse and maintain sobriety.
9. **Educational and Vocational Assistance:** This can help individuals rebuild their lives and reintegrate into society post-treatment.
10. **Regular Monitoring:** Regular check-ups or monitoring by healthcare providers can help catch and address any relapses quickly.

The effectiveness of treatment depends on the individual's willingness to participate and the appropriateness of the treatment approach to their specific situation. It is also crucial to remember that recovery is a journey that can include setbacks. A relapse does not mean failure; it is an opportunity to re-evaluate and adjust the treatment approach. Seeking professional help from a healthcare provider or addiction specialist is an important first step in addressing alcohol addiction.

How to treat nicotine addiction?

Treating nicotine addiction typically involves a combination of therapies, including behavioral support and medication. The goal is to help the individual manage withdrawal symptoms and cravings, and to develop strategies to prevent relapse. Here are the key components of nicotine addiction treatment:

1. **Nicotine Replacement Therapy (NRT):** NRT provides nicotine in a controlled way without the harmful chemicals found in tobacco. It helps to reduce withdrawal symptoms and cravings. NRT products include nicotine gum, patches, lozenges, inhalers, and nasal sprays.
2. **Prescription Medications:**
   - **Varenicline (Chantix):** This medication works by blocking nicotine receptors in the brain, reducing cravings and withdrawal symptoms. It also reduces the satisfaction that people usually experience when they smoke.
   - **Bupropion (Zyban):** An antidepressant that helps reduce nicotine cravings and withdrawal symptoms.
3. **Behavioral Therapies:**
   - **Cognitive-Behavioral Therapy (CBT):** Helps identify and change thinking patterns that contribute to nicotine use and develop coping strategies.
   - **Motivational Interviewing:** Focuses on increasing the individual's motivation to quit and helping them to resolve ambivalence about stopping smoking.
4. **Support Groups and Counseling:** These provide emotional support and practical advice from others who have successfully quit smoking. Group counseling can be particularly effective.
5. **Digital and Telehealth Interventions:** Apps and online programs can offer support and resources for quitting, often including tracking features, educational material, and community support.
6. **Lifestyle Changes:**
   - **Stress Management Techniques:** Since many people smoke as a way to handle stress, learning new stress management techniques can be very helpful.
   - **Physical Activity:** Exercise can reduce nicotine cravings and withdrawal symptoms.
   - **Dietary Adjustments:** Certain foods and drinks can make cigarettes taste better or worse, and adjusting diet can help reduce cravings.
7. **Education and Awareness:** Understanding the risks of smoking and the benefits of quitting can increase motivation.
8. **Trigger Avoidance and Management:** Identifying and avoiding situations or emotions that trigger the urge to smoke is crucial.
9. **Relapse Prevention Planning:** Developing strategies to handle situations that might lead to smoking again.
10. **Gradual Reduction Strategy:** For some, gradually reducing cigarette consumption before quitting completely can be an effective approach.

It is important to note that quitting smoking is often a challenging process, and many people have multiple attempts before they quit for good. Each attempt is a learning experience, not a failure. Professional guidance from healthcare providers can significantly enhance the chances of success, offering personalized advice and support. Combining medication with behavioral therapy is generally more effective than using either approach alone.

How to treat marijuana addiction?

Treating marijuana addiction, also known as cannabis use disorder, involves a multi-faceted approach, as there are no FDA-approved medications specifically for this condition. The treatment typically focuses on behavioral therapies and supportive interventions. Here are the key components of marijuana addiction treatment:

1. **Cognitive-Behavioral Therapy (CBT):** CBT is effective in helping individuals identify and modify their thoughts and behaviors related to marijuana use. It also teaches coping skills to manage potential triggers and prevent relapse.
2. **Motivational Enhancement Therapy (MET):** This approach helps to resolve ambivalence about quitting and encourages intrinsic motivation to change marijuana use behavior.
3. **Contingency Management (CM):** This strategy uses a voucher-based system or other rewards to reinforce abstinence from marijuana use.
4. **Group Therapy and Support Groups:** Peer support groups can provide a sense of community and support. While there are no specific groups for marijuana addiction, broad substance misuse groups like Narcotics Anonymous can be helpful.
5. **Individual Counseling:** This can be beneficial for addressing personal issues related to marijuana use, including any underlying psychological or social problems.

6. **Family Therapy:** Involving family members in treatment can improve communication and support systems, which are important for recovery.
7. **Outpatient Treatment Programs:** These programs allow individuals to continue with their daily lives while receiving regular treatment and support.
8. **Inpatient or Residential Treatment Programs:** For more severe cases, or when the individual has not been successful with outpatient treatment, residential treatment may be necessary.
9. **Dual Diagnosis Treatment:** If there are co-occurring mental health conditions, such as anxiety or depression, it is important to treat these alongside the marijuana addiction.
10. **Lifestyle Changes and Holistic Approaches:** Regular exercise, stress management techniques, a balanced diet, and activities that promote overall well-being can support recovery.
11. **Relapse Prevention Education:** Learning how to deal with triggers and cravings and developing a plan to handle potential relapses are crucial aspects of treatment.
12. **Aftercare Planning:** Ongoing support after the completion of a treatment program, such as continued therapy or support groups, is important to maintain sobriety.

It is important to recognize that the effectiveness of different treatment approaches can vary from person to person. The decision on which treatment to pursue should be made in consultation with a healthcare provider or addiction specialist. Recovery from marijuana addiction is a personal journey, and it often requires a combination of treatments and continued support.

How to treat opiate addiction?

Treating opiate addiction, also known as opioid use disorder, is multifaceted and typically involves a combination of medication-assisted treatment (MAT), behavioral therapies, and supportive services. The approach is often individualized, based on the severity of the addiction, the specific opioids used, and the individual's overall health and personal circumstances. Here are the key components of opiate addiction treatment:

1. **Medication-Assisted Treatment (MAT):** MAT is considered the gold standard for treating opiate addiction and involves the use of medications to reduce cravings and withdrawal symptoms. Common medications include:
   - **Methadone:** A long-acting opioid agonist that reduces cravings and withdrawal symptoms without producing the euphoria associated with other opioids.
   - **Buprenorphine (Suboxone, Subutex):** A partial opioid agonist that relieves cravings and withdrawal symptoms. It has a ceiling effect, reducing the risk of misuse and dependency.
   - **Naltrexone (Vivitrol):** An opioid antagonist that blocks the effects of opioids. It is non-addictive and does not lead to physical dependence.
2. **Behavioral Therapies:**
   - **Cognitive-Behavioral Therapy (CBT):** Helps individuals recognize and change behaviors and thought patterns associated with opioid use, and develop coping strategies.
   - **Contingency Management (CM):** Uses a system of rewards for behaviors such as staying drug-free.
   - **Motivational Interviewing (MI):** Increases motivation to change and supports efforts to engage in treatment.
3. **Detoxification:** Medically supervised detox can safely manage the acute physical symptoms of withdrawal that occur when stopping opioid use. This is often the first step in treatment.
4. **Group Therapy and Support Groups:** Support groups like Narcotics Anonymous (NA) or other peer support programs can provide shared experiences and mutual support.
5. **Dual Diagnosis Treatment:** If there are co-occurring mental health disorders such as depression, anxiety, or PTSD, these should be treated simultaneously.
6. **Family Therapy and Support:** Involving family members can provide additional support and help in repairing and strengthening family relationships.
7. **Aftercare Planning:** Ongoing support, such as continued therapy or participation in support groups, is crucial to maintain long-term recovery and prevent relapse.
8. **Lifestyle Changes and Holistic Treatments:** Activities that promote overall well-being, such as exercise, nutritional counseling, meditation, and yoga, can complement the primary treatment approaches.

9. **Inpatient or Residential Treatment:** For those with severe addiction or who have not succeeded with outpatient treatment, inpatient programs offer a structured environment to focus on recovery.
10. **Outpatient Treatment Programs:** These programs allow individuals to live at home while receiving regular treatment, which can include counseling and medication management.
11. **Relapse Prevention Education:** Learning to recognize triggers, manage stress, and cope with cravings is a key part of treatment.
12. **Employment and Educational Support:** Assisting individuals in finding employment or continuing their education can be an important part of reintegrating into society and maintaining sobriety.

Effective treatment for opiate addiction often requires a long-term approach, with ongoing monitoring and adjustments to treatment as needed. Each individual's journey to recovery is unique, and treatment plans should be tailored to their specific needs. It is important for individuals struggling with opioid use disorder to seek professional help and to know that recovery is possible with the right treatment and support.

How to treat heroin addiction?

Treating heroin addiction, a form of opioid use disorder, involves a comprehensive approach that combines medication, behavioral therapies, and support services. This approach is often tailored to the individual's specific needs and circumstances. Here are the key components of heroin addiction treatment:

1. **Medication-Assisted Treatment (MAT):** MAT is a core component for treating heroin addiction and involves medications that help reduce cravings and withdrawal symptoms. Common medications include:
   - **Methadone:** A long-acting opioid agonist that reduces cravings and withdrawal symptoms, and blocks the euphoric effects of heroin.
   - **Buprenorphine (Suboxone, Subutex):** A partial opioid agonist that eases withdrawal symptoms and cravings without producing the same high as heroin.
   - **Naltrexone (Vivitrol):** An opioid antagonist that blocks opioid receptors and prevents heroin from producing euphoric effects.
2. **Behavioral Therapies:**
   - **Cognitive-Behavioral Therapy (CBT):** Helps patients recognize, avoid, and cope with situations in which they are most likely to use heroin.
   - **Contingency Management (CM):** Provides tangible rewards for maintaining sobriety.
   - **Motivational Interviewing (MI):** Enhances the individual's motivation to change their drug-using behavior.
3. **Detoxification:** Medically supervised detox can help manage withdrawal symptoms in a safe environment. It is typically the first step in treatment.
4. **Inpatient or Residential Treatment Programs:** These provide an immersive, structured environment for individuals with severe addiction, offering intensive care and support.
5. **Outpatient Treatment Programs:** These allow individuals to receive treatment while living at home, which can include therapy sessions and medication management.
6. **Support Groups and Peer Support:** Groups like Narcotics Anonymous (NA) offer community support and a space to share experiences and coping strategies.
7. **Dual Diagnosis Treatment:** Co-occurring mental health disorders such as depression or anxiety should be treated alongside the addiction.
8. **Family Therapy and Support:** Involving family members in the treatment process can help improve communication, address family dynamics contributing to the addiction, and strengthen the support network.
9. **Lifestyle Changes and Holistic Therapies:** Incorporating healthy habits like regular exercise, a balanced diet, stress management techniques, and activities like yoga or meditation can support recovery.
10. **Relapse Prevention Planning:** Developing strategies to deal with triggers and high-risk situations is crucial for maintaining long-term sobriety.
11. **Aftercare and Continued Support:** Ongoing therapy, support groups, and regular check-ins

with healthcare providers are important to prevent relapse.

12. **Vocational and Educational Support:** Assistance in finding employment or engaging in educational opportunities can help individuals reintegrate into society and build a stable, substance-free life.

Recovery from heroin addiction is a long-term process that often involves multiple attempts and continuous effort. It is important to remember that relapse can be part of the recovery journey and does not mean failure. Adjusting treatment strategies as needed and maintaining ongoing support are crucial for long-term recovery.

It is essential for individuals struggling with heroin addiction to seek professional help. Treatment should be started as soon as possible, and individuals should be encouraged to explore different treatment options to find what works best for their specific situation. With the right treatment and support, recovery from heroin addiction is achievable.

What are the uses of naltrexone?

Naltrexone is a medication primarily used in the management of alcohol and opioid dependence. It belongs to a class of drugs known as opioid antagonists and works by blocking the effects of opioids and alcohol at the receptor level in the brain. Here are the primary uses of naltrexone:

1. **Treatment of Alcohol Dependence:** Naltrexone helps reduce the craving for alcohol and the pleasurable effects associated with drinking. It is often prescribed as part of a comprehensive treatment plan that includes counseling and support. Naltrexone can help reduce the likelihood of relapse in people who have stopped drinking alcohol.

2. **Prevention of Opioid Relapse:** For individuals recovering from opioid addiction, naltrexone blocks the euphoric and sedative effects of opioids such as heroin, morphine, and codeine. This reduces the risk of relapse, as the use of opioids will not produce the desired effects. It is important to note that a person must be opioid-free for a minimum period (typically 7-10 days) before starting naltrexone to avoid precipitating withdrawal symptoms.

3. **Extended-Release Injectable Form:** Naltrexone is available as an extended-release injectable (known as Vivitrol), which is administered once a month. This form is used for treating both opioid and alcohol dependence and is beneficial for patients who have difficulty adhering to daily medication regimens.

It is important to note that naltrexone is not a cure for addiction but is used as part of a broader treatment plan that includes psychological support and lifestyle changes. It does not alleviate withdrawal symptoms or treat co-occurring mental health disorders.

Before starting naltrexone, patients should discuss their medical history with a healthcare provider, as naltrexone may not be suitable for everyone, particularly those with liver disease or acute hepatitis. Regular monitoring by a healthcare provider is also important during treatment with naltrexone to ensure its effectiveness and to manage any potential side effects.

Patients should also be aware that while on naltrexone, they will be more sensitive to lower doses of opioids, which increases the risk of opioid overdose if they attempt to overcome the blockade by taking large amounts of opioids. This risk is especially high if naltrexone treatment is discontinued.

Naltrexone is most effective when used as part of a comprehensive treatment program that includes behavioral therapy and support from healthcare professionals, family, and peer support groups. The goal is to help individuals in recovery build a foundation for long-term sobriety and to address underlying issues related to their substance use disorder.

What is the genetic influence on addiction?

The genetic influence on addiction is a significant and complex area of research. Genetics can play a considerable role in the likelihood of developing an addiction, but it is essential to understand that addiction is a multifactorial condition, influenced by a mix of genetic, environmental, and personal factors. Here are some key points:

1. **Genetic Predisposition:** Studies have shown that genetics can account for about 40% to 60% of the risk for addiction. This means that if a person has family members who have struggled with addiction, they may be at a higher risk themselves.

2. **Specific Genetic Factors:** Scientists have identified certain genes that may influence addiction. For example, variations in genes that affect the function of neurotransmitters like dopamine and serotonin can influence how an individual responds to substances. This response can increase the likelihood of developing an addiction.

3. **Environmental Interactions:** Genetics do not act in isolation. Environmental factors such as exposure to drugs or alcohol, stress, and social or family dynamics can significantly impact whether an individual with a genetic predisposition will develop an addiction.
4. **Types of Substances:** The influence of genetics may vary depending on the type of substance. For instance, the genetic factors involved in alcohol addiction may be different from those in opioid addiction.
5. **Behavioral Addictions:** Genetic factors may also play a role in behavioral addictions (like gambling or internet addiction), although research in this area is less developed compared to substance addictions.
6. **Epigenetics:** Recent studies in epigenetics (how genes are expressed) suggest that environmental factors can alter the way genes are expressed, which can influence the risk of addiction. This field is providing new insights into how the interaction between genetics and environment affects addiction risk.
7. **Prevention and Treatment:** Understanding the genetic factors in addiction can help in developing targeted prevention strategies and personalized treatment approaches, including pharmacogenomics (using genetic information to guide medication choices).

In summary, while genetics play a significant role in the risk of addiction, they are just one part of a complex interplay of factors. Addiction is not solely determined by genetics, and having a genetic predisposition to addiction does not mean that an individual will inevitably become addicted. Environmental and personal factors are also crucial in determining the overall risk.

What is the prognosis of addictive disorders?

The prognosis of addictive disorders varies widely and is influenced by several factors including the type of addiction, the individual's circumstances, and the presence of any co-occurring mental health disorders. Here are some key aspects to consider:

1. **Type of Substance or Behavior:** The prognosis can vary depending on the substance or behavior involved in the addiction. For example, recovery from opioid addiction might have different challenges and success rates compared to alcohol addiction.
2. **Severity and Duration of Addiction:** Generally, longer and more severe addictive behaviors are associated with a more challenging recovery process. Early intervention often leads to a better prognosis.
3. **Co-occurring Disorders:** The presence of co-occurring mental health issues, such as depression, anxiety, or schizophrenia, can complicate the recovery process and may require integrated treatment addressing both the addiction and the mental health disorder.
4. **Support Systems:** A strong support system, including family, friends, and support groups, can significantly improve the prognosis. Social isolation or a lack of support can hinder recovery.
5. **Access to Treatment:** Access to comprehensive treatment, including medical, psychological, and social support services, is critical for a positive outcome. Treatment approaches can include medication-assisted treatment (MAT), behavioral therapies, and counseling.
6. **Compliance with Treatment:** Adherence to treatment plans, including regular attendance at therapy sessions and, where applicable, taking prescribed medications as directed, is crucial for a favorable prognosis.
7. **Relapse Rates:** Relapse is common in the journey to recovery and should be considered a part of the process rather than a failure. The rates of relapse can vary, and relapse prevention is an important aspect of treatment.
8. **Lifestyle Changes:** Long-term recovery often requires significant lifestyle changes, such as avoiding triggers, changing social circles, and adopting healthier coping mechanisms. The willingness and ability to make these changes can influence the prognosis.
9. **Personal Motivation and Readiness to Change:** The individual's motivation to recover and readiness to engage in the recovery process are critical determinants of the prognosis.
10. **Chronic Nature of Addiction:** It is important to recognize that addiction is often a chronic condition, and managing it may require ongoing effort and treatment over a lifetime.

In conclusion, while addiction is a challenging and often chronic disorder, recovery is possible. The prognosis for addictive disorders is influenced by a variety of factors, and individual outcomes can vary significantly. With appropriate treatment and support, many people with addiction disorders can achieve long-term recovery.

What are the causes of death in addiction?

Addiction can lead to various causes of death, largely dependent on the nature of the addiction and related behaviors. Here are some of the primary causes of death associated with addiction:

1. **Overdose:** This is one of the most common causes of death in individuals with substance use disorders, especially for those using opioids, heroin, or prescription painkillers. Overdose occurs when a person consumes a toxic amount of a substance, leading to life-threatening symptoms or death.
2. **Accidents and Injuries:** Impaired judgment and coordination due to substance use can increase the risk of accidents, such as motor vehicle crashes, falls, or other types of injuries that can be fatal.
3. **Suicide:** Addiction is strongly linked to an increased risk of suicide. Substances can exacerbate mental health issues like depression or anxiety and can impair judgment, leading to an increased risk of suicide.
4. **Physical Health Complications:** Long-term substance abuse can lead to numerous health complications that can be fatal. These include liver disease (especially related to alcohol and certain drugs), heart disease, respiratory failure, kidney damage, and infectious diseases such as HIV/AIDS and hepatitis, often due to needle sharing.
5. **Withdrawal Complications:** In some cases, withdrawal from substances, particularly alcohol and benzodiazepines, can be life-threatening if not properly managed.
6. **Homicide and Violence:** Substance abuse can increase the risk of becoming involved in violent situations, including homicide, either as a perpetrator or a victim, often due to impaired judgment or involvement in illegal activities.
7. **Health Deterioration Due to Lifestyle:** Substance addiction often leads to a neglect of personal health and well-being, resulting in poor nutrition, lack of exercise, and neglect of chronic health conditions, which can contribute to premature death.
8. **Cancer:** Certain substances, including alcohol and tobacco, are linked to an increased risk of various cancers.
9. **Mental Health Deterioration:** Chronic substance use can exacerbate or lead to mental health disorders, some of which can be debilitating or life-threatening if not properly treated.
10. **Infection and Sepsis:** Intravenous drug use can increase the risk of infections, including skin infections, bloodstream infections, and endocarditis (an infection of the heart lining), which can be fatal.
11. **Alcohol Poisoning:** For those addicted to alcohol, acute alcohol poisoning can be a risk, especially in cases of binge drinking, leading to potentially fatal respiratory depression, coma, and organ failure.
12. **Drug Interactions and Contaminations:** The use of street drugs, which may be contaminated or mixed with other dangerous substances, can lead to unexpected toxic reactions and death. Additionally, combining different substances, including prescription medications, can have fatal effects.

It is important to note that the risk of these causes of death can be significantly reduced through effective treatment and recovery support. Addressing addiction is not only about stopping the substance use but also involves managing the associated physical, psychological, and social issues to improve overall health and reduce the risk of these fatal outcomes.

What is hypoglycaemia?

Hypoglycaemia refers to a condition where there is an abnormally low level of glucose (sugar) in the blood. Glucose is the main source of energy for the body's cells and is particularly crucial for brain function. Here are key aspects of Hypoglycaemia:

1. **Causes:** It is most commonly associated with diabetes treatment, where it can occur due to taking too much insulin or other diabetes medications, not eating enough carbohydrates, delaying or missing a meal, or exercising more than usual. However, Hypoglycaemia can also occur in people without diabetes due to a variety of reasons like excessive alcohol consumption,

certain medications, severe illnesses, hormonal deficiencies, or prolonged fasting.

2. **Symptoms:** Symptoms of Hypoglycaemia can vary from person to person but often include feeling shaky, sweaty, hungry, tired, anxious or irritable, dizzy or light-headed, and having a fast heartbeat. Severe Hypoglycaemia can lead to confusion, blurred vision, seizures, loss of consciousness, and in extreme cases, death.
3. **Diagnosis:** Hypoglycaemia is diagnosed based on the presence of the characteristic symptoms (often referred to as Whipple's triad) and a blood sugar level below the normal range. A healthcare provider may also conduct tests to determine the underlying cause if it is not clear.
4. **Treatment:** Immediate treatment for Hypoglycaemia involves consuming fast-acting carbohydrates, such as glucose tablets, sugar, honey, or fruit juice, to raise blood sugar levels quickly. It is important for people at risk of Hypoglycaemia, particularly those with diabetes, to carry something sweet with them at all times.
5. **Prevention:** For those with diabetes, managing blood sugar levels through regular monitoring, proper medication dosing, and following a balanced diet and exercise regime is crucial in preventing Hypoglycaemia. Those without diabetes who experience Hypoglycaemia need to address the underlying cause to prevent recurrence.
6. **Severe Hypoglycaemia:** In cases of severe Hypoglycaemia, where an individual may be unable to treat themselves, medical intervention is necessary. This can include the administration of intravenous glucose or an injection of glucagon.

Understanding the signs and symptoms of hypoglycaemia and knowing how to treat and prevent it are crucial, especially for those with diabetes or other risk factors. Regular medical check-ups and proper management of underlying conditions are important for minimizing the risk of hypoglycaemia.

What are the causes of hypoglycaemia?

Hypoglycaemia, the condition characterized by abnormally low blood glucose levels, can be caused by various factors, especially in individuals with diabetes. However, it can also occur in people without diabetes. Here are some of the primary causes:

1. **Diabetes-Related Causes:**
   - **Excessive Use of Insulin or Diabetes Medication:** This is the most common cause in people with diabetes. Taking too much insulin or other blood glucose-lowering medications can cause blood sugar to drop too low.
   - **Irregular Eating Habits:** Skipping meals, eating less than usual, or delaying meals can lead to Hypoglycaemia, especially if diabetes medications are not adjusted accordingly.
   - **Excessive Physical Activity:** Unusually intense or prolonged exercise can deplete glucose levels, leading to Hypoglycaemia, particularly if the person with diabetes does not adjust their food intake or medication dose.
   - **Alcohol Consumption:** Drinking alcohol, especially on an empty stomach, can interfere with the liver's ability to release glucose, increasing the risk of Hypoglycaemia.
2. **Non-Diabetic Causes:**
   - **Reactive Hypoglycaemia:** This occurs a few hours after eating and is thought to be the result of excessive insulin release triggered by the meal.
   - **Fasting Hypoglycaemia:** Caused by a lack of food, this form of Hypoglycaemia can be due to a variety of reasons, including prolonged fasting or malnutrition.
   - **Medications:** Besides diabetes medications, other drugs, like certain antibiotics, antiarrhythmic agents, or pentamidine, can induce Hypoglycaemia.
   - **Alcohol:** Excessive alcohol consumption without eating can block the liver from releasing stored glucose into the bloodstream, leading to Hypoglycaemia.
   - **Severe Illnesses:** Liver, kidney, or heart failure, as well as sepsis, can cause Hypoglycaemia.
   - **Hormonal Deficiencies:** In rare cases, deficiencies in hormones, such as cortisol (from the adrenal glands) or glucagon (from the pancreas), which regulate glucose levels, can lead to Hypoglycaemia.
   - **Insulinoma:** A rare pancreatic tumor that secretes insulin can cause Hypoglycaemia.

- Post-Gastric Bypass Hypoglycaemia: Some people who have undergone gastric bypass surgery may experience postprandial Hypoglycaemia.

3. **Other Factors:**
   - **Certain Medical Conditions:** Conditions such as anorexia or hepatic, adrenal, or kidney disorders can lead to Hypoglycaemia.
   - **Congenital Enzyme Deficiencies:** Rare genetic enzyme deficiencies can affect the body's ability to maintain normal glucose levels.

It is important for individuals experiencing symptoms of Hypoglycaemia to seek medical evaluation to determine the underlying cause and appropriate treatment. For those with diabetes, it is crucial to manage their condition carefully under the guidance of a healthcare provider to prevent Hypoglycaemia.

What is the treatment of hypoglycaemia?

The treatment of Hypoglycaemia largely depends on its severity and the individual's consciousness level. Here is a breakdown of the typical treatment approaches:

1. **Mild to Moderate Hypoglycaemia:**
   - **Immediate Consumption of Fast-Acting Carbohydrates:** The initial step is to consume 15-20 grams of fast-acting carbohydrates. Examples include glucose tablets or gel, fruit juice, regular (not diet) soda, honey, or sugar. Candy can be used, but chocolate or candy with fat digests more slowly and is less effective in the immediate situation.
   - **Recheck Blood Glucose Levels:** After 15 minutes, blood glucose levels should be rechecked. If they remain low (usually below 70 mg/dL or the target range set by a healthcare provider), the person should consume another 15-20 grams of fast-acting carbohydrates.
   - **Follow-up with a Snack or Meal:** Once blood glucose levels are back to normal, if it is going to be an hour or more before the next meal, a snack that includes carbohydrates and protein (like crackers with cheese or peanut butter) should be eaten to stabilize blood glucose levels.
2. **Severe Hypoglycaemia:**
   - **Glucagon Administration:** Severe Hypoglycaemia, especially if it leads to unconsciousness or inability to swallow, requires the administration of glucagon. Glucagon is a hormone that raises blood glucose levels and can be given as an injection or nasal spray. Family members, friends, and co-workers should be trained on how to administer glucagon in case of an emergency.
   - **Medical Attention:** After glucagon administration, emergency medical help should be sought immediately. The individual will need medical evaluation and monitoring to ensure recovery and to address the underlying cause of the severe Hypoglycaemia.
3. **Prevention and Long-term Management:**
   - **Adjusting Diabetes Management Regimen:** For those with diabetes, it is crucial to work with a healthcare provider to adjust the diabetes management plan to prevent future episodes. This might include changes in medication types or doses, meal planning, and exercise routines.
   - **Education and Self-Monitoring:** Education on recognizing early signs of Hypoglycaemia and regular monitoring of blood glucose levels are essential, especially for people with diabetes.
4. **Lifestyle Modifications:**
   - **Regular Meals and Snacks:** Eating regular meals and snacks with the right balance of carbohydrates, fats, and proteins can help maintain stable blood sugar levels.
   - **Avoiding Alcohol on an Empty Stomach:** For those who drink alcohol, it is important to avoid consuming it on an empty stomach, as alcohol can increase the risk of Hypoglycaemia.
5. **Medical Review:**
   - **Review of Medications and Health Status:** Regular medical reviews are essential to ensure that any medications being taken are not contributing to hypoglycemic episodes. This is also important to manage any other health conditions that might affect blood glucose levels.
6. **Wearing a Medical Alert Bracelet:**
   - Identification: People with a high risk of Hypoglycaemia should consider wearing a medical alert bracelet or carrying an identification card that notifies others of their condition in case of an emergency.

Remember, the approach to treating Hypoglycaemia can vary based on individual circumstances, and what works for one person may not be appropriate for another. It is important for individuals, especially those with diabetes, to have a clear plan developed with their healthcare provider for managing Hypoglycaemia.

How to assess and treat hyponatremia?

Hyponatremia, a condition characterized by low sodium levels in the blood, requires careful assessment and management due to its potentially serious complications. Here is how it is generally assessed and treated:

Assessment of Hyponatremia

1. **Symptom Evaluation:** Symptoms can range from mild to severe and include nausea, headache, confusion, lethargy, fatigue, muscle weakness, seizures, and in severe cases, coma.
2. **Medical History and Physical Examination:** A thorough medical history (including medication use, water intake, and any recent changes in health) and physical examination are crucial to determine potential causes and severity.
3. **Laboratory Tests: These typically include:**
   - **Serum Sodium Test:** To confirm low sodium levels.
   - **Serum Osmolality Test:** To determine if the hyponatremia is hypotonic (most common type), isotonic, or hypertonic.
   - **Urine Tests:** Urine osmolality and urine sodium levels help identify the cause of hyponatremia.
4. **Assessment of Volume Status:** This involves evaluating whether the patient is hypovolemic (low volume), euvolemic (normal volume), or hyper-volemic (excess volume), as treatment varies based on the volume status.

Treatment of Hyponatremia

1. **Addressing the Underlying Cause:** The primary cause of hyponatremia (like heart failure, kidney problems, or medication side effects) needs to be identified and treated.
2. **Fluid Management:**
   - **Fluid Restriction:** Often used in euvolemic and hypervolemic hyponatremia (e.g., in cases related to heart failure, liver disease, or SIADH - Syndrome of Inappropriate Antidiuretic Hormone Secretion).
   - **Fluid Administration:** In hypovolemic hyponatremia, administering saline solution can be necessary.
3. **Medications:**
   - **Vasopressin Receptor Antagonists (Vaptans):** These can be used in certain types of euvolemic and hypervolemic hyponatremia.
   - **Diuretics:** May be used in hypervolemic hyponatremia to reduce fluid overload.
4. **Monitoring and Adjusting Treatment:** Careful monitoring of serum sodium levels and the patient's response to treatment is crucial. Rapid correction of sodium levels can be dangerous (leading to a risk of osmotic demyelination syndrome), so the rate of correction is typically gradual and carefully controlled.
5. **Dietary Changes:** Dietary advice may include limiting water intake and adjusting the intake of dietary salt.
6. **Severe or Symptomatic Hyponatremia:**
   - **Emergency Treatment:** In cases of severe hyponatremia (sodium level less than 120 mmol/L) or if severe symptoms are present (like seizures), more rapid correction of sodium levels may be required, often in an intensive care setting.

Special Considerations

- **Rate of Sodium Correction:** The rate of correction should typically not exceed 10 mmol/L in 24 hours to avoid the risk of osmotic demyelination syndrome, a serious neurological condition.
- **Chronic vs Acute Hyponatremia:** The approach to treatment can vary depending on whether hyponatremia developed slowly (chronic) or quickly (acute). Chronic hyponatremia requires more cautious correction.
- **Regular Monitoring:** Continuous monitoring of serum sodium levels and overall health status is essential during the treatment of hyponatremia.
- **Intravenous Treatment:** In some cases, especially in acute or severe hyponatremia, intravenous hypertonic saline may be administered.
- **Prevention:** Ongoing management of underlying medical conditions and careful medication management can help prevent recurrent hyponatremia.

Conclusion

The assessment and treatment of hyponatremia are complex and should be guided by a healthcare professional, as the condition can vary significantly from person to person. The key to effective management is identifying the underlying cause, careful correction of sodium levels to avoid rapid shifts, and ongoing monitoring. It is also important to educate patients, especially those with risk factors for hyponatremia, about the signs and symptoms of the condition and when to seek medical attention.

What are the principal causes of Hyponatremia?

Hyponatremia, characterized by low sodium levels in the blood, can result from various causes. Understanding these causes is crucial for effective treatment and management. The principal causes of hyponatremia are often categorized based on the patient's fluid status - whether they are hypovolemic (low fluid volume), euvolemic (normal fluid volume), or hypervolemic (high fluid volume):

1. **Hypovolemic Hyponatremia:**
   - **Dehydration:** Loss of body fluids through excessive sweating, diarrhea, or vomiting can lead to hyponatremia.
   - **Diuretics:** The use of diuretics can cause both sodium and water loss, leading to hyponatremia.
   - **Adrenal Insufficiency:** Conditions like Addison's disease, where the adrenal glands do not produce enough hormones, can lead to sodium loss.
   - **Third-Space Fluid Shifts:** Fluid loss into the body spaces (e.g., due to burns, pancreatitis) can result in hyponatremia.
2. **Euvolemic Hyponatremia:**
   - **SIADH (Syndrome of Inappropriate Antidiuretic Hormone Secretion):** This condition leads to excessive retention of water without significant salt loss, diluting the blood sodium. It can be caused by certain medications, lung diseases, central nervous system disorders, or cancer.
   - **Hypothyroidism:** Underactive thyroid can disrupt the body's balance of sodium and fluids.
   - **Psychogenic Polydipsia:** Excessive water drinking, often seen in mental health disorders, can dilute the sodium in the body.
   - **Certain Medications:** Some drugs, like SSRIs (selective serotonin reuptake inhibitors) and antiepileptics, can cause euvolemic hyponatremia.
3. **Hypervolemic Hyponatremia:**
   - **Heart Failure:** Reduced heart function can lead to fluid and sodium retention.
   - **Liver Cirrhosis:** Liver dysfunction can disrupt fluid and sodium balance, leading to fluid accumulation in the body.
   - **Kidney Disease:** Chronic kidney disease can impair the kidneys' ability to excrete water, leading to fluid overload and diluted sodium levels.
   - **Nephrotic Syndrome:** A kidney disorder causing excessive protein loss in urine can result in low blood sodium.
4. **Other Factors:**
   - **Older Age:** Older adults are at higher risk due to factors like a higher likelihood of taking medications that affect sodium levels and a decreased ability to regulate fluid and sodium balance.
   - **Hormonal Imbalances:** Conditions affecting hormonal balance, such as adrenal or pituitary gland disorders, can impact sodium levels.
   - **Dietary Factors:** Extremely low sodium intake or excessive water intake can lead to hyponatremia.

It is important to identify the specific cause of hyponatremia in each individual, as the treatment approach can vary significantly depending on the underlying reason. Medical evaluation typically involves a combination of physical examination, medical history review, and laboratory tests to determine the cause and guide appropriate treatment.

What is the pathology of hyponatremia?

The pathology of hyponatremia, or low sodium concentration in the blood, is a complex process that involves various mechanisms and factors. Sodium is vital for numerous bodily functions, including maintaining fluid balance, transmitting nerve signals, and muscle function. In hyponatremia, the pathology often revolves around the balance between water and sodium in the body. Here is a breakdown of the key pathological aspects:

1. **Disrupted Water-Sodium Balance:** Hyponatremia typically occurs when there is an imbalance in the body's water levels relative to sodium. This can happen due to either an excess of water or a loss of sodium, or a combination of both.

2. **Osmoregulation and Antidiuretic Hormone (ADH):**

   - **ADH Role:** The release of ADH (vasopressin) from the pituitary gland plays a crucial role in hyponatremia. ADH is released in response to increased plasma osmolality (concentration) or decreased blood volume and acts on the kidneys to conserve water.

   - **Inappropriate ADH Secretion:** In conditions like SIADH (Syndrome of Inappropriate Antidiuretic Hormone Secretion), excessive ADH is released, leading to water retention and dilutional hyponatremia.

3. **Hypovolemic Hyponatremia:** This occurs due to a loss of both sodium and water, but with a relatively greater loss of sodium. Causes can include gastrointestinal losses (vomiting, diarrhea), renal losses (use of diuretics), and skin losses (excessive sweating).

4. **Euvolemic Hyponatremia:** Here, total body water increases without a significant change in total body sodium. SIADH is a common cause, as well as conditions like hypothyroidism and glucocorticoid deficiency.

5. **Hypervolemic Hyponatremia:** This involves both an increase in total body water and sodium, but with a disproportionately larger increase in water. Common causes include heart failure, liver cirrhosis, and renal disease.

6. **Cellular Effects:** In hyponatremia, the low extracellular sodium concentration leads to a relative excess of water outside the cells. Water moves into cells to balance the osmotic difference, causing cellular swelling. This is particularly dangerous in the brain, leading to cerebral edema, increased intracranial pressure, and potentially life-threatening complications like brain stem herniation.

7. **Hormonal and Renal Responses:** The body's hormonal (like renin-angiotensin-aldosterone system) and renal responses to perceived volume status also play a role in the development and perpetuation of hyponatremia.

8. **Dietary and Lifestyle Factors:** Diet, water intake, and medications can contribute to the pathology, especially in susceptible individuals.

In conclusion, the pathology of hyponatremia involves a complex interplay of factors affecting water and sodium balance. The exact pathophysiological mechanism depends on the underlying cause of the hyponatremia, which is why accurate diagnosis and identification of the cause are essential for effective treatment.

What is Syndrome of Inappropriate Antidiuretic hormone (ADH) Secretion-a cause of hyponatremia?

Syndrome of Inappropriate Antidiuretic Hormone Secretion (SIADH) is a condition characterized by the excessive release of antidiuretic hormone (ADH), also known as vasopressin, from the posterior pituitary gland or other sources. This syndrome is a common cause of hyponatremia, which is an abnormally low concentration of sodium in the blood. Here is an overview of SIADH:

Pathophysiology

1. **Excessive ADH Secretion:** In SIADH, there is inappropriate and continued secretion of ADH despite normal or low plasma osmolality. ADH acts on the kidneys to increase water reabsorption, leading to dilutional hyponatremia.

2. **Euvolemic Hyponatremia:** Patients with SIADH typically exhibit euvolemic hyponatremia, meaning they have normal fluid volume status, as the excess water retention does not lead to significant edema or hypervolemia.

3. **Impaired Water Excretion:** The body's ability to excrete dilute urine is impaired, leading to water retention and dilution of blood sodium levels.

Causes

SIADH can be caused by a variety of conditions:

- **Malignancies:** Particularly small cell lung cancer, which can produce ADH.

- **Pulmonary Disorders:** Such as pneumonia, tuberculosis, or acute respiratory failure.

- **Central Nervous System Disorders:** Including meningitis, encephalitis, brain tumors, head trauma, or stroke.

- **Medications:** Certain drugs, like antidepressants (SSRIs), antipsychotics, and anticonvulsants, can stimulate ADH secretion.

- **Postoperative State:** Particularly after surgeries involving general anesthesia.

- **Idiopathic:** In some cases, the cause of SIADH is unknown.

Clinical Features

1. **Symptoms of Hyponatremia:** Including headache, nausea, vomiting, muscle cramps, lethargy, confusion, seizures, and in severe cases, coma.
2. **No Edema or Dehydration:** Unlike other conditions that cause hyponatremia, patients with SIADH do not exhibit signs of fluid overload (like edema) or dehydration.

Diagnosis

1. **Low Plasma Sodium Level:** Indicative of hyponatremia.
2. **Low Plasma Osmolality:** Due to dilution from retained water.
3. **High Urine Osmolality:** Despite the low blood sodium and osmolality, indicating that the kidneys are inappropriately concentrating urine.
4. **High Urine Sodium Excretion:** Despite the low blood sodium.
5. **Clinical Evaluation:** To rule out other causes of euvolemic hyponatremia, such as hypothyroidism, adrenal insufficiency, or diuretic use.

Treatment

1. **Fluid Restriction:** The mainstay of treatment is fluid restriction to decrease water intake.
2. **Salt and Fluid Administration:** In some cases, salt tablets or hypertonic saline solution may be used, especially if hyponatremia is severe or symptomatic.
3. **Medications:**
   - **Vasopressin Receptor Antagonists:** These drugs, also known as "vaptans," work by blocking the effect of ADH on the kidneys, increasing water excretion without losing sodium.
   - **Diuretics:** In some cases, loop diuretics may be used to increase water excretion.
4. **Treatment of Underlying Cause:** If an underlying cause for SIADH is identified, such as a tumor or infection, treating that condition is crucial.
5. **Monitoring:** Careful monitoring of sodium levels, fluid balance, and overall clinical status is essential to prevent rapid correction of sodium, which can lead to osmotic demyelination syndrome, a serious neurological condition.

Special Considerations

- **Slow Correction of Sodium Levels:** Rapid correction of sodium levels in chronic hyponatremia can be dangerous. The recommended rate of correction is generally no more than 8-10 mmol/L in the first 24 hours.
- **Chronic Management:** In cases where SIADH is chronic or the underlying cause cannot be corrected, long-term management strategies, including lifestyle modifications and regular monitoring, are important.
- **Patient Education:** Educating patients about the importance of fluid restriction and the signs and symptoms of hyponatremia is crucial, especially in chronic SIADH.

SIADH represents a complex interplay between hormone regulation, fluid balance, and electrolyte levels. Its management requires a careful and often multidisciplinary approach, particularly in cases where the underlying cause is not readily identifiable or treatable.

What are the Symptoms and Signs of hyponatremia?

Hyponatremia, a condition characterized by low sodium levels in the blood, can manifest with a range of symptoms and signs, varying from mild to severe based on the rapidity and degree of the sodium decrease. Here are the common symptoms and signs associated with hyponatremia:

Mild to Moderate Hyponatremia

- **Nausea and Malaise:** A general feeling of discomfort or unease.
- **Headache:** Can range from mild to severe.
- **Fatigue or Weakness:** General physical weakness and a lack of energy.
- **Muscle Cramps or Spasms:** Especially in the extremities.
- **Irritability or Restlessness:** Mood changes and agitation.
- **Dizziness or Light-headedness:** Especially upon standing (orthostatic changes).

Severe Hyponatremia

- **Confusion and Disorientation:** Trouble with thinking, attention, concentration, and memory.
- **Seizures:** Uncontrolled electrical disturbances in the brain.
- **Stupor or Coma:** Severe impairment or loss of consciousness.

- **Vomiting:** Which can exacerbate the hyponatremia.

Neurological Signs (due to Brain Swelling)

- **Altered Mental Status:** Including confusion, hallucinations, or decreased alertness.
- **Ataxia:** Lack of muscle coordination, which might affect speech, eye movements, the ability to swallow, walking, picking up objects, and other voluntary movements.
- **Severe Headaches:** Resulting from brain swelling.
- **Respiratory Arrest:** In extreme cases, due to brain stem herniation.

Variable Signs Depending on the Underlying Cause

- **Signs of Fluid Overload:** Such as swelling or edema, ascites, or pulmonary congestion in hypervolemic hyponatremia (often seen in heart failure, liver disease, or kidney disease).
- **Signs of Dehydration:** Such as dry mucous membranes, low blood pressure, and tachycardia in hypovolemic hyponatremia.

Special Considerations

- **Rate of Onset:** Acute hyponatremia (developing in less than 48 hours) often presents with more severe neurological symptoms due to the rapid change affecting the brain.
- **Chronic Hyponatremia:** When the decrease in sodium levels occurs gradually over time (more than 48 hours), the symptoms might be milder or less noticeable, as the body has time to adapt to the change.

Prompt recognition and treatment of hyponatremia are important, especially in severe cases, due to the risk of serious complications like cerebral edema and brain stem herniation. If hyponatremia is suspected, especially with neurological symptoms, immediate medical attention is necessary.

How to diagnose hyponatremia?

Diagnosing hyponatremia, which is defined as a serum sodium concentration below 135 mmol/L, involves a combination of clinical assessment, laboratory tests, and evaluation of the patient's medical history and symptoms. Here is a step-by-step approach to diagnosing hyponatremia:

1. Clinical Assessment

- **Symptom Evaluation:** Assess for signs and symptoms of hyponatremia, which can range from nausea and malaise to severe confusion, seizures, and coma, depending on the severity.
- **Medical History:** Review the patient's medical history, including any chronic conditions, recent hospitalizations, surgeries, or changes in health status.
- **Medication Review:** Certain medications, such as diuretics, antidepressants, and antipsychotics, can contribute to hyponatremia.
- **Dietary and Fluid Intake:** Assess the patient's fluid and salt intake, including the use of over-the-counter medications that might affect sodium levels.

2. Laboratory Tests

- **Serum Sodium Level:** Confirm low serum sodium concentration (below 135 mmol/L).
- **Serum Osmolality:** Differentiates between true hyponatremia (hypo-osmolar) and pseudohyponatremia (normal or high osmolality). Pseudohyponatremia can occur in hyperlipidemia or hyperproteinemia.
- **Urine Osmolality and Sodium:** Helps in determining the cause of hyponatremia. High urine osmolality suggests the kidney is responding to ADH and conserving water, while urine sodium helps differentiate between different types of hyponatremia (e.g., renal vs non-renal causes).
- **Glucose Level:** High blood glucose can lead to "translocational" hyponatremia due to osmotic effects, where water moves from the intracellular to the extracellular space, diluting sodium.
- **Blood Urea Nitrogen (BUN) and Creatinine:** Assess kidney function, which can affect sodium balance.
- **Other Tests:** Depending on the suspected cause, additional tests such as thyroid function tests, cortisol levels, and a full blood count might be conducted.

3. Assessment of Volume Status

- **Physical Examination:** Evaluate the patient for signs of dehydration (e.g., dry mucous membranes, decreased skin turgor), fluid overload (e.g., edema, ascites), or euvolemia.
- **Blood Pressure and Heart Rate:** Can provide clues about the patient's volume status.

4. Identifying the Cause

- **Categorizing Hyponatremia:** Based on urine osmolality and urine sodium, along with clinical assessment, hyponatremia can be categorized as hypovolemic, euvolemic, or hypervolemic, each of which has different potential causes.

- **Investigating Underlying Conditions:** Explore potential causes such as heart failure, liver disease, renal disease, SIADH, adrenal insufficiency, hypothyroidism, and others.

5. Monitoring and Re-evaluation

- **Continuous Monitoring:** In severe cases, continuous monitoring of sodium levels and overall health status is crucial, especially during treatment.
- **Response to Therapy:** Observing how the sodium level responds to initial management can also provide diagnostic clues.

Special Considerations

- **Rapid vs Gradual Onset:** Distinguishing between acute and chronic hyponatremia is important for management, as the risk of complications like osmotic demyelination varies.
- **Severity:** Severe or symptomatic hyponatremia, particularly with neurological symptoms, is a medical emergency requiring prompt treatment.

Accurate diagnosis of hyponatremia is essential for effective treatment and management. It is a complex condition that requires a systematic approach to determine the underlying cause and guide appropriate therapy.

What is the Treatment of hyponatremia?

The treatment of hyponatremia, a condition characterized by low sodium levels in the blood, must be tailored to the individual based on the severity of the condition, the rate at which it developed, the underlying cause, and the patient's overall health status. Here is an overview of the general treatment approaches:

1. Treat the Underlying Cause

- **Addressing the Root Cause:** Whether it is medication-induced, due to a medical condition like heart failure, liver disease, SIADH, or dehydration, treating the underlying cause is crucial.

2. Fluid Management

- **Fluid Restriction:** Often the first step in treating mild to moderate cases, especially in euvolemic or hypervolemic hyponatremia (e.g., SIADH).
- **Fluid Administration:** In cases of hypovolemic hyponatremia, intravenous saline solution (isotonic or hypertonic, depending on the severity) may be administered to replenish sodium levels.

3. Medication Adjustments

- **Adjusting Diuretics:** In hypervolemic hyponatremia, modifying the use of diuretics can be beneficial.
- **Vasopressin Receptor Antagonists (Vaptans):** Used particularly in euvolemic and hypervolemic cases (like SIADH) to block the action of ADH and promote water excretion without losing sodium.
- **Mineralocorticoids:** In cases related to adrenal insufficiency.

4. Monitoring Sodium Levels

- **Careful Correction:** Rapid correction of sodium can lead to serious complications like osmotic demyelination syndrome. The goal is usually to increase sodium levels by no more than 8-10 mmol/L in the first 24 hours.
- **Continuous Monitoring:** Frequent monitoring of serum sodium levels, especially during the initial phase of treatment, is critical.

5. Severe or Symptomatic Hyponatremia

- **Emergency Treatment:** Severe hyponatremia (sodium levels less than 120 mmol/L) or symptomatic cases (especially with neurological symptoms) require prompt and more aggressive treatment, often in a hospital setting.
- **Intravenous Hypertonic Saline:** May be used to rapidly increase sodium levels in acute or severe cases.

6. Dietary Modifications

- **Sodium and Fluid Intake:** Adjusting dietary sodium and fluid intake can be part of long-term management, especially in chronic or recurrent cases.

7. Treatment of SIADH

- **Fluid Restriction and Medication:** In addition to fluid restriction, medications such as vaptans or adjustments in current medications causing SIADH may be needed.

8. Special Considerations for Chronic Hyponatremia

- **Gradual Correction:** Chronic hyponatremia should be corrected more slowly than acute hyponatremia to minimize the risk of osmotic demyelination syndrome.

Conclusion

The treatment of hyponatremia requires a careful and individualized approach to safely correct the sodium imbalance while addressing the underlying cause. Overly rapid correction of sodium levels can be dangerous, and ongoing monitoring is essential during the treatment process. Medical professionals often manage severe or complicated cases of hyponatremia in a hospital setting to ensure proper care and monitoring.

What is hypothyroidism?

Hypothyroidism is a common endocrine disorder where the thyroid gland does not produce enough thyroid hormones. The thyroid, a butterfly-shaped gland in the front of the neck, plays a crucial role in regulating metabolism and energy use in the body. Thyroid hormones, mainly thyroxine (T4) and triiodothyronine (T3), influence the function of many of the body's organs. When these hormone levels are too low, it can affect numerous bodily functions.

Causes of Hypothyroidism

1. **Hashimoto's Thyroiditis:** An autoimmune disorder where the body's immune system attacks thyroid tissue. It is the most common cause in countries with sufficient iodine intake.
2. **Iodine Deficiency:** Essential for thyroid hormone production, iodine deficiency is a common cause of hypothyroidism in areas where iodine is lacking in the diet.
3. **Thyroid Surgery or Radiation Therapy:** Removal of the thyroid or radiation treatment for conditions such as hyperthyroidism or thyroid cancer can lead to hypothyroidism.
4. **Certain Medications:** Some drugs, such as lithium and amiodarone, can affect thyroid function.
5. **Congenital Hypothyroidism:** Some babies are born with a dysfunctional or absent thyroid gland.
6. **Pituitary or Hypothalamic Disease:** Rarely, a disorder of the pituitary gland or hypothalamus can interfere with thyroid hormone production.

Symptoms of Hypothyroidism

Symptoms develop slowly, often over several years, and can include:

- Fatigue and Weakness
- Weight Gain
- Cold Intolerance
- Dry Skin and Hair
- Hair Loss
- Constipation
- Depression
- Memory and Concentration Difficulties
- Menstrual Irregularities in Women
- Elevated Blood Cholesterol Level
- Muscle Aches and Stiffness

Diagnosis

Diagnosis of hypothyroidism typically involves:

- **Medical History and Physical Exam:** Looking for symptoms and physical signs like dry skin, swelling, and slower reflexes.
- **Blood Tests:** The most definitive way to diagnose hypothyroidism is through blood tests that measure Thyroid-Stimulating Hormone (TSH) and Thyroxine (T4) levels. High levels of TSH and low levels of T4 indicate hypothyroidism.

Treatment

- **Thyroid Hormone Replacement Therapy:** The standard treatment is synthetic thyroxine (levothyroxine), which is taken orally and restores normal hormone levels, reversing the symptoms of hypothyroidism.
- **Regular Monitoring:** Treatment often requires lifelong medication and regular monitoring of thyroid function tests to adjust the dosage of levothyroxine correctly.

Managing Hypothyroidism

- **Regular Follow-up:** Regular follow-up with a healthcare provider is important to ensure that thyroid hormone levels remain within the target range.
- **Lifestyle Adjustments:** Healthy diet and regular exercise can help manage symptoms and improve overall health.

Conclusion

Hypothyroidism is a common condition, especially among women and older adults, and can significantly impact quality of life if left untreated. With proper diagnosis and treatment, however, most people with hypothyroidism can lead normal, healthy lives.

What are types of hypothyroidism?

Hypothyroidism, characterized by an underactive thyroid gland, can be classified into several types based on different criteria, such as the cause, the level at which the dysfunction occurs, and the time of onset. Here are the main types:

1. Primary Hypothyroidism

- **Cause:** The dysfunction occurs directly in the thyroid gland. It is the most common type.
- **Common Causes:** Hashimoto's thyroiditis (an autoimmune disease), iodine deficiency, thyroidectomy (surgical removal of the thyroid gland), or radiation treatment to the thyroid.

2. Secondary Hypothyroidism

- **Cause:** The pituitary gland fails to produce enough Thyroid-Stimulating Hormone (TSH), which is necessary to stimulate the thyroid gland.
- **Common Causes:** Pituitary gland disorders or tumors.

3. Tertiary Hypothyroidism

- **Cause:** Dysfunction in the hypothalamus, leading to inadequate production of Thyrotropin-Releasing Hormone (TRH), which stimulates the pituitary gland to produce TSH.
- **Common Causes:** Hypothalamic disease or injury.

4. Congenital Hypothyroidism

- **Occurrence:** Present at birth.
- **Cause:** The thyroid gland is absent, underdeveloped, or located in the wrong place. It can also result from genetic defects affecting hormone production.

5. Subclinical Hypothyroidism

- **Characteristics:** Mild form where blood levels of thyroid hormones are normal, but TSH is slightly elevated.
- **Symptoms:** Often few or no symptoms are noticed.

6. Autoimmune Hypothyroidism

- **Example:** Hashimoto's thyroiditis.
- **Mechanism:** The immune system mistakenly attacks the thyroid gland, gradually destroying its ability to produce hormones.

7. Iatrogenic Hypothyroidism

- **Cause:** Resulting from medical treatment, such as radioactive iodine therapy or surgery for hyperthyroidism or thyroid cancer.

8. Central Hypothyroidism

- **Encompasses:** Both secondary and tertiary hypothyroidism.
- **Cause:** Problems with the pituitary gland or hypothalamus.

9. Transient Hypothyroidism

- **Occurrence:** Temporary reduction in thyroid function.
- **Causes:** Conditions like thyroiditis (inflammation of the thyroid gland) or certain medications.

Conclusion

Each type of hypothyroidism has distinct causes and may require different approaches to diagnosis and treatment. Understanding the specific type is crucial for effective management. Primary hypothyroidism is the most common and is typically treated with thyroid hormone replacement therapy. Secondary and tertiary forms may require additional treatments to address the underlying pituitary or hypothalamic dysfunction.

What is Subclinical Hypothyroidism?

Subclinical hypothyroidism is a form of mild thyroid failure, characterized by elevated levels of Thyroid-Stimulating Hormone (TSH) with normal levels of the thyroid hormones thyroxine (T4) and triiodothyronine (T3). This condition indicates that the thyroid is beginning to struggle to maintain adequate hormone levels. Here are key points about subclinical hypothyroidism:

Characteristics

- **Laboratory Findings:** Normal thyroid hormone levels (T4 and T3) but elevated TSH levels.
- **Asymptomatic or Mild Symptoms:** Many individuals do not experience noticeable symptoms, or symptoms may be very subtle.

Causes

- Similar to overt hypothyroidism, including autoimmune thyroiditis (such as Hashimoto's thyroiditis), iodine deficiency, and effects of certain medications.
- Can also be a transient response to non-thyroidal illness, surgery, or medications.

Risk Factors

- More common in women, particularly older women.
- Risk increases with age.
- Family history of thyroid disease.
- Presence of autoimmune diseases.

Significance

- **Indicator of Early Thyroid Failure:** It may progress to overt hypothyroidism, where thyroid hormone levels fall below the normal range.
- **Cardiovascular Risk:** Some studies suggest a link between subclinical hypothyroidism and increased risk of heart disease, though this is still a subject of research.

Diagnosis

- **Blood Tests:** Diagnosis is based on blood tests measuring TSH and thyroid hormone levels.
- **Symptom Evaluation:** Although many individuals are asymptomatic, a careful review of subtle symptoms can be part of the evaluation.

Treatment

- **Controversial and Individualized:** Treatment decisions are based on factors like TSH levels, symptom presence, patient age, and risk factors for heart disease and osteoporosis.
- **Levothyroxine Therapy:** Some patients may benefit from low-dose levothyroxine therapy, especially if TSH is consistently elevated, or if there are symptoms suggestive of hypothyroidism.
- **Regular Monitoring:** Regular follow-up and monitoring of TSH levels are essential to determine if and when treatment should be started or adjusted.

Management

- **Lifestyle and Diet:** General health measures, including a balanced diet and regular exercise.
- **Monitoring for Progression:** Regular thyroid function tests to monitor for progression to overt hypothyroidism.

In conclusion, subclinical hypothyroidism is a mild form of thyroid dysfunction, often requiring careful monitoring and sometimes treatment, especially in cases with higher risks for progression or complications. The management and treatment are tailored to individual needs and risk factors.

What is Irritable bowel syndrome (IBS)?

Irritable Bowel Syndrome (IBS) is a common gastro-intestinal disorder characterized by a group of symptoms that typically occur together. These symptoms can vary in severity and duration from person to person, and the exact cause of IBS is not fully understood. Here is an overview:

Key Characteristics

- **Symptom Patterns:** IBS symptoms include abdominal pain, bloating, and changes in bowel habits - such as diarrhea, constipation, or alternating between the two.
- **Chronic Condition:** IBS is a long-term, chronic condition, but many individuals can manage symptoms through diet, lifestyle, and treatment.

Common Symptoms

- **Abdominal Pain and Cramping:** Often relieved by defecation.
- **Altered Bowel Habits:** Diarrhea (IBS-D), constipation (IBS-C), or a mix of both (IBS-M).
- **Bloating and Gas:** A feeling of fullness or swelling in the abdomen.
- **Food Intolerance:** Certain foods may trigger symptoms.
- **Fatigue and Difficulty Sleeping:** Not directly a bowel symptom but often reported.

Causes and Triggers

- **Muscle Contractions in the Intestine:** Abnormalities in intestinal muscle contractions can cause pain, diarrhea, or constipation.
- **Nervous System Abnormalities:** Poor coordination between the brain and the intestines can cause the body to overreact to normal digestive processes, resulting in pain, diarrhea, or constipation.
- **Severe Infection:** IBS can develop after a severe bout of diarrhea (gastroenteritis) caused by bacteria or a virus.
- **Changes in Gut Microbiota:** Variations in the bacteria in the gut may be a factor.
- **Food Sensitivities:** Certain foods can trigger IBS symptoms.
- **Stress:** While not a direct cause, stress can exacerbate symptoms.

Diagnosis

- **No Specific Test:** IBS is often diagnosed based on symptoms and by ruling out other conditions.
- **Criteria:** The Rome IV criteria are often used to diagnose IBS.
- **Tests:** Tests to rule out other conditions may include blood tests, stool tests, and colonoscopy.

Treatment

- **Dietary Changes:** Including high-fiber diet, gluten-free diet, or low FODMAP diet.
- **Medications:** Laxatives for constipation, antidiarrheal medications for diarrhea, antispasmodics for pain relief, and sometimes antidepressants.
- **Probiotics:** May help some people by changing the gut microbiota.
- **Stress Management:** Techniques like counseling, regular exercise, and meditation.

Management

- **Lifestyle Changes:** Regular exercise, improved sleep habits, and dietary modifications can help manage symptoms.
- **Patient Education:** Understanding the condition and recognizing triggers.

IBS is a complex and often frustrating condition, as symptoms can be unpredictable and impact quality of life. However, with appropriate management, many people with IBS find effective ways to reduce their symptoms and live comfortably.

What is migraine in general?

Migraine is a neurological condition characterized by intense, debilitating headaches, often accompanied by other symptoms. It is more than just a typical headache; migraines have specific features and can significantly impact the quality of life of those affected. Here is a general overview:

Characteristics of Migraine

- **Type of Pain:** Typically, the pain is throbbing or pulsating, and often one-sided (unilateral), but can affect both sides.
- **Intensity and Duration:** Migraine headaches are usually moderate to severe in intensity, lasting anywhere from 4 to 72 hours if untreated.
- **Frequency:** The frequency of attacks varies widely among individuals, ranging from several times a week to once every few months.

Common Symptoms

- **Headache Phase:** Intense throbbing or pulsing sensation, often on one side of the head.
- **Aura:** About one-third of people with migraine experience an 'aura' before the headache, which can include visual disturbances (like flashes of light, blind spots), sensory changes (such as tingling), or speech difficulties.
- **Other Associated Symptoms:** Nausea, vomiting, sensitivity to light (photophobia), sound (phonophobia), and sometimes smells (osmophobia).
- **Prodrome Phase:** Subtle changes that signal the onset of a migraine, such as mood changes, food cravings, neck stiffness, increased thirst and urination, and frequent yawning.
- **Postdrome Phase:** After the headache, a person may feel drained, confused, or exhausted for up to a day.

Triggers

- **Environmental and Lifestyle Factors:** These can include stress, changes in sleep patterns, certain foods and drinks, weather changes, bright or flashing lights, and hormonal changes in women.
- **Genetic Predisposition:** Migraine often runs in families, suggesting a genetic component.

Types of Migraine

- **Migraine Without Aura:** The most common type, not preceded by aura.
- **Migraine With Aura:** Preceded by visual or other sensory disturbances.
- **Chronic Migraine:** Defined as a headache occurring on 15 or more days a month for more than three months, of which at least eight days are with migraine.
- **Other Variants:** Including hemiplegic migraine (causing temporary paralysis on one side of the body) and retinal migraine (affecting vision in one eye).

Diagnosis

- **Clinical Diagnosis:** Based on medical history, symptoms, and by ruling out other causes.
- **Criteria:** Diagnosis typically follows the criteria set by the International Headache Society.

- **Tests:** There are no specific tests for migraine, but tests like MRI or CT scans may be used to rule out other conditions.

Treatment and Management

- **Acute Treatments:** Aim to stop or reduce the severity of a migraine attack. These include over-the-counter pain relievers and prescription medications like triptans.
- **Preventive Treatments:** Medications or therapies used regularly to reduce the frequency, severity, and length of migraines.
- **Lifestyle Adjustments:** Stress management, avoiding known triggers, maintaining a regular sleep schedule, and regular exercise.
- **Alternative Therapies:** Biofeedback, acupuncture, and cognitive-behavioral therapy can be helpful for some people.

Conclusion

Migraine is a complex and individual condition with varying presentations and requires a personalized approach to management and treatment. Understanding triggers and effective treatment strategies can significantly improve the quality of life for those living with migraines.

What is Treatment of migraine?

The treatment of migraine involves a combination of lifestyle modifications, acute (abortive) treatments to alleviate symptoms during an attack, and preventive (prophylactic) treatments to reduce the frequency and severity of migraines. The approach to treating migraine is tailored to the individual's specific needs, the frequency and severity of their migraines, and any other coexisting medical conditions. Here is an overview:

Acute Treatments

- **Pain Relievers:** Over-the-counter medications such as ibuprofen, aspirin, or acetaminophen can be effective for mild migraine attacks.
- **Triptans:** Prescription drugs like sumatriptan and rizatriptan, which are specifically designed for migraines. They work by constricting blood vessels and blocking pain pathways in the brain.
- **Ergots:** Ergotamine and caffeine combination drugs are less effective than triptans but can be helpful for some patients, especially those with prolonged migraine attacks.
- **Anti-Nausea Medications:** Often prescribed along with other migraine medications to relieve nausea and vomiting associated with migraines.
- **Ditans and Gepants:** Newer classes of drugs specifically for acute migraine treatment, useful especially for patients who cannot take triptans.

Preventive Treatments

- **Medication:** Daily preventive medications may be recommended for those who have frequent or severe migraines. These can include cardiovascular drugs (beta-blockers and calcium channel blockers), antidepressants, anti-seizure drugs, and CGRP (calcitonin gene-related peptide) monoclonal antibodies.
- **Onabotulinumtoxina (Botox) Injections:** Approved for the treatment of chronic migraines.
- **Lifestyle Modifications:** Regular exercise, adequate sleep, hydration, stress management, and avoiding known triggers.
- **Dietary Changes:** Identifying and avoiding foods that trigger migraines. Some people benefit from a diet that avoids chocolate, cheese, alcohol, and other known triggers.

Complementary and Alternative Medicine

- **Acupuncture:** Some patients find relief from migraine symptoms through acupuncture.
- **Biofeedback and Relaxation Techniques:** Stress-reduction strategies can be effective in preventing migraines.
- **Herbs and Supplements:** Magnesium, riboflavin (vitamin B2), and coenzyme Q10 have been shown to help prevent migraines in some people.

Lifestyle and Home Remedies

- **Regular Sleep Patterns:** Going to bed and waking up at the same time every day.
- **Hydration:** Drinking plenty of water to avoid dehydration, which can trigger migraines.
- **Exercise:** Regular aerobic exercise can reduce the frequency and intensity of migraines.

Treatment Plan

- **Individualized Approach:** The treatment plan should be tailored to the individual's migraine pattern, severity, and any other existing health conditions.
- **Regular Follow-up:** Regular follow-ups with a healthcare provider are important to assess the effectiveness of the treatment and make adjustments as necessary.

Conclusion

Effective migraine management often requires a multi-faceted approach, combining medical treatments with lifestyle changes and alternative therapies. It is important for individuals to work closely with their healthcare providers to develop a treatment plan that effectively manages their migraines.

What is Migraine vs headache?

Migraine and headache are often confused, but they are distinct conditions. Understanding the differences between them is important for effective treatment and management. Here is a comparison:

Headache

- **Definition:** A headache is a pain in any region of the head. Headaches may occur on one or both sides of the head, be isolated to a certain location, radiate across the head from one point, or have a viselike quality.
- **Types:** Includes tension headaches, cluster headaches, sinus headaches, and others.
- **Symptoms:** Usually characterized by a constant ache or pressure around the head, particularly at the temples or back of the head and neck. Not typically accompanied by other symptoms.
- **Causes:** Can be caused by a variety of factors, including stress, tension, dehydration, eye strain, or certain medical conditions.
- **Treatment:** Often treated with over-the-counter pain medications such as ibuprofen or acetaminophen. Lifestyle changes like stress management and hydration can also help.

Migraine

- **Definition:** Migraine is a neurological condition that can cause multiple symptoms. It is frequently characterized by intense, debilitating headaches.
- **Symptoms:** Symptoms may include nausea, vomiting, difficulty speaking, numbness or tingling, and sensitivity to light and sound. Migraines often have a pulsating, throbbing pain on one side of the head.
- **Phases:** Can have distinct phases, including prodrome, aura, attack, and postdrome.
    - o **Prodrome:** Subtle changes one or two days before the migraine.
    - o **Aura:** Visual or other sensory disturbances that precede or accompany the migraine.
    - o **Attack Phase:** Period of the actual migraine headache.
    - o **Postdrome:** After the attack, feeling drained or washed out.
- **Triggers:** Can be triggered by a variety of factors, including hormonal changes, certain foods and drinks, stress, and exercise.
- **Treatment:** Treatment is more complex and may include over-the-counter pain relief drugs, triptans, and preventive medications. Lifestyle adjustments and identifying triggers are key parts of management.

Key Differences

1. **Symptom Severity:** Migraines are typically more severe than a regular headache and can be debilitating.
2. **Associated Symptoms:** Migraines often come with symptoms like nausea, visual disturbances (aura), and sensitivity to light and sound, which are not usually present with a regular headache.
3. **Triggers and Causes:** Migraines have specific triggers, and the condition is often hereditary, whereas headaches can have a variety of everyday causes.
4. **Treatment and Management:** Migraine treatment is typically more specialized and may include prescription medication and lifestyle changes to avoid triggers.

In summary, while all migraines can be classified as headaches, not all headaches are migraines. Migraines are a specific type of headache with distinct features and require more targeted treatment. Understanding the type of headache is crucial for effective treatment and relief.

What is tension headache?

A tension headache is the most common type of headache, characterized by mild to moderate pain, tightness, or pressure around the forehead or back of the head and neck. Unlike migraines, tension headaches typically don't cause nausea, vomiting, or sensitivity to light and sound. They can be episodic or chronic and have various triggers and treatments:

Characteristics

- **Pain Quality:** Often described as a constant, dull ache on both sides of the head, a sensation of tightness or pressure across the forehead, or a feeling like a tight band around the head.

- **Location:** Usually occurs in the forehead, temples, back of the head, and neck.
- **Duration:** Can last from 30 minutes to several days. Episodic tension headaches occur less than 15 days per month, while chronic tension headaches occur more frequently.

Causes and Triggers

- **Stress:** The most common trigger.
- **Muscle Strain:** Often related to poor posture or tension in the muscles of the neck and scalp.
- **Eye Strain:** Due to prolonged computer use or inadequate lighting.
- **Fatigue:** Lack of sleep or irregular sleeping patterns.
- **Environmental Factors:** Such as noise or bright lights.
- **Diet and Lifestyle:** Skipping meals, dehydration, caffeine withdrawal, alcohol, and smoking can contribute.

Symptoms

- **Pain:** Generally mild to moderate, but can be intense.
- **Headache Type:** Usually a pressing or tightening, non-pulsating pain.
- **No Aura:** Unlike migraines, tension headaches do not have an aura phase.
- **No Severe Gastrointestinal Symptoms:** Rarely causes nausea or vomiting.

Diagnosis

- **Clinical Diagnosis:** Based on symptoms and medical history.
- **Ruling Out Other Causes:** Sometimes imaging tests are used to rule out other causes if the headache pattern changes or if symptoms are unusual.

Treatment

- **Over-the-Counter Pain Relievers:** Such as ibuprofen, aspirin, or acetaminophen.
- **Stress Management:** Techniques like meditation, relaxation training, or biofeedback.
- **Improving Posture:** Especially when working at a desk or computer.
- **Regular Exercise:** To relieve muscle tension.
- **Heat Therapy:** Applying a heat pack or warm cloth to the neck or back of the head.
- **Massage:** To relieve muscle tension.

Prevention

- **Lifestyle Adjustments:** Regular sleep, healthy eating habits, staying hydrated, and regular physical activity.
- **Ergonomics:** Proper posture and ergonomic adjustments in the workplace.
- **Stress Reduction:** Regular relaxation and stress management techniques.

Tension headaches, while generally not as debilitating as migraines, can significantly impact daily life, especially when chronic. Understanding and managing triggers, along with appropriate treatment, can greatly help in reducing their frequency and severity.

Who gets tension headaches?

Tension headaches are very common and can affect anyone, but certain factors may increase the likelihood of experiencing them:

Age and Gender

- **Adults and Adolescents:** Tension headaches are more commonly reported in adults and adolescents, though they can occur at any age.
- **More Common in Women:** Studies show that women are more likely than men to experience tension headaches.

Lifestyle Factors

- **Stress:** People with high levels of stress or those going through significant life changes are more prone to tension headaches.
- **Poor Posture:** Individuals with poor posture, especially when sitting for long periods (e.g., office workers, students), are at higher risk.
- **Sleep Issues:** Those with irregular sleep patterns, insomnia, or sleep disorders may experience more frequent tension headaches.
- **Eye Strain:** Prolonged computer use or extended periods of focusing on close tasks can lead to eye strain, a common trigger.
- **Diet and Hydration:** Skipping meals, dehydration, and certain dietary habits can play a role.

Medical and Psychological Factors

- **Muscle Strain:** Chronic neck or shoulder muscle strain, possibly due to injury or repetitive motion, can contribute.
- **Mental Health Conditions:** Anxiety and depression are associated with a higher incidence of tension headaches.
- **Other Headaches:** Individuals who experience migraines or other types of headaches may also be susceptible to tension headaches.

Environmental Factors

- **Workplace and Home Environment:** Poor ergonomics at work or home, bright lights, and loud noise can be triggers.
- **Weather Changes:** Some people report tension headaches during changes in weather or barometric pressure.

It is important to note that tension headaches are a common health issue and can affect anyone, regardless of their background or lifestyle. However, by identifying and managing potential triggers and risk factors, individuals can often reduce the frequency and severity of these headaches. Regular exercise, stress management techniques, maintaining good posture, ensuring proper hydration and nutrition, and having a regular sleep schedule are all beneficial practices in preventing tension headaches.

What are cluster headaches?

Cluster headaches are a rare but extremely painful type of headache that occurs in cyclical patterns or clusters. An intense burning or piercing pain behind or around one eye, often accompanied by other symptoms on the same side of the face, marks them. Here is an overview:

Characteristics

- **Severe Pain:** Typically described as sharp, penetrating, or burning. The pain is usually located around or behind one eye, but can radiate to other areas of the face, head, neck, and shoulders.
- **One-Sided:** The pain is almost always unilateral, affecting the same side of the head during a cluster period.
- **Short Duration but Frequent:** Attacks typically last between 15 minutes and 3 hours and can occur several times a day.
- **Cluster Periods:** These headaches occur in groups, or "clusters," often at the same time of day or night for several weeks or months, followed by remission periods when the headaches stop.
- **Sudden Onset:** They can begin quickly without warning, often at the same time each day.

Associated Symptoms

- **Restlessness:** Unlike migraine sufferers who prefer to lie down, those with cluster headaches are often restless.
- **Eye Symptoms:** Redness, watering, or swelling of the eye on the affected side.
- **Nasal Congestion:** Runny or stuffy nose on the affected side.
- **Facial Sweating:** Often on the affected side.
- **Horner Syndrome:** In some cases, symptoms like drooping eyelid (ptosis) and decreased pupil size (miosis) can occur on the affected side.
- **Sensitivity:** Some individuals experience sensitivity to light or sound, though these are less common than with migraines.

Triggers

- **Alcohol:** Especially during a cluster period.
- **Cigarette Smoking:** Many people with cluster headaches are smokers, though quitting smoking does not always improve the condition.
- **Histamine or Nitroglycerin:** Can trigger attacks in susceptible individuals.
- **Seasonal Changes:** Attacks can have a seasonal pattern.

Diagnosis

- **Clinical Assessment:** Based on the distinctive pattern and symptoms. There are no specific tests for cluster headaches.
- **Ruling Out Other Conditions:** Imaging tests like MRI can rule out other causes of the pain.

Treatment

- **Abortive Therapies:** High-flow oxygen therapy and sumatriptan injections are common and effective treatments to abort an attack.
- **Preventive Medications:** Verapamil, a calcium channel blocker, is often used. Corticosteroids and lithium are other options.
- **Nerve Block:** An occipital nerve block can provide temporary relief for some people.
- **Lifestyle Adjustments:** Avoiding alcohol and smoking, maintaining a regular sleep schedule, and managing stress.

Management

- **Rapid Treatment:** Due to the intensity and rapid onset of pain, fast-acting treatments are preferred.
- **Chronic Management:** In chronic cases, where remission periods are short or nonexistent, ongoing preventive medication may be necessary.
- **Supportive Care:** The extreme pain of cluster headaches can be distressing, and psychological support or counseling may be beneficial.

Conclusion

Cluster headaches, though not as common as other types of headaches, are among the most painful. Effective management often requires a combination of lifestyle changes, abortive treatments during attacks, and preventive strategies during cluster periods. Due to their intensity and potential impact on quality of life, it is important for individuals with cluster headaches to work closely with healthcare providers to develop an effective treatment plan.

What is the best treatment for acute cluster headaches?

The treatment of acute cluster headaches focuses on quickly relieving the intense pain that characterizes these attacks. Since cluster headaches come on suddenly and are of relatively short duration but extreme intensity, the effectiveness of treatment depends on how quickly it can provide relief. The most effective treatments are:

1. High-Flow Oxygen Therapy

- **How it is Administered:** Through a face mask at a flow rate of 7 to 15 liters per minute for 15 to 20 minutes.
- **Effectiveness:** It can provide significant relief within 15 minutes for many patients. This method is safe and can be repeated if necessary.

2. Triptans

- **Sumatriptan (Injection):** Subcutaneous sumatriptan injections are often the first line of pharmaceutical treatment. The injectable form is preferred over oral tablets due to its rapid onset of action.
- **Sumatriptan (Nasal Spray):** Can be effective and may be an alternative for those who do not wish to use injections.
- **Zolmitriptan (Nasal Spray):** Another effective option for some patients.

3. Dihydroergotamine (DHE)

- **Form:** Available as an injection or nasal spray.
- **Usage:** It can be effective, especially when other treatments fail, but it has more contraindications and side effects compared to triptans.

4. Local Anesthetics

- **Lidocaine (Nasal Spray):** An intranasal application of local anesthetic can be effective for some people.

5. Octreotide

- **Alternative:** For patients who cannot use triptans or oxygen, subcutaneous injections of the synthetic hormone octreotide might provide relief.

Considerations and Precautions

- **Rapid Administration:** Due to the rapid onset and severe pain of cluster headaches, treatments that act quickly are preferred.
- **Patient Preference and Medical History:** Choice of treatment may depend on the patient's medical history, comorbid conditions, and personal preferences.
- **Preventive Treatment:** While these treatments are for acute attacks, patients often need preventive treatments during a cluster period to reduce the frequency and severity of attacks.
- **Professional Guidance:** Patients should work closely with healthcare providers to choose the most appropriate and effective treatment.

It is important to note that while these treatments can be highly effective in managing acute cluster headache attacks, they may not work for everyone. Individual responses can vary, and it might take some trial and error to find the most effective treatment for a particular individual. Regular follow-up with a healthcare provider is essential to monitor the condition and adjust treatment as necessary.

Why Psychiatrists have a major role in headache treatment?

Psychiatrists can play a significant role in the treatment of headaches, particularly when these headaches are chronic or have a significant impact on the patient's mental health and quality of life. The connection between mental health and headaches, especially tension-type headaches and migraines, is well-established. Here are some reasons why psychiatrists are important in headache treatment:

1. **Comorbidity with Mental Health Disorders:** Headaches, particularly migraines, are often comorbid with mental health conditions such as depression, anxiety, and bipolar disorder.

Managing these psychiatric conditions can be crucial in the effective treatment of headaches.

2. **Stress and Psychological Factors:** Psychological factors, including stress, anxiety, and mood disorders, can trigger or worsen headaches. Psychiatrists are skilled in addressing these issues, which can be vital for headache management.

3. **Behavioral Treatment Approaches:** Techniques such as cognitive-behavioral therapy (CBT) can be effective in managing headaches. These approaches, often used by psychiatrists, help patients modify their pain perception, cope with stress, and alter behaviors that might trigger headaches.

4. **Medication Management:** Psychiatrists are experienced in prescribing medications that can treat both headaches and psychiatric conditions. For example, certain antidepressants and antiepileptic drugs are used in the prevention of migraines and also treat mood disorders.

5. **Biofeedback and Relaxation Techniques:** Psychiatrists or psychologists trained in these techniques can teach patients methods to control certain body responses related to stress and pain, which can be beneficial for headache sufferers.

6. **Chronic Pain Management:** For those with chronic headache conditions, psychiatrists can help in developing strategies for coping with chronic pain, which can include managing expectations, developing coping strategies, and addressing any related psychological issues.

7. **Holistic Approach:** Psychiatrists often take a holistic approach to patient care, which can be particularly beneficial in treating conditions like headaches that can be influenced by a wide range of physical, psychological, and environmental factors.

8. **Patient Education and Support:** Educating patients about the relationship between mental health and headaches, and providing support for lifestyle changes can be an important part of treatment.

In summary, the role of psychiatrists in headache treatment is multifaceted, addressing both the physical and psychological aspects of headache management. Their involvement can be particularly beneficial for patients who have not responded to conventional headache treatments or those whose headaches are significantly impacting their mental health and daily functioning.

What are Physical disorders mimicking mental disorders?

Various physical disorders can present symptoms that closely mimic those of mental disorders. This overlap can sometimes lead to misdiagnosis or delayed diagnosis of the underlying physical condition. It is crucial for healthcare providers to consider these possibilities, especially when mental health symptoms appear suddenly or without a clear psychological cause. Here are some examples:

1. **Thyroid Disorders:** Both hypothyroidism and hyperthyroidism can mimic symptoms of mental disorders. Hypothyroidism can present with symptoms similar to depression, such as fatigue, low mood, and cognitive slowing. Hyperthyroidism may mimic anxiety disorders, with symptoms like nervousness, irritability, and sleep disturbances.

2. **Neurological Disorders:** Conditions such as epilepsy, brain tumors, multiple sclerosis, and Parkinson's disease can sometimes present with symptoms resembling psychiatric disorders, including mood swings, cognitive changes, and hallucinations.

3. **Vitamin Deficiencies:** Deficiencies in certain vitamins, such as B12, D, and folate, can lead to symptoms of depression, anxiety, and cognitive impairment.

4. **Endocrine Disorders:** Disorders such as Cushing's disease (caused by high cortisol levels) and Addison's disease (characterized by low levels of cortisol and aldosterone) can cause symptoms like fatigue, mood swings, and depression.

5. **Chronic Fatigue Syndrome:** Characterized by extreme fatigue, this syndrome can also involve cognitive impairments and mood disturbances, which can be mistaken for a psychiatric disorder.

6. **Fibromyalgia:** This chronic pain disorder is often associated with symptoms such as fatigue, sleep disturbances, and cognitive difficulties, which can overlap with those of depression and anxiety disorders.

7. **Lyme Disease:** Chronic Lyme disease can lead to neurological and cognitive issues, including memory problems, mood swings, and fatigue, which can mimic mental health disorders.

8. **Cardiac Arrhythmias:** Some heart rhythm disorders can cause symptoms like palpitations, shortness of breath, and dizziness, which might be mistaken for panic attacks.
9. **Hormonal Imbalances:** Fluctuations in hormones, particularly during periods like menopause or postpartum, can cause mood swings, anxiety, and depression-like symptoms.
10. **Sleep Disorders:** Conditions such as obstructive sleep apnea and insomnia can lead to symptoms of fatigue, cognitive impairment, and mood disturbances, mimicking conditions like depression and anxiety.

Importance of Comprehensive Evaluation

Given the potential for overlap, a thorough medical evaluation including detailed history, physical examination, and appropriate laboratory tests is essential when mental disorder symptoms are present. This helps ensure accurate diagnosis and treatment, addressing both physical and mental health needs of the patient. Collaboration between medical and mental health professionals is often key in these cases, ensuring a holistic approach to patient care.

What is faith healing?

Faith healing refers to the practice of prayer and gestures (such as laying on of hands) that are believed by some to elicit divine intervention in physical and spiritual healing. It is often associated with religious belief, where faith is placed in a higher power to heal illness and improve health conditions. Here is a more detailed overview:

Characteristics

- **Based on Belief and Spirituality:** Central to faith healing is the belief in a higher power or divine force that can intervene in human suffering and illness.
- **Practices:** Can include prayer, anointing with oil, laying on of hands, or participation in religious rituals.
- **Diverse Traditions:** Present in various forms across different religions and cultures.

Religious Context

- **Christianity:** Some Christian denominations practice faith healing, with instances reported in Pentecostal and Charismatic movements.
- **Other Religions:** Similar concepts of spiritual healing are found in many other religious traditions worldwide.

Controversies and Criticisms

- **Lack of Scientific Evidence:** The effectiveness of faith healing has not been proven in controlled scientific studies, and it remains a controversial topic.
- **Risk of Medical Neglect:** Concerns arise when individuals rely solely on faith healing, avoiding or delaying conventional medical treatment for serious conditions.
- **Ethical and Legal Issues:** Particularly in cases involving minors, where parents may refuse medical treatment for their children in favor of faith healing.

Psychological Aspects

- **Placebo Effect:** Some argue that faith healing can induce a placebo effect, where the belief in treatment can bring about real changes in health.
- **Mental and Emotional Support:** For believers, faith healing can offer comfort, community support, and a sense of hope.

Integration with Conventional Medicine

- **Holistic Approach:** Some advocate for integrating faith healing with conventional medical treatments, respecting the patient's cultural and religious beliefs while ensuring they receive appropriate medical care.

Conclusion

Faith healing is a complex and multifaceted practice deeply rooted in religious and cultural beliefs. While it plays a significant role in the lives of many individuals, it is important to balance these practices with evidence-based medical care, especially in cases of serious illness. The integration of spiritual care with conventional medicine can be a valuable approach in holistic patient care, acknowledging the importance of spiritual and emotional well-being in overall health.

What to do for tardive dyskinesia?

Tardive dyskinesia (TD) is a side effect that can occur with long-term use of antipsychotic medications and certain other drugs. Involuntary, repetitive movements that can include grimacing, tongue movements, lip smacking, puckering, and pursing of the lips, or rapid eye blinking characterize it. Managing TD involves several steps:

1. Consult a Healthcare Professional

- **Medication Review:** Discuss all current medications with a doctor, as TD is often related to certain medications, particularly older antipsychotics.

- **Diagnosis:** It is important to get a proper diagnosis to rule out other conditions that may have similar symptoms.

2. Adjust Medication

- **Reduce or Discontinue:** The doctor may suggest lowering the dose or discontinuing the causative medication. However, this should only be done under medical supervision, as abrupt changes can worsen symptoms or cause other complications.
- **Switch Medications:** In some cases, switching to a different type of antipsychotic or medication can help.

3. Medications for Tardive Dyskinesia

- **VMAT2 Inhibitors:** Medications like valbenazine (Ingrezza) and deutetrabenazine (Austedo) are approved by the FDA specifically for treating TD and can be effective in reducing symptoms.
- **Other Treatments:** Some anticholinergic medications, benzodiazepines, or botulinum toxin injections may be used in specific cases.

4. Supportive Therapies

- **Physical Therapy:** Can help manage symptoms and improve voluntary muscle control.
- **Speech Therapy:** If speech or swallowing is affected.
- **Occupational Therapy:** To assist with daily activities that may be affected by TD.

5. Lifestyle Modifications

- **Exercise:** Regular physical activity can improve overall well-being and help in managing symptoms.
- **Stress Management:** Techniques like meditation, deep breathing, or yoga can be beneficial.

6. Regular Monitoring

- **Follow-up Appointments:** Regular check-ups are important to monitor the condition and adjust treatment plans as needed.

7. Education and Support

- **Understanding the Condition:** Educate yourself about TD, its symptoms, and treatment options.
- **Support Groups:** Joining a support group can provide emotional support and coping strategies.

Conclusion

Managing tardive dyskinesia is a collaborative process that involves careful medication management, supportive therapies, and lifestyle adjustments. It is crucial to work closely with healthcare providers to find the most effective treatment plan and to regularly monitor the condition for any changes or improvements. Remember, changes in medication should always be done under medical supervision.

What to do for benzodiazepine addiction?

Benzodiazepine addiction is a serious condition that requires a comprehensive treatment approach. Benzodiazepines, commonly prescribed for anxiety, insomnia, and other conditions, can be highly addictive, especially with long-term use or misuse. Here is a guide on what to do if you or someone you know is struggling with benzodiazepine addiction:

1. Seek Professional Help

- **Consult a Healthcare Professional:** The first step is to talk to a doctor or addiction specialist who can assess the situation and recommend a treatment plan.
- **Addiction Specialist or Psychiatrist:** They can provide specialized care for addiction and any underlying mental health conditions.

2. Tapering Off Medication

- **Gradual Reduction:** Abruptly stopping benzodiazepines can be dangerous. A doctor will typically recommend a gradual tapering off schedule to safely reduce dependency.
- **Medical Supervision:** This process should always be done under medical supervision to manage withdrawal symptoms and complications.

3. Treatment Programs

- **Inpatient Treatment:** For severe addiction, inpatient programs can provide intensive care and monitoring.
- **Outpatient Treatment:** Allows individuals to live at home while attending treatment sessions. This can include therapy, counseling, and medical check-ups.

4. Therapy and Counseling

- **Cognitive Behavioral Therapy (CBT):** Effective in treating addiction and any co-occurring anxiety or depression.
- **Group Therapy:** Offers support from others who are facing similar challenges.
- **Family Therapy:** Can help improve family dynamics and support systems.

5. Support Groups

- 12-Step Programs like Narcotics Anonymous (NA) or non-12-step groups can provide community support and ongoing encouragement.

6. Addressing Underlying Issues

- **Mental Health Treatment:** If the benzodiazepines were initially prescribed for an anxiety disorder or other mental health issue, alternative treatments should be explored.
- **Lifestyle Changes:** Stress management, regular exercise, and a healthy diet can improve overall well-being and aid recovery.

7. Relapse Prevention

- **Education:** Understanding the nature of addiction and triggers for relapse.
- **Ongoing Support:** Regular follow-up with healthcare providers and continued participation in therapy or support groups.

8. Self-Care

- **Mindfulness and Relaxation Techniques:** Practices like meditation, yoga, and deep breathing can help manage stress and anxiety without medication.

9. Legal and Ethical Considerations

- **Prescription Management:** Working with a doctor to ensure responsible use of medications in the future.

Conclusion

Recovering from benzodiazepine addiction is a challenging but achievable goal. It requires a commitment to a comprehensive treatment plan and often involves a combination of medical supervision, therapy, lifestyle changes, and support. Patience and perseverance are key, as recovery can be a gradual process. It is also crucial to maintain open communication with healthcare providers and to build a strong support network of family, friends, and support groups.

What is schizophrenia in general?

Schizophrenia is a chronic and severe mental health disorder that affects a person's thinking, feeling, and behavior. It is characterized by a range of psychological symptoms, which can be divided into positive, negative, and cognitive symptoms. Schizophrenia is often misunderstood, and it is important to note that it is a complex condition with varying presentations and degrees of severity.

Key Characteristics

1. **Positive Symptoms:** Represent a distortion of normal functions. These include:
   - **Hallucinations:** Seeing, hearing, or feeling things that are not there, with auditory hallucinations (hearing voices) being the most common.
   - **Delusions:** False beliefs that are not based in reality, such as believing that one is being persecuted or monitored, or that they have extraordinary powers or identity.
   - **Disorganized Thinking and Speech:** Including incoherence or irrelevant responses during conversation.
   - **Disorganized or Abnormal Motor Behavior:** This can range from childlike silliness to unpredictable agitation.
2. **Negative Symptoms:** Represent a reduction or loss of normal functions. These include:
   - **Reduced Emotional Expression:** A lack of facial expressions, eye contact, and changes in voice tone.
   - **Avolition:** Decreased motivation to initiate and perform purposeful activities.
   - **Anhedonia:** Inability to experience pleasure from activities usually found enjoyable.
   - **Alogia:** Reduced speech output.
3. **Cognitive Symptoms:** These involve problems with thought processes. These include:
   - **Poor Executive Functioning:** Difficulty in understanding information and using it to make decisions.
   - **Trouble Focusing or Paying Attention.**
   - **Memory Problems:** Particularly with working memory.

Causes

The exact cause of schizophrenia is not known, but it is believed to be a combination of genetics, brain chemistry, and environment. Risk factors include a family history of schizophrenia, certain prenatal factors (like exposure to viruses or malnutrition in the womb), and psychosocial factors.

Onset

Symptoms typically manifest in late adolescence to early adulthood, although they can start at any age. It is more common in men.

Diagnosis

Diagnosis is based on observed behavior, reported experiences, and, in some cases, brain imaging or blood tests to rule out other conditions.

Treatment

Treatment typically involves antipsychotic medications and psychotherapy, such as cognitive-behavioral therapy or supportive therapy. Treatment plans are often long-term and may include social rehabilitation and support services.

Living with Schizophrenia

With proper treatment, many people with schizophrenia can lead fulfilling and productive lives. It is crucial for individuals with schizophrenia to have access to comprehensive medical care, social support, and rehabilitation services. Stigma and misunderstanding about schizophrenia remain significant barriers to both diagnosis and treatment, underscoring the need for public education and support for those affected by the disorder and their families.

What is prevalence of schizophrenia?

The prevalence of schizophrenia, which refers to how common the disorder is within a population at a given time, is relatively consistent worldwide. Here are some key points regarding its prevalence:

1. **Global Prevalence:** Schizophrenia affects about 0.5% to 1% of the global population. This percentage translates to approximately 20 to 40 million people worldwide, though the exact number can vary.
2. **Gender Differences:** Schizophrenia occurs at similar rates in men and women, although the age of onset often differs. Men typically show symptoms in their late teens to early 20s, while women often develop the disorder in their late 20s to early 30s.
3. **Geographical Variation:** The prevalence of schizophrenia is fairly uniform across different countries and cultures, suggesting that genetic and biological factors play a significant role in its development.
4. **Onset Age:** Schizophrenia usually first presents in late adolescence to early adulthood, but it can begin at any age. The onset tends to be earlier in men than in women.
5. **Chronicity:** Schizophrenia is a chronic condition, and its prevalence at any given time reflects both new cases and those who have been living with the condition, sometimes for many years.
6. **Impact of Socioeconomic Factors:** While schizophrenia affects all socioeconomic groups, its prevalence is higher in populations facing poverty, social disadvantage, or in urban environments. This correlation may reflect both the stress of living in such environments and barriers to accessing mental health care.
7. **Lifetime Risk:** The lifetime risk of developing schizophrenia is generally estimated at around 1%, meaning that about 1 in 100 people will develop schizophrenia at some point in their life.

Understanding the prevalence of schizophrenia is important for public health planning and resource allocation. It is a complex disorder with significant implications for affected individuals, their families, and society, requiring adequate healthcare services and support systems.

What are the issues in treatment of schizophrenia?

The treatment of schizophrenia presents several challenges and issues, largely due to the complexity and variability of the disorder. Here are some key issues that are often encountered in the treatment of schizophrenia:

1. **Adherence to Medication:** One of the biggest challenges is ensuring patients adhere to their prescribed medication regimen. Non-adherence can be due to factors like side effects, lack of insight into the illness, forgetfulness, or misunderstanding the need for continuous treatment.
2. **Side Effects of Antipsychotic Medications:** Many antipsychotic drugs, especially older ones, can have significant side effects, such as weight gain, diabetes, movement disorders (like tardive dyskinesia), and sedation. These side effects can impact a patient's willingness to continue medication.
3. **Access to Healthcare:** There can be barriers to accessing quality mental health care, including a shortage of mental health professionals, socioeconomic barriers, and stigma associated with mental illness.
4. **Comorbid Conditions:** Patients with schizophrenia often have comorbid conditions, including substance abuse disorders, depression, and anxiety, which can complicate treatment.
5. **Cognitive Impairment:** Schizophrenia is often accompanied by cognitive deficits that can affect memory, attention, and executive functioning.

These impairments can make it difficult for patients to manage their treatment and adhere to medication schedules.

6. **Psychotherapy Challenges:** Engaging patients in psychotherapy can be challenging, particularly those with severe symptoms, such as paranoia or severe cognitive deficits.

7. **Early Intervention:** Early diagnosis and treatment of schizophrenia can greatly improve long-term outcomes, but early symptoms can be subtle and easily missed.

8. **Holistic and Long-term Care:** Effective treatment of schizophrenia requires a holistic approach that addresses not only the symptoms but also the social, occupational, and educational needs of the individual. Long-term care planning is essential but can be challenging to implement.

9. **Social Stigma:** Stigma surrounding schizophrenia can affect patients' willingness to seek and adhere to treatment and can impact the support they receive from the community and healthcare systems.

10. **Lack of Resources and Support:** There is often a lack of necessary resources and support systems for individuals with schizophrenia, including housing, employment assistance, and community-based programs.

11. **Treatment Resistance:** Some patients may be resistant to standard antipsychotic medications, requiring alternative treatment strategies.

Addressing these issues requires a coordinated effort among healthcare providers, patients, families, and support systems. It involves not only the management of symptoms through medication and therapy but also providing comprehensive support services to address the various challenges faced by individuals with schizophrenia.

What is rehabilitation in schizophrenia?

Rehabilitation in schizophrenia is an integral part of the management and treatment plan for individuals living with the condition. It encompasses a range of strategies and services aimed at helping patients lead more productive and fulfilling lives. Rehabilitation goes beyond the treatment of symptoms and focuses on the improvement of functioning and quality of life. Here is an overview:

Goals of Rehabilitation

- **Social Skills Training:** Improving interpersonal communication and social interactions.
- **Vocational Rehabilitation:** Assisting with job training and employment opportunities.
- **Educational Support:** Helping patients continue or return to their educational pursuits.
- **Living Skills:** Assisting in developing skills for daily living, such as cooking, budgeting, and personal hygiene.
- **Community Integration:** Encouraging and facilitating participation in community activities.

Components of Rehabilitation

1. **Psychosocial Rehabilitation:** Focuses on improving patients' social functioning and helping them integrate into their communities. This can include group therapy, social skills training, and community-based activities.

2. **Cognitive Remediation:** Designed to improve cognitive functions such as memory, attention, and problem-solving skills, which are often affected in schizophrenia.

3. **Supported Employment/Education Programs:** These programs help individuals with schizophrenia find and maintain employment or continue their education, providing necessary support and accommodations.

4. **Family Education and Support:** Involves educating family members about schizophrenia and providing them with skills and support to better assist their loved ones.

5. **Peer Support and Self-Help Groups:** Facilitates connections with others who have similar experiences, offering mutual support and sharing of coping strategies.

6. **Case Management:** Case managers can help coordinate various aspects of care, including medical, social, and vocational services.

7. **Housing Support:** Assistance in finding and maintaining stable housing, which is crucial for overall well-being.

8. **Life Skills Training:** Focusing on developing skills necessary for independent living.

Challenges in Rehabilitation

- **Stigma and Discrimination:** Can hinder the reintegration of individuals with schizophrenia into society.

- **Resource Availability:** Access to comprehensive rehabilitation services can be limited, especially in under-resourced areas.
- **Individualization of Care:** Rehabilitation plans need to be tailored to each individual's needs, preferences, and level of illness.

Conclusion

Rehabilitation in schizophrenia is about empowering individuals to live as independently as possible and achieve their personal goals. It is a multidimensional approach that requires the collaboration of healthcare providers, patients, families, and community services. Effective rehabilitation can significantly improve the quality of life for people with schizophrenia, helping them to lead more satisfying and autonomous lives.

When to hospitalise in schizophrenia?

Hospitalization in schizophrenia is typically considered under specific circumstances, particularly when there is an immediate risk to the safety of the patient or others, or when the symptoms are so severe that outpatient care is insufficient. Here are some common situations when hospitalization might be necessary:

1. Risk of Harm

- **Suicidal Ideation or Attempts:** If the patient expresses thoughts of harming themselves or has attempted suicide.
- **Homicidal Ideation:** Thoughts or plans to harm others.
- **Severe Self-Neglect:** Inability to care for oneself, leading to serious health risks.

2. Severe Psychotic Symptoms

- **Acute Psychosis:** Experiencing severe hallucinations or delusions that significantly impair reality testing and lead to dangerous behaviors.
- **Extreme Paranoia:** Which might result in aggressive or defensive behaviors.

3. Inability to Care for Self

- **Lack of Basic Self-Care:** When a patient is unable to attend to basic needs like eating, hygiene, or taking medication.
- **Inability to Communicate Needs:** If the patient is unable to communicate effectively, either due to severe disorganization in thinking or due to being mute.

4. Severe Deterioration of Mental Status

- **Rapid Decline in Functioning:** Marked worsening of symptoms or sudden behavioral changes.
- **Catatonia:** Severe catatonic symptoms, such as immobility or excessive, pointless motor activity, which can be dangerous.

5. Medication Management

- **Adjustment of Medication:** In cases where medication needs to be adjusted or monitored closely due to severe side effects or ineffectiveness.
- **Non-compliance with Medication:** When a patient is unable or unwilling to take medication as prescribed, and it is leading to a significant deterioration in their condition.

6. Lack of Support at Home

- **Inadequate Support System:** If the patient's living situation does not provide the support necessary to manage their condition safely.
- **Caregiver Burnout:** When the stress of caregiving impacts the ability of caregivers to provide necessary support.

7. Legal Reasons

- **Involuntary Commitment:** In some cases, legal criteria may be met for involuntary commitment if the individual poses a danger to themselves or others and refuses voluntary treatment.

Making the Decision

- **Assessment by Professionals:** mental health professionals based on a comprehensive assessment of the patient's condition generally make Decisions about hospitalization.
- **Involvement of Family and Caregivers:** The patient's family and caregivers are often involved in the decision-making process, providing valuable insight into the patient's recent behavior and functioning.

Conclusion

Hospitalization in schizophrenia is a significant step, typically reserved for situations where more intensive treatment is required than can be provided on an outpatient basis. The goal is to stabilize the patient's condition, ensure safety, and make necessary adjustments in treatment. After stabilization, the focus shifts to establishing a viable plan for continued treatment and support post-discharge, which may include adjustments in medication, ongoing therapy, and community-based services to support reintegration and continued recovery.

How to interpret violence among mentally ill patients?

Interpreting violence among individuals with mental illness requires a nuanced understanding of the complex interplay between mental health conditions and violent behavior. It is a sensitive area that involves addressing misconceptions, recognizing risk factors, and providing appropriate interventions. Here are key points to consider:

1. Challenge Myths and Stereotypes

- **Not All Mentally Ill Individuals are Violent:** Most people with mental illness are not violent. It is crucial to challenge the stereotype that equates mental illness with a propensity for violence.
- **Media Representation:** Media often disproportionately represents mentally ill individuals as violent, which can perpetuate stigma and misunderstanding.

2. Understand the Risk Factors

- **Certain Conditions:** Some severe mental health conditions, such as certain types of schizophrenia, bipolar disorder during manic phases, and severe depression, might have a slightly increased risk of associated violent behavior.
- **Comorbidity with Substance Abuse:** Substance abuse significantly increases the risk of violent behavior in individuals with and without mental illness.
- **History of Violence:** Past violent behavior is a strong predictor of future violence, regardless of mental illness.
- **Situational Factors:** Environmental stressors, lack of social support, and victimization can increase the risk of violent behavior.

3. Look Beyond Mental Illness

- **Contextual Factors:** It is important to consider the individual's environment, stressors, and history, rather than attributing violent behavior solely to mental illness.
- **Personal History:** Experiences of trauma, abuse, or neglect can be relevant factors.

4. Assessing Threats of Violence

- **Professional Evaluation:** Mental health professionals should assess threats of violence, taking into account the individual's history, current symptoms, and situational factors.
- **Risk Assessment Tools:** Structured tools can assist in evaluating the likelihood of violent behavior.

5. Effective Intervention Strategies

- **Treatment Compliance:** Ensuring adherence to psychiatric treatment and medications can help in managing symptoms that might be related to aggression.
- **Addressing Comorbid Conditions:** Treating substance abuse and other comorbid conditions is crucial.
- **Therapeutic Approaches:** Anger management, cognitive behavioral therapy, and other therapeutic strategies can be effective.

6. Provide Support and Education

- **Family and Community Education:** Educating family members and the community about mental illness and violence can help reduce stigma and misunderstanding.
- **Support Systems:** Strong support networks, including family, healthcare providers, and community resources, can play a significant role in prevention.

Conclusion

Interpreting violence in mentally ill patients requires a careful, individualized approach. It is important to balance public safety concerns with compassionate care and to avoid broad generalizations that stigmatize mental illness. Most importantly, effective treatment and support for mental health conditions are key in reducing the risk of violence and helping individuals lead stable, productive lives.

What is substance-induced mood disorder (SIMD)?

Substance-Induced Mood Disorder (SIMD) is a mental health condition characterized by mood disturbances that are directly caused by the effects of substances such as drugs, medications, or toxins. This disorder can present as a major depressive episode, a manic episode, a mixed episode, or a hypomanic episode, and is directly related to the intake, use, or withdrawal of various substances.

Key Features of SIMD

1. **Mood Disturbance:** The individual experiences significant depression, elevated, expansive, or irritable mood that is atypical for them and directly related to substance use.
2. **Substance Link:** The mood disorder is a direct consequence of substance use. This can be due to:

- **Intoxication:** Mood symptoms that occur during or shortly after direct use of the substance.
- **Withdrawal:** Mood symptoms that occur in response to the cessation or reduction in heavy and prolonged substance use.

3. **Types of Substances Involved:**
   - **Alcohol:** Can cause depressive or manic symptoms.
   - **Prescription Medications:** Such as corticosteroids, hormonal medications, and certain antihypertensive drugs.
   - **Illicit Drugs:** Including stimulants (like cocaine and amphetamines), hallucinogens, and opioids.
   - **Toxins:** Exposure to certain toxins and heavy metals can also lead to mood disturbances.

Symptoms

- **Depressive Symptoms:** Sadness, hopelessness, loss of interest in activities, changes in appetite, sleep disturbances, fatigue, and in severe cases, suicidal thoughts.
- **Manic Symptoms:** Elevated or irritable mood, grandiosity, decreased need for sleep, talkativeness, racing thoughts, distractibility, increased goal-directed activity, and excessive involvement in risky behaviors.

Diagnosis

- **Exclusion of Primary Mood Disorder:** It is important to distinguish SIMD from primary mood disorders. The key is the timing of substance use and the onset of symptoms.
- **History and Evaluation:** A thorough history of substance use, medical history, and psychiatric evaluation is essential.

Treatment

- **Substance Cessation:** The first step in treatment is typically to stop the use of the causative substance.
- **Symptomatic Treatment:** Address the mood symptoms, which might involve the use of medication and psychotherapy, depending on the severity and nature of the symptoms.
- **Detoxification and Rehabilitation:** For substance abuse issues, detoxification under medical supervision followed by rehabilitation may be necessary.
- **Addressing Underlying Issues:** It is important to treat any underlying psychiatric conditions and to provide support for issues related to substance abuse, such as stress, trauma, or social problems.

Prognosis

- The prognosis of SIMD is generally favorable if the substance use disorder is effectively treated and the individual avoids further substance abuse. Mood symptoms often improve significantly with abstinence, though some individuals may require ongoing treatment for mood stabilization.

Prevention

- Educating patients about the potential mood-altering effects of certain substances and medications can help in prevention. Additionally, regular monitoring of patients who are prescribed potentially mood-altering medications can enable early detection and intervention.

In conclusion, Substance-Induced Mood Disorder is a significant mental health condition that requires comprehensive treatment addressing both the mood disorder and the substance use issue. Early intervention and integrated treatment approaches are key to effective management and recovery.

What is the most common substance induced mood disorder?

The most common Substance-Induced Mood Disorder (SIMD) typically results from substances that are widely used and have significant mood-altering effects. The prevalence of a specific SIMD often reflects the prevalence of use of the substance itself in the general population. Among the various substances that can induce mood disorders, the following are commonly implicated:

1. **Alcohol:** Alcohol-Induced Mood Disorder is one of the most common forms of SIMD. Alcohol is a central nervous system depressant and can lead to depressive symptoms during intoxication and withdrawal. Chronic alcohol use is particularly associated with an increased risk of depression.
2. **Stimulants:** Including cocaine and amphetamines. These substances can induce manic-like symptoms during intoxication and depressive symptoms during withdrawal. Stimulant-induced mood disorders are often characterized by significant mood swings corresponding to the cycle of use and abstinence.
3. **Cannabis:** While traditionally thought to be less likely to cause mood disorders, emerging evidence

suggests that heavy and prolonged cannabis use, especially with high potency strains, can be associated with mood disturbances.

4. **Opioids:** Long-term use of opioids, including prescription pain relievers and heroin, can lead to depressive symptoms, particularly during withdrawal.

5. **Benzodiazepines:** Chronic use and withdrawal from benzodiazepines (commonly prescribed for anxiety and insomnia) can cause significant mood disturbances, including depressive symptoms.

6. **Prescription Medications:** Certain prescription medications, such as corticosteroids, can induce mood symptoms, particularly manic or hypomanic episodes.

It is important to note that while these substances are commonly associated with mood disorders, the development of SIMD depends on various factors, including the amount and duration of substance use, individual vulnerability, and the presence of co-occurring psychiatric disorders. The diagnosis and treatment of SIMD require a comprehensive approach that addresses both the mood disorder and the underlying substance use issue.

How long will the effects of SIMD last?

The duration of the effects of a Substance-Induced Mood Disorder (SIMD) can vary widely depending on several factors. These include the type of substance involved, the duration and amount of substance use, individual susceptibility, and whether there are co-occurring mental health disorders. Here is a general overview:

1. During Intoxication or Withdrawal

- **Short-Term Effects:** For many substances, mood disturbance symptoms may manifest during periods of acute intoxication or withdrawal. In these cases, symptoms often resolve within days to a few weeks after the substance is metabolized and cleared from the body.

- **Withdrawal Period:** For substances with withdrawal syndromes (such as alcohol, opioids, and benzodiazepines), mood symptoms can be particularly pronounced and may last for days to weeks after cessation of use.

2. Chronic Use

- **Longer Duration:** In cases of prolonged or chronic use, especially with substances like alcohol or prescription medications, mood disturbances may last longer, even after the substance is discontinued.

- **Neurochemical Changes:** Chronic substance use can lead to changes in brain chemistry that might prolong mood symptoms, even after cessation of use.

3. Individual Factors

- **Metabolism and Health:** Individual differences in metabolism and overall physical health can affect how quickly a substance and its effects are cleared from the body.

- **Psychological and Environmental Factors:** Pre-existing mental health conditions, psychological resilience, and environmental stressors can also influence the duration and severity of SIMD.

4. Persistent Effects in Some Cases

- **Prolonged Recovery:** In some cases, particularly where there has been long-term heavy use of the substance, recovery from SIMD may take months, and there may be a need for ongoing treatment and support.

5. Post-Acute Withdrawal Syndrome (PAWS)

- **Extended Symptoms:** Some individuals may experience PAWS, where mood and other symptoms persist or recur for several months or even longer after stopping substance use.

6. Treatment and Support

- **Psychiatric and Psychological Support:** Ongoing psychiatric care, therapy, and support groups can be crucial in managing prolonged symptoms and facilitating recovery.

- **Medication Management:** In some cases, medications may be used to manage persistent mood symptoms or to treat underlying or co-occurring mental health disorders.

Conclusion

The duration of SIMD effects is highly individual and depends on a complex interplay of factors. In many cases, symptoms resolve with the cessation of substance use and appropriate treatment, but some individuals may experience longer-lasting effects that require extended care. Early intervention and comprehensive treatment are key to improving outcomes in SIMD.

How can I take care of myself from SIMD?

Taking care of yourself when dealing with a substance-induced mood disorder involves a multifaceted approach, focusing on both physical and mental health. It's important to consult healthcare professionals for personalized advice, but here are some general guidelines:

1. **Seek Professional Help:** Consult a mental health professional or a healthcare provider specializing in addiction and mood disorders. They can provide a diagnosis, treatment options, and ongoing support.
2. **Substance Abuse Treatment:** If substance use is ongoing, consider undergoing detoxification and rehabilitation programs. These programs help in managing withdrawal symptoms and reducing the risk of relapse.
3. **Therapy and Counseling:** Psychotherapy, such as Cognitive Behavioral Therapy (CBT), can be effective. It helps in identifying and changing negative thought patterns and behaviors associated with substance use.
4. **Medication Management:** If prescribed, take medications as directed by your healthcare provider. This may include mood stabilizers, antidepressants, or medications for substance abuse treatment.
5. **Support Groups:** Participating in support groups like Alcoholics Anonymous (AA) or Narcotics Anonymous (NA) can provide peer support and coping strategies.
6. **Healthy Lifestyle Choices:** Adopting a healthy diet, regular physical activity, and adequate sleep can improve mood and overall well-being.
7. **Stress Management Techniques:** Techniques such as mindfulness, meditation, yoga, and deep breathing exercises can help in managing stress and emotional upheaval.
8. **Avoid Triggers:** Identify and avoid situations, places, or people that trigger the urge to use substances.
9. **Build a Support Network:** Maintain close connections with family and friends who support your recovery. Having a strong support system is crucial.
10. **Continued Monitoring and Follow-up:** Regular follow-up with healthcare providers is important for monitoring progress and addressing any challenges promptly.

Remember, recovery is a journey, and it's okay to seek help and support along the way. Each person's path to recovery is unique, so it's important to find what works best for you.

What is chronic pain?

Chronic pain is a complex medical condition characterized by persistent pain that lasts for weeks, months, or even years beyond the usual recovery period of an injury or illness, or pain associated with a chronic health condition. Unlike acute pain, which is a normal sensation triggered in the nervous system to alert you to possible injury and the need to take care of yourself, chronic pain is different. Here are some key aspects of chronic pain:

1. **Duration:** Chronic pain is defined as pain that lasts for 12 weeks or longer, even after the injury or illness that caused the initial pain has healed or gone away.
2. **Causes:** It can be caused by a variety of conditions, including chronic diseases (like arthritis or diabetes), injuries that have not healed properly, nerve damage, fibromyalgia, migraines, and many others. In some cases, the exact cause of chronic pain is unknown.
3. **Impact on Quality of Life:** It can significantly impact a person's quality of life, leading to decreased mobility, reduced flexibility, strength, and endurance, which can make it difficult to carry out daily activities and enjoy life.
4. **Psychological Effects:** Chronic pain is often associated with psychological effects, such as depression, anxiety, and changes in mood. The constant discomfort can affect sleep, energy levels, and mental health.
5. **Treatment:** Managing chronic pain often requires a multidisciplinary approach. This can include medication, physical therapy, psychological counseling, lifestyle changes like diet and exercise, and sometimes complementary therapies like acupuncture or massage.
6. **Pain Management:** It is important to work with healthcare professionals to develop a pain management plan. This can include learning pain management techniques, physical therapy exercises, and ways to manage the psychological aspects of chronic pain.
7. **Personalized Care:** Because chronic pain is a personal experience and varies widely from one person to another, treatment plans are highly individualized.
8. **Chronic Pain Syndromes:** There are specific chronic pain syndromes, like Complex Regional Pain Syndrome (CRPS), which have their own set of symptoms and treatment approaches.

Understanding and managing chronic pain is a challenging and ongoing process. If you are dealing with chronic pain, it is important to seek the advice of healthcare professionals who can help tailor a treatment plan to your specific needs.

How to evaluate chronic pain?

Evaluating chronic pain involves a comprehensive approach, as chronic pain is a complex and highly individual experience. Healthcare providers typically use a combination of methods to assess and understand a patient's pain. Here are the key steps involved in evaluating chronic pain:

1. **Medical History:** This includes discussing the patient's overall health, previous illnesses, injuries, and surgeries. The healthcare provider will inquire about when the pain started, what it feels like, and if there were any triggering events.
2. **Pain Description:** Patients are often asked to describe their pain in detail, including the location, intensity, quality (sharp, dull, throbbing, burning, etc.), duration, and what makes it better or worse. Pain scales or charts might be used to rate the intensity.
3. **Physical Examination:** A thorough physical exam helps in identifying any underlying causes of the pain. This may include checking for areas of tenderness, swelling, limited mobility, and other signs of pain.
4. **Pain Diaries or Journals:** Patients might be asked to keep a pain diary, recording when pain occurs, its intensity, and potential triggers. This can help identify patterns and factors that exacerbate or relieve pain.
5. **Psychological Evaluation:** Since chronic pain often affects mental health, and vice versa, an assessment of the patient's emotional well-being is crucial. This might involve discussing stress, anxiety, depression, and how the pain impacts daily life.
6. **Diagnostic Tests:** Depending on the suspected cause of the pain, various tests such as blood tests, X-rays, MRI scans, CT scans, or nerve conduction studies may be recommended to rule out or confirm specific conditions.
7. **Functional Impact Assessment:** Evaluating how pain affects the patient's ability to perform daily activities, work, hobbies, and social interactions.
8. **Review of Previous Treatments:** Discussing what treatments the patient has tried in the past, including medications, therapies, surgeries, and how effective they were.
9. **Multidisciplinary Approach:** Often, a team of healthcare providers including doctors, physical therapists, psychologists, and pain specialists collaborate to evaluate and treat chronic pain.
10. **Patient Education and Communication:** Providing information about chronic pain and encouraging an open dialogue about pain experiences and treatment expectations.
11. **Referral to Specialists:** If needed, patients may be referred to specialists such as rheumatologists, neurologists, orthopedists, or pain management specialists for more specific evaluations.

The goal of chronic pain evaluation is not only to determine the cause of the pain but also to understand its impact on the individual's life and to develop a comprehensive, personalized treatment plan.

Are there some treatments for depression that are not antidepressants?

Yes, there are several treatments for depression that do not involve antidepressants. It is important to note that the effectiveness of these treatments can vary depending on the individual, and they are often used in combination with each other for better results. Here are some common non-pharmacological treatments for depression:

1. **Psychotherapy:**
    - **Cognitive Behavioral Therapy (CBT):** Helps patients identify and change negative thinking and behavior patterns.
    - **Interpersonal Therapy (IPT):** Focuses on improving personal relationships and communication patterns.
    - **Dialectical Behavior Therapy (DBT):** Combines strategies of CBT with mindfulness and acceptance.
    - **Psychodynamic Therapy:** Explores past experiences and emotions.
2. **Lifestyle Changes:**
    - **Regular Exercise:** Physical activity can boost mood and mental health.
    - **Healthy Diet:** Nutritional psychiatry studies how diet affects mental health.
    - **Adequate Sleep:** Improving sleep can have a positive impact on mood.

3. **Mindfulness and Stress Reduction Techniques:**
   - Practices like meditation, yoga, and deep breathing exercises can reduce stress and improve mental well-being.
4. **Light Therapy:**
   - Especially useful in Seasonal Affective Disorder (SAD), light therapy involves exposure to a bright light that mimics natural outdoor light.
5. **Brain Stimulation Therapies:**
   - **Electroconvulsive Therapy (ECT):** Used for severe depression, particularly when other treatments have failed.
   - **Transcranial Magnetic Stimulation (TMS):** Uses magnetic fields to stimulate nerve cells in the brain.
6. **Support Groups:**
   - Sharing experiences and learning from others who are facing similar challenges can be very helpful.
7. **Alternative Medicine:**
   - Some people find relief with acupuncture, herbal supplements (like St. John's Wort, SAMe), though these should be used with caution and under the guidance of a healthcare provider.
8. **Art and Music Therapy:**
   - Engaging in creative activities can provide an outlet for expression and improve mood.

It is crucial to consult with a healthcare provider before starting any new treatment for depression, especially to understand the potential benefits and risks associated with each option. Treatment plans are often tailored to the individual, taking into account the severity of the depression, personal preferences, and any other health concerns.

What is new about catatonia?

Recent research on catatonia has brought forward new insights and perspectives, particularly in understanding its underlying brain mechanisms and its manifestation in different populations, such as children and adolescents.

A systematic review published in 2024 focused on the brain mechanisms underlying catatonia. This research employed various neuroimaging techniques, including structural and functional MRI, to study catatonia. The findings indicated numerous brain changes, especially in fronto-parietal and limbic regions, the thalamus, and the striatum. There were also observations of abnormalities in the orbitofrontal, medial prefrontal, and motor cortices, as well as in the cerebellum and brainstem. These studies highlighted structural, functional, perfusion, and metabolic cortico-subcortical abnormalities in catatonia. However, there is considerable heterogeneity in these studies, suggesting a need for cautious interpretation and further research to better understand the neural motor and psychomotor mechanisms underlying catatonia .

Another significant development is the recognition of catatonia in children and adolescents with neurodevelopmental disorders, including autism spectrum disorder. Recent literature suggests that the diagnosis and clinical management of catatonia in these populations require a more nuanced approach. Researchers have proposed new concepts for understanding catatonia in relation to the baseline status of an individual, emphasizing the need for a measure that considers previous complex and underlying motor, medical, functional, and neurobehavioral symptoms. This approach aims to provide a practical tool for clinicians and researchers working with this underserved and high-risk population .

These advancements in understanding catatonia's brain mechanisms and its manifestation in neurodevelopmental disorders represent significant steps forward in diagnosing and managing this complex condition. The integration of these new insights into clinical practice could improve the care and treatment of individuals with catatonia.

What is therapeutic recreation?

Therapeutic recreation, also known as recreational therapy, is a type of therapy that uses recreational activities as a means to rehabilitate or improve the physical, mental, and emotional well-being of individuals. It is based on the idea that engaging in enjoyable and meaningful leisure activities can be healing and beneficial in various ways. Here are some key aspects of therapeutic recreation:

1. **Targeted Populations:** It is often used for individuals with disabilities, injuries, or illnesses, including mental health conditions. The therapy is tailored to meet the needs of each individual.
2. **Activities Used:** Therapeutic recreation can involve a wide range of activities, such as arts and crafts, sports, games, dance, music, outdoor adventures, and more. The activities are chosen based on the interests, abilities, and needs of the individual.
3. **Goals and Benefits:** The primary goal is to improve the overall quality of life and well-being of the participants. This can include enhancing physical abilities, building confidence, improving

social skills, managing stress, and fostering a sense of achievement and enjoyment.

4. **Therapeutic Process:** Recreational therapists work with individuals to set specific goals and create a plan that incorporates various activities. They also evaluate the progress and make adjustments as necessary.
5. **Settings:** Therapeutic recreation can be offered in various settings, including hospitals, rehabilitation centers, nursing homes, community centers, and schools.
6. **Professional Involvement:** It is typically facilitated by certified recreational therapists who have specialized training in understanding how leisure and recreation impact health and well-being.

Therapeutic recreation is recognized as a valuable component of comprehensive healthcare and rehabilitation programs, as it addresses the whole person – mind, body, and spirit.

How to manage common sleep problems?

Managing common sleep problems involves a combination of good sleep hygiene and lifestyle adjustments. Here are some general tips:

1. **Regular Schedule:** Maintain a consistent sleep schedule, even on weekends.
2. **Relaxation Techniques:** Practice relaxation methods before bed, like deep breathing or meditation.
3. **Comfortable Sleep Environment:** Ensure your bedroom is dark, quiet, and cool.
4. **Limit Screen Time:** Reduce exposure to screens before bedtime, as the blue light can interfere with sleep.
5. **Avoid Stimulants:** Limit caffeine and nicotine, especially in the evening.
6. **Physical Activity:** Regular exercise can promote better sleep, but avoid vigorous activities close to bedtime.
7. **Mindful Eating:** Avoid large meals, alcohol, and too many fluids before sleep.
8. **Manage Stress:** Try to address stressors with techniques like journaling or counseling.

Types of common sleep problems:

Common sleep problems include a variety of conditions that can affect the quality, timing, and duration of sleep. Some of the most common types are:

1. **Insomnia:** Difficulty falling asleep or staying asleep. People with insomnia may wake up too early and not feel refreshed after sleeping.
2. **Sleep Apnea:** A serious sleep disorder where breathing repeatedly stops and starts during sleep. Common symptoms include loud snoring and feeling tired even after a full night's sleep.
3. **Restless Legs Syndrome (RLS):** An uncomfortable sensation in the legs with a compulsive urge to move them, often occurring in the evening or night, which can impair the ability to fall asleep.
4. **Narcolepsy:** A chronic neurological disorder that affects the brain's ability to control sleep-wake cycles. People with narcolepsy may experience excessive daytime sleepiness and sudden attacks of sleep.
5. **Circadian Rhythm Disorders:** Problems with the sleep-wake cycle, leading to sleep at unusual times. These disorders can result from a mismatch between a person's internal sleep-wake clock and the external environment.
6. **Parasomnias:** Abnormal behaviors during sleep, such as sleepwalking, sleep talking, nightmares, and night terrors.
7. **Snoring:** Breathing through a partially closed airway during sleep, causing a vibrating sound. While snoring is common and usually not a serious problem, it can be a nuisance for bed partners and sometimes indicates a more serious condition like sleep apnea.
8. **Delayed Sleep Phase Syndrome (DSPS):** A disorder where a person's sleep is delayed by two hours or more beyond what is considered a conventional bedtime, leading to difficulty in waking up at a desired time.
9. **Bruxism:** Involuntarily grinding or clenching of the teeth while sleeping, which can lead to jaw pain, headaches, and other problems.
10. **Hypersomnia:** Excessive sleepiness during the day, even after long periods of sleep at night. People with hypersomnia might have difficulty waking up and feel disoriented.

Each of these conditions can significantly impact a person's quality of life and may require different treatment approaches. If you suspect you have a sleep disorder, it is important to consult a healthcare provider for a proper diagnosis and treatment plan.

What is dystonia?

Dystonia is a neurological movement disorder charac-terized by involuntary muscle contractions, which cause repetitive or twisting movements. It is a condition that can affect just one muscle, a group of muscles, or muscles throughout the body, leading to abnormal postures and movements.

Types of Dystonia:

Dystonia can be classified based on various factors:

1. **By Affected Regions:**
   - **Focal Dystonia:** Involves a single area of the body, such as the neck (cervical dystonia), eyelids (blepharospasm), or hand (writer's cramp).
   - **Segmental Dystonia:** Affects two or more adjacent parts of the body.
   - **Multifocal Dystonia:** Involves multiple non-adjacent parts of the body.
   - **Generalized Dystonia:** Affects most or all of the body.
2. **By Age of Onset:**
   - **Childhood-Onset:** Begins in childhood, often more severe and likely to spread to other parts of the body.
   - **Adult-Onset:** Typically affects one or two regions of the body and is less likely to progress.
3. **By Cause:**
   - **Primary Dystonia:** Caused directly by a problem in the nervous system and not related to another medical issue.
   - **Secondary Dystonia:** Results from another disease or condition (like stroke, brain injury, or Parkinson's disease) or due to certain medications.

Symptoms:

Symptoms of dystonia can vary greatly depending on the type of dystonia. Common signs include:

- Involuntary muscle contractions.
- Twisting or repetitive movements.
- Abnormal postures.
- Tremor.
- Pain and discomfort.
- Fatigue due to constant muscle contraction.

Causes:

The exact cause of dystonia is often unknown, but it is thought to result from improper signaling in the brain. It can be related to:

- Genetic mutations, particularly in primary dystonia.
- Brain injuries or trauma.
- Stroke.
- Infections.
- Reactions to certain medications.
- Diseases of the nervous system, such as Parkinson's disease.

Diagnosis:

Diagnosing dystonia can be challenging and usually involves:

- Medical history evaluation.
- Neurological examination.
- Blood and urine tests to rule out other conditions.
- Imaging studies like MRI or CT scans.
- Genetic testing, particularly if there is a family history suggesting a genetic component.

Treatment:

While there is no cure for dystonia, treatments focus on relieving symptoms and improving quality of life:

1. **Medications:** These can include muscle relaxants, drugs to treat Parkinson's disease (if applicable), or medications that affect neurotransmitters.
2. **Botulinum Toxin Injections:** For focal dystonias, injections of botulinum toxin can be effective in reducing muscle contractions and improving abnormal postures.
3. **Physical Therapy:** Can help maintain or improve mobility, strength, and balance.
4. **Occupational Therapy:** Assists individuals in managing daily activities and adapting to living with dystonia.
5. **Speech Therapy:** Particularly helpful if dystonia affects the vocal cords or speech muscles.
6. **Deep Brain Stimulation (DBS):** In severe cases, particularly for generalized or segmental dystonia,

DBS, a surgical procedure that implants a device to stimulate specific areas of the brain, may be considered.

7. **Stress Management and Support:** Techniques to manage stress and support groups can be beneficial for coping with the psychological aspects of living with a chronic condition.

It is important for individuals with dystonia to work closely with a healthcare team to tailor a treatment plan that addresses their specific symptoms and needs. Regular monitoring and adjustments in therapy are often necessary.

What are Somatoform Disorders?

Somatoform disorders, also known as Somatic Symptom and Related Disorders, are a group of psychological conditions where a person experiences physical symptoms that are inconsistent with or cannot be fully explained by any underlying medical or neurological condition. These symptoms are not intentionally produced or feigned; they are real to the patient and often cause significant distress and impairment in daily functioning.

Types of Somatoform Disorders:

1. **Somatic Symptom Disorder:** This involves having one or more chronic physical symptoms, such as pain or fatigue, which cause significant emotional distress and difficulty in daily functioning. The individual often has excessive thoughts, feelings, or behaviors related to the symptoms.

2. **Illness Anxiety Disorder:** Formerly known as hypochondriasis, this disorder involves a preoccupation with having or acquiring a serious, undiagnosed medical illness despite few or no symptoms and consistently negative medical evaluations.

3. **Conversion Disorder (Functional Neurological Symptom Disorder):** Characterized by neurological symptoms (like paralysis, blindness, or movement disorders) that cannot be explained by medical evaluation. These symptoms suggest a neurological condition but are believed to be a response to psychological conflict or stress.

4. **Factitious Disorder:** Although not technically a somatoform disorder, it is closely related. In factitious disorder, a person deliberately fabricates or induces symptoms of illness in themselves (or in others, as in Factitious Disorder Imposed on Another, previously known as Munchausen Syndrome by Proxy) for emotional reasons such as a desire for attention or sympathy. This is different from somatoform disorders, where the symptom production is not intentional.

5. **Other Specified Somatic Symptom and Related Disorder:** This category includes conditions with somatic symptoms that do not meet full criteria for any of the specific disorders but still cause significant distress or impairment.

6. **Psychological Factors Affecting Other Medical Conditions:** This involves psychological or behavioral factors that exacerbate or influence a medical condition.

Causes:

The exact cause of somatoform disorders is unknown, but a combination of genetic, biological, psychological, and environmental factors may contribute. This can include:

- A history of trauma or significant stress.
- Learned behavior (for example, attention received for physical complaints in childhood).
- Increased sensitivity to pain or other sensations.
- Psychological factors linked to unconscious conflicts or stress.
- Family history of somatic symptoms or related disorders.

Diagnosis:

Diagnosing somatoform disorders is challenging and often involves ruling out medical conditions that could explain the symptoms. It usually requires:

- Detailed medical history and physical examination.
- Consideration of the patient's psychological state and stressors.
- Collaboration between medical and mental health professionals.

Treatment:

Treatment focuses on improving quality of life and may include:

- Psychotherapy, especially cognitive-behavioral therapy (CBT), to help change thinking and behavior patterns.
- Medication, such as antidepressants, for associated symptoms like depression or anxiety.
- Stress reduction techniques and coping strategies.
- Regular follow-up and coordination of care between healthcare providers.

It is important to approach treatment of somatoform disorders with sensitivity and understanding, as patients are often frustrated and feel misunderstood after multiple medical evaluations without clear answers. A compassionate, multidisciplinary approach is key to successful management.

What is cognitive therapy?

Cognitive therapy, often referred to as cognitive-behavioral therapy (CBT), is a type of psychotherapeutic treatment that helps patients understand the thoughts and feelings that influence behaviors. It is commonly used to treat a wide range of disorders, including phobias, addiction, depression, and anxiety.

Key Principles of Cognitive Therapy:

1. **Identification of Negative Thoughts:** Cognitive therapy revolves around the concept that our thoughts, not external events, create our moods. It focuses on identifying and challenging negative and often irrational thoughts (known as cognitive distortions).
2. **Challenge and Change Unhelpful Patterns:** Once these thoughts are identified, the therapy aims to challenge and change unhelpful thinking patterns and beliefs, replacing them with more realistic, positive thoughts.
3. **Behavioral Change:** It also involves changing behaviors that result from distorted thinking. This might include facing fears instead of avoiding them, or practicing new skills to cope with difficult situations.
4. **Problem-Solving:** Cognitive therapy often teaches patients problem-solving skills to help them cope with difficult situations.
5. **Goal-Oriented:** Therapy is usually goal-oriented and focused on the present. Patients and therapists work together to set goals and work methodically to achieve them.

Techniques Used in Cognitive Therapy:

1. **Cognitive Restructuring:** Learning to recognize and dispute irrational or maladaptive thoughts.
2. **Behavioral Experiments:** Testing out the beliefs in real-life situations to see if they hold true.
3. **Mindfulness and Relaxation Techniques:** To reduce stress and improve awareness of thoughts and feelings.
4. **Exposure Therapy:** Particularly for treating phobias and anxiety disorders, where the patient is exposed to the feared object or context without any danger, in order to overcome their anxiety.
5. **Homework Assignments:** Practical exercises to practice skills outside of therapy sessions.

Applications of Cognitive Therapy:

Cognitive therapy is used to treat a variety of mental health conditions, including:

- Depression and bipolar disorder.
- Anxiety disorders (such as panic attacks, social anxiety, generalized anxiety disorder).
- Phobias.
- Obsessive-compulsive disorder (OCD).
- Post-traumatic stress disorder (PTSD).
- Eating disorders.
- Substance abuse and addiction.
- Personality disorders.

Effectiveness:

Numerous studies have found cognitive therapy to be effective for a wide range of mental illnesses. It can be as effective as antidepressants for some individuals with depression and anxiety disorders. Additionally, combining cognitive therapy with medication therapy can be particularly effective for certain conditions.

Cognitive therapy offers a hands-on, practical approach to problem-solving. Its goal is to change patterns of thinking or behavior that are behind people's difficulties, and so change the way they feel. It is usually more focused on the present and is a shorter-term treatment compared to other types of psychotherapy.

What are types of suicidal behaviors?

Suicidal behavior encompasses a range of actions related to self-harm and suicide. Understanding these behaviors is crucial for prevention and intervention efforts. The types of suicidal behaviors are typically classified into the following categories:

1. **Suicidal Ideation:** This refers to thoughts about wanting to take one's own life. Suicidal ideation can vary greatly in terms of its severity, frequency, and degree of planning. It can range from fleeting thoughts to detailed planning.
2. **Suicide Plan:** This involves the formulation of a specific method through which one intends to take their own life. Having a suicide plan is a more

serious indication of suicidal risk, as it suggests a higher level of intent.

3. **Suicide Attempt:** This is an act of self-harm with at least some intent to end one's life. Suicide attempts can vary in terms of lethality and intent. An attempt could be a more serious effort to die, or it might be a less lethal method or a cry for help.
4. **Interrupted Suicide Attempt:** This occurs when a person begins to take action to kill themselves but stops or is stopped by another person before they inflict fatal harm.
5. **Aborted Suicide Attempt:** This is when a person begins to take action to kill themselves but stops themselves before they engage in the behavior (e.g., they decide not to go through with it at the last moment).
6. **Suicide Gesture:** These are actions that look like a suicide attempt but are usually a cry for help rather than an actual attempt to die. The intent is more about expressing distress or calling for attention rather than a genuine desire to end one's life.
7. **Completed Suicide:** This refers to successfully taking one's own life.

It is important to note that suicidal thoughts and behaviors are often symptoms of underlying issues, such as mental health disorders (like depression, bipolar disorder, and schizophrenia), traumatic stress, substance abuse, or significant life crises. Early intervention, appropriate mental health treatment, and support from friends, family, and healthcare professionals can significantly reduce the risk of suicide.

If someone exhibits any form of suicidal behavior, it is critical to take it seriously and seek immediate professional help. Suicidal behaviors are a sign of extreme distress and should never be dismissed or ignored.

What to do in case of suicidal patient?

If you are dealing with a suicidal patient or someone who is expressing suicidal thoughts or intentions, it is crucial to act promptly and compassionately to ensure their safety and get them the help they need. Here are steps to follow:

1. **Stay Calm and Supportive:** Approach the situation calmly and non-judgmentally. Show empathy and understanding. It is important to listen to them and validate their feelings, rather than dismissing or challenging their emotions.
2. **Ensure Immediate Safety:** Ask if they have a plan for suicide and if they have the means to carry it out (like access to weapons, pills, etc.). If they have a specific plan and the means to execute it, they are at a higher risk and immediate action is required.
3. **Do Not Leave Them Alone:** Stay with the person or ensure they are in a secure and supervised environment. If you are not physically with them, try to get someone who is close to their location to be with them.
4. **Seek Professional Help Immediately:** Contact emergency services or take the person to the nearest emergency room. If you are not sure about the local emergency services, call a suicide hotline for guidance.
5. **Remove Means of Self-Harm:** If it is safe to do so, remove any objects that could be used for self-harm, such as firearms, drugs, sharp objects, or ropes.
6. **Listen Attentively:** Allow them to express their feelings and thoughts. Sometimes, just having someone to listen to them can reduce the intensity of their suicidal feelings.
7. **Avoid Arguing or Challenging Their Feelings:** Do not try to argue them out of suicide or challenge their feelings. Avoid saying things like "You have so much to live for" or "Think about how this will hurt your family."
8. **Encourage Professional Help:** Encourage them to seek help from a mental health professional. Offer to help them find a therapist or counselor, and assist them in setting up an appointment.
9. **Follow-up:** After the immediate crisis has passed, continue to be a source of support. Check in on them regularly, encourage them to stick with treatment, and be there to listen.
10. **Be Prepared with Resources:** Have contact information for emergency services, local crisis centers, and suicide hotlines readily available.

Remember, if you are not a mental health professional, your role is to provide support and get the person to professional help, not to try to counsel or treat them yourself. Dealing with a suicidal individual can be emotionally draining, so make sure you also seek support for yourself if needed.

What are self-Harming Behaviors?

Self-harming behaviors refer to various actions that people undertake to intentionally inflict pain or injury upon themselves, often as a coping mechanism to deal with overwhelming emotions, stress, or trauma. These behaviors are usually a symptom of deeper psychological distress and are not typically intended as suicide attempts, although they can increase the risk of accidental or deliberate suicide. It is important to understand that self-harm is often a sign of underlying issues that need professional attention.

Common Forms of Self-Harm:

1. **Cutting:** The most widely recognized form of self-harm, involving making cuts or scratches on the body with sharp objects.
2. **Burning:** Using fire or hot objects to burn the skin.
3. **Hitting or Punching:** This includes hitting oneself or objects to cause pain or injury.
4. **Piercing the Skin with Sharp Objects:** Apart from cutting, this can include sticking pins, needles, or other sharp objects into the skin.
5. **Hair Pulling:** Known as trichotillomania, it involves pulling out one's hair, leading to hair loss and bald spots.
6. **Skin Picking:** Repeatedly picking at or severely scratching the skin, leading to sores and scars. This is also known as dermatillomania or excoriation disorder.
7. **Bone Breaking:** Deliberately breaking one's own bones.
8. **Poisoning or Ingesting Harmful Substances:** This includes consuming substances that are not meant for ingestion or are toxic.
9. **Interfering with Wound Healing:** Deliberately preventing wounds from healing, often to maintain a visible sign of distress or to re-experience the pain of injury.

Causes of Self-Harming Behaviors:

Self-harm is complex and can be caused by a variety of factors, including:

- **Emotional Distress:** To cope with or express emotions they cannot put into words, distract from emotional pain, or relieve emotional numbness.
- **Psychological Pain:** As a physical manifestation of internal psychological pain.
- **Trauma or Abuse:** As a response to trauma, including sexual, physical, or emotional abuse.
- **Mental Health Disorders:** Associated with various mental health conditions like borderline personality disorder, depression, anxiety disorders, and eating disorders.
- **Control:** As a means to exert control over one's own body when they feel they can't control other aspects of their life.
- **Self-Punishment:** Due to feelings of guilt, worthlessness, or self-hatred.
- **Seeking Sensation:** In cases where individuals feel disconnected or numb, self-harm might be a way to feel something tangible.

Recognizing Self-Harm:

Recognizing self-harm can be challenging as individuals often go to great lengths to hide their behavior. Signs may include:

- Unexplained cuts, bruises, burns, or other injuries.
- Wearing long sleeves or pants even in hot weather to cover injuries.
- Secrecy, such as insisting on privacy in the bathroom or bedroom.
- Hoarding sharp objects.
- Frequent reports of accidental injury.
- Emotional and behavioral signs like mood swings, withdrawal, or depression.

Treatment and Support:

Treatment for self-harming behaviors often involves addressing the underlying psychological issues:

1. **Psychotherapy:** Such as cognitive-behavioral therapy (CBT), dialectical behavior therapy (DBT), or psychodynamic therapy, can help individuals understand and manage their emotions and reduce self-harming behaviors.
2. **Medication:** May be prescribed to treat underlying mental health conditions like depression or anxiety.
3. **Support Groups:** Can provide a sense of community and understanding, as well as strategies for coping.

4. **Family Therapy:** Can be helpful in cases where family dynamics play a role in the individual's distress.

5. **Skill Development:** Learning healthier coping mechanisms to deal with emotional distress, such as stress management techniques, emotional regulation strategies, and communication skills.

If you suspect someone is self-harming, approach the subject with care and compassion, avoiding judgment or criticism. Encourage them to seek professional help. If the person is a minor, it is important to notify a responsible adult, such as a parent or school counselor, who can intervene appropriately.

What is a psychological autopsy and how can it help?

A psychological autopsy is a postmortem investigation into a person's mental state prior to their death, primarily used in cases where the cause of death is suspected to be suicide. This process involves gathering and analyzing information from various sources to understand the deceased person's psychological, emotional, and mental health status leading up to their death. The goal is to reconstruct the deceased person's mental state by examining factors such as their thoughts, feelings, and behaviors, as well as the circumstances of their death.

How Psychological Autopsies are Conducted:

1. **Interviews:** Conducting detailed interviews with family members, friends, co-workers, and healthcare providers who knew the deceased.

2. **Review of Documents:** Examining personal documents like diaries, letters, emails, or social media posts, as well as medical records, psychiatric treatment records, and any notes left by the deceased.

3. **Analysis of the Death Scene:** Gathering information from the scene of death, including the method used, and any notes or evidence left behind.

4. **Review of Coroner or Medical Examiner Reports:** Including autopsy findings, toxicology reports, and death scene investigation results.

How Psychological Autopsies Can Help:

1. **Determining the Cause of Death:** Helps in determining whether a death was due to suicide, accident, natural causes, or homicide, particularly in cases where the cause of death is unclear.

2. **Understanding Suicide and Prevention:** Provides insights into why individuals may commit suicide, which can inform suicide prevention strategies, interventions, and policies.

3. **Legal and Insurance Purposes:** Can be used in legal cases (e.g., to determine the fulfilment of insurance policies that may not cover suicide) and in helping authorities make informed decisions about the death.

4. **Closure for Families:** Can provide closure for grieving families by helping them understand the mental state and possible reasons behind their loved one's actions.

5. **Research and Education:** Contributes to research in the field of mental health and suicide prevention by providing valuable data on risk factors and warning signs of suicide.

6. **Guiding Public Health Strategies:** Helps in developing targeted mental health interventions and public health strategies to prevent suicides.

While a psychological autopsy can provide valuable insights, it is important to note that it has limitations. Reconstructing a person's mental state retrospectively can be challenging, and conclusions are based on interpretations of the collected data, which might not always fully represent the deceased person's experiences or intentions. Despite these challenges, psychological autopsies remain a significant tool in understanding and preventing suicides and in providing closure to those affected by the loss.

What are the signs and symptoms of Parkinson's disease?

Parkinson's disease is a progressive neurological disorder that primarily affects movement. It develops gradually, sometimes starting with barely noticeable tremors in just one hand. While tremors are a well-known sign of Parkinson's, the disorder also commonly causes stiffness or slowing of movement. The symptoms and their severity can vary greatly among individuals.

Early Signs and Symptoms:

1. **Tremor:** A slight tremor or shaking in a finger, thumb, hand, or chin is often one of the first signs. The tremor usually happens when the limb is at rest and stops during movement.

2. **Bradykinesia (Slowed Movement):** Over time, Parkinson's disease may slow movement, making simple tasks difficult and time-consuming. Steps may become shorter when walking, or it may be hard to get out of a chair.

3. **Rigid Muscles:** Muscle stiffness can occur in any part of the body. The stiff muscles can be painful and limit the range of motion.

4. **Impaired Posture and Balance:** Posture may become stooped, or there may be balance problems as a result of Parkinson's disease.

5. **Loss of Automatic Movements:** Decreased ability to perform unconscious movements, including blinking, smiling, or swinging the arms when walking.

6. **Speech Changes:** Speech may become soft, quick, slur, or hesitate before talking. The usual inflection and modulation of speech may also become more monotonous.

7. **Writing Changes:** Writing may appear small and become more difficult to do.

Later Stages Symptoms:

As the disease progresses, these symptoms may worsen:

- Increased Tremors and Muscle Stiffness.
- Greater Slowness of Movements.
- Balance Problems Becoming More Pronounced, leading to increased falls.
- Cognitive Issues and Dementia may develop in the later stages.
- Emotional Changes, such as increased depression or anxiety.
- Swallowing Difficulties.
- Sleep Disturbances.
- Bladder Problems or constipation.
- Sensory Symptoms, such as pain or a decrease in sense of smell.

Non-Motor Symptoms:

Parkinson's also includes a range of non-motor symptoms that can affect quality of life:

- **Mood Disorders:** Depression and anxiety.
- **Cognitive Impairment:** Problems with attention, planning, and problem-solving.
- **Autonomic Dysfunction:** Blood pressure changes, sweating, and urinary urgency.
- **Sleep Disorders:** Including REM sleep behavior disorder and insomnia.
- Fatigue and loss of energy.

It is important to note that these symptoms can also be caused by other conditions. If someone is experiencing these symptoms, they should consult a healthcare provider for a thorough evaluation. While there is no cure for Parkinson's disease, treatments are available to help manage symptoms. These treatments may include medication, lifestyle changes, physical therapy, and in some cases, surgery. The approach to treatment is tailored to the individual's symptoms and can significantly improve quality of life.

What are the causes of Parkinson's disease?

The exact causes of Parkinson's disease are not fully understood, but the condition is believed to result from a combination of genetic and environmental factors. Here is an overview of the known and suspected causes:

1. **Loss of Dopamine-Producing Neurons:** Parkinson's disease primarily involves the gradual loss of neurons in a part of the brain called the substantia nigra. These neurons produce dopamine, a neurotransmitter that plays a key role in regulating movement, emotional responses, and other functions. The reduction in dopamine levels leads to the movement symptoms characteristic of Parkinson's.

2. **Genetic Factors:** While most cases of Parkinson's appear to be sporadic, meaning they occur randomly, about 10 to 15 percent of cases are familial, indicating a genetic contribution. Certain genetic mutations have been identified that can increase the risk of Parkinson's, but these are relatively rare.

3. **Environmental Triggers:** Exposure to certain toxins or environmental factors may increase the risk of Parkinson's disease. These include exposure to pesticides, herbicides, and heavy metals, although the risk from these factors is relatively low.

4. **Age:** Parkinson's disease predominantly affects older adults, typically developing after the age of 60. The risk increases with age.

5. **Sex:** Men are more likely to develop Parkinson's disease than women, although the reasons for this sex difference are not entirely clear.

6. **Oxidative Stress and Mitochondrial Dysfunction:** Damage to cells from oxidative stress and the dysfunction of mitochondria, the energy-producing components of cells, are believed to contribute to neuron death in Parkinson's disease.

7. **Lewy Bodies:** These abnormal clumps of protein (alpha-synuclein) found in the brains of people with Parkinson's are a hallmark of the disease. However, it is not completely understood how these Lewy bodies contribute to the death of dopamine-producing neurons.

8. **Head Trauma:** Some research suggests that repeated head injuries or trauma may be linked to a higher risk of developing Parkinson's disease later in life.

9. **Other Neurochemical Changes:** Apart from dopamine, other neurotransmitters like norepinephrine, which regulates the autonomic nervous system, are also affected in Parkinson's disease, contributing to the non-motor symptoms.

10. **Autoimmune Factors:** Recent research suggests that there might be an autoimmune component to Parkinson's, where the body's immune system mistakenly attacks the brain's neurons.

Despite ongoing research, the exact cause of Parkinson's in most individuals remains unknown. It is likely that a combination of genetic predisposition and environmental factors work together to cause the disease. Early detection and management are key to improving the quality of life for individuals with Parkinson's disease.

What is the difference between Parkinson's dementia and Alzheimer's dementia?

Parkinson's dementia and Alzheimer's dementia are both neurodegenerative disorders that lead to cognitive decline, but they have different underlying causes, symptom profiles, and progressions. Understanding these differences is important for diagnosis and management.

Parkinson's Dementia:

1. **Underlying Cause:** Parkinson's dementia develops in the later stages of Parkinson's disease, a disorder primarily affecting motor function due to the loss of dopamine-producing neurons in the brain. Cognitive symptoms arise as the disease progresses.

2. **Symptoms:** Initially, Parkinson's disease presents with motor symptoms such as tremors, stiffness, and slow movements. Cognitive impairment, when it occurs, typically involves executive dysfunction (problems with planning, decision-making), difficulty in multitasking, slowed thinking, and problems with attention and concentration. Memory impairment can occur but is not usually an early symptom.

3. **Progression:** Cognitive decline in Parkinson's dementia tends to occur several years after the onset of motor symptoms. The speed of progression can vary.

4. **Associated Features:** Parkinson's dementia is often accompanied by physical symptoms of Parkinson's disease, such as tremors, rigidity, and bradykinesia (slow movements). There may also be sleep disturbances, visual hallucinations, and changes in mood and behavior.

Alzheimer's Dementia:

1. **Underlying Cause:** Alzheimer's disease is primarily a disorder of the brain characterized by the accumulation of amyloid plaques and tau tangles, leading to the death of brain cells. It is the most common cause of dementia.

2. **Symptoms:** The hallmark symptom of Alzheimer's dementia is memory loss, especially difficulty remembering newly learned information. As Alzheimer's advances, symptoms include confusion, disorientation, difficulty in speaking and writing, and changes in mood and behavior.

3. **Progression:** Alzheimer's disease typically begins with mild memory loss and progresses to severe brain impairment. The course of the disease can span several years, and the progression rate varies among individuals.

4. **Associated Features:** In the later stages, individuals with Alzheimer's may experience a decline in physical functions, such as walking or swallowing, but these typically occur after significant cognitive decline.

Key Differences:

- **Primary Symptoms:** Parkinson's dementia typically starts with motor symptoms followed by cognitive decline, whereas Alzheimer's begins with memory problems leading to a broader cognitive and behavioral impairment.

- **Nature of Cognitive Impairment:** Parkinson's dementia is more characterized by executive dysfunction, whereas Alzheimer's predominantly affects memory, especially in the early stages.

- **Underlying Pathology:** Parkinson's involves the loss of dopamine-producing neurons and the presence of Lewy bodies, while Alzheimer's is marked by amyloid plaques and tau tangles.

- **Progression:** The progression of cognitive decline relative to the onset of the disease differs. Parkinson's dementia occurs in the later stages of Parkinson's disease, while in Alzheimer's, cognitive decline is often the first and most prominent feature.

Proper diagnosis by a healthcare professional, often involving neuroimaging and neuropsychological testing, is crucial for distinguishing between these types of dementia, as it can influence the management and treatment approach.

What are the end stages of Parkinson's Disease?

The end stages of Parkinson's Disease represent the most advanced phase of this progressive neurological disorder. During these stages, symptoms become more severe and can significantly impact the individual's quality of life and ability to perform daily activities. Key characteristics of the end stages of Parkinson's Disease include:

1. **Severe Motor Symptoms:** Tremors, rigidity, and bradykinesia (slowness of movement) are more pronounced. Patients may experience great difficulty with movement or become completely immobile.
2. **Increased Risk of Falls:** Due to a combination of balance problems, rigidity, and impaired motor coordination, there is a high risk of falls, which can lead to injuries.
3. **Dependence in Daily Activities:** Individuals often require assistance with daily activities such as dressing, eating, bathing, and mobility. This is due to a combination of motor symptoms and decreased dexterity.
4. **Cognitive Decline:** Parkinson's dementia may occur, characterized by memory impairment, difficulty with attention and concentration, executive dysfunction, and, in some cases, hallucinations and delusions.
5. **Communication Difficulties:** Speech becomes more affected, often becoming very soft, monotone, or slurred. This can make communication challenging.
6. **Swallowing Difficulties:** Dysphagia, or difficulty swallowing, becomes more common, increasing the risk of choking and aspiration pneumonia.
7. **Nutritional Concerns:** Due to swallowing difficulties and decreased appetite, there may be significant weight loss and malnutrition.
8. **Increased Risk of Infections:** The risk of infections, particularly respiratory infections like pneumonia, is increased due to immobility and swallowing difficulties.
9. **Psychological Symptoms:** Depression and anxiety can be significant in the advanced stages, affecting the individual's quality of life.
10. **Need for Comprehensive Care:** As Parkinson's disease progresses to its advanced stages, the need for comprehensive medical and supportive care increases. This may include home care services, nursing care, or hospice care, focusing on maintaining comfort and quality of life.
11. **Medication Management:** Medications may need more frequent adjustments to manage symptoms as effectively as possible. However, individuals might also experience increased sensitivity to medication side effects.

During these stages, the focus of care often shifts towards palliative care, emphasizing comfort and quality of life. It is crucial to have a supportive network in place, including healthcare providers, family, and caregivers, to address the complex needs of individuals in the end stages of Parkinson's Disease. This care is not only about managing physical symptoms but also providing emotional and psychological support.

What is the treatment of Parkinson's disease?

The treatment of Parkinson's disease is primarily focused on managing symptoms, as there is currently no cure for the condition. The treatment plan for Parkinson's disease is tailored to each individual's symptoms and may involve a combination of medication, lifestyle changes, physical therapy, and in some cases, surgical interventions. Here is an overview of the treatment options:

Medications:

1. **Levodopa/Carbidopa:** The most effective Parkinson's disease treatment. Levodopa is converted into dopamine in the brain, while carbidopa prevents levodopa from converting into dopamine outside the brain, reducing side effects and allowing more levodopa to reach the brain.
2. **Dopamine Agonists:** Mimic the effects of dopamine in the brain and can be used alone or with Levodopa.
3. **MAO-B Inhibitors:** These medications, such as selegiline and rasagiline, help prevent the breakdown of brain dopamine by inhibiting the enzyme monoamine oxidase B (MAO).

4. **Catechol O-Methyltransferase (COMT) Inhibitors:** Such as entacapone and tolcapone, prolong the effect of levodopa by blocking an enzyme that breaks down dopamine.

5. **Anticholinergics**: These drugs, such as trihexyphenidyl and benztropine, help control tremors and rigidity, especially in younger patients, but can have cognitive side effects in the elderly.

6. **Amantadine:** Can be used to provide short-term relief of symptoms in early-stage Parkinson's or to help control involuntary movements (dyskinesias) in later stages.

Surgical Treatments:

1. **Deep Brain Stimulation (DBS):** Involves surgically implanting a neurostimulator to send electrical impulses to specific parts of the brain. DBS is most often offered to individuals whose symptoms cannot be adequately controlled with medications.

2. **Other surgical procedures:** Such as pallidotomy and thalamotomy, are less common and involve destroying small parts of brain tissue responsible for Parkinson's symptoms.

Lifestyle and Home Remedies:

1. **Healthy Diet:** Including high fiber foods to prevent constipation and ensuring balanced nutrition.

2. **Regular Exercise:** Helps maintain muscle tone, flexibility, and balance. Activities like walking, swimming, yoga, or tai chi can be particularly beneficial.

3. **Physical Therapy:** Can help improve mobility, range of mot ion, and balance.

4. **Occupational Therapy:** Helps with daily activities and recommends modifications to the living environment to ensure safety and independence.

5. **Speech Therapy:** For those experiencing speech difficulties.

Alternative Medicine:

1. **Mind-Body Therapies:** Such as meditation, yoga, and tai chi, may help improve overall well-being and reduce stress.

2. **Supplements and Vitamins:** Some individuals find relief with certain supplements, but it is important to consult with a healthcare provider before starting any new supplement.

3. **Acupuncture:** Some patients report improvement in symptoms and overall well-being.

Supportive Therapies:

1. **Support Groups:** Can provide emotional support and practical advice for living with Parkinson's disease.

2. **Counseling or Psychotherapy:** For dealing with the emotional and psychological aspects of living with a chronic illness.

It is important for individuals with Parkinson's disease to work closely with their healthcare team, including neurologists, primary care providers, and other specialists, to create a personalized treatment plan. This team approach is crucial for managing the complex and evolving symptoms of Parkinson's disease.

What are Indications for EEG in psychiatric practice?

Electroencephalography (EEG) is a non-invasive test that measures electrical activity in the brain. It is widely used in neurology, but it also has several applications in psychiatric practice. The indications for EEG in psychiatry include:

1. **Differential Diagnosis of Psychiatric Disorders and Neurological Conditions:** EEG can help distinguish between psychiatric conditions and neurological disorders that may present with similar symptoms, such as epilepsy, which can sometimes manifest as psychogenic non-epileptic seizures (PNES) that resemble psychiatric conditions.

2. **Assessment of Treatment-Resistant Psychiatric Disorders:** In cases where psychiatric conditions, particularly depression or schizophrenia, are resistant to standard treatments, EEG can be used to assess for potential neurological contributions to the disorder.

3. **Diagnosis of Delirium and Dementia:** EEG can be helpful in differentiating between delirium and dementia, as these conditions may have overlapping symptoms but different EEG patterns.

4. **Evaluating Cognitive Disorders:** EEG can help assess the severity and progression of cognitive

impairments in conditions like Alzheimer's disease and other forms of dementia.

5. **Monitoring the Effects of Psychiatric Medications:** Some medications used in psychiatry can have effects on brain activity. EEG can be used to monitor these effects, particularly if there are concerns about medication-induced seizures or other neurological side effects.

6. **Diagnosis and Monitoring of Catatonia:** EEG can assist in the diagnosis of catatonia, a state of psychomotor disturbance that can occur in severe psychiatric disorders. It can help differentiate catatonic states from other conditions, such as non-convulsive status epilepticus.

7. **Evaluation of Sleep Disorders:** Since many psychiatric disorders are associated with sleep disturbances, EEG, particularly as part of a polysomnography study, can be useful in diagnosing and understanding sleep disorders.

8. **Quantitative EEG (qEEG) for Treatment Planning:** qEEG, which involves the statistical analysis of EEG data, can sometimes be used to guide treatment planning. It may provide information about the functional state of the brain that can inform decisions about medications or other treatments.

9. **Investigation of Psychogenic Seizures:** EEG is crucial in differentiating between epileptic seizures and psychogenic non-epileptic seizures (PNES), which are psychological in origin.

10. **Research Purposes:** EEG is a valuable tool in psychiatric research, helping to explore the neurophysiological basis of psychiatric disorders and the effects of various psychiatric treatments.

It is important to note that while EEG can provide valuable information, it should be used as part of a comprehensive psychiatric assessment and not as the sole diagnostic tool. The interpretation of EEG results should be done by a qualified professional, as the readings can be complex and are best understood in the context of the individual's overall clinical picture.

What is alcohol withdrawal (AW)?

Alcohol withdrawal (AW) refers to a range of symptoms that can occur when a person who has been drinking heavily for weeks, months, or years suddenly stops or significantly reduces their alcohol consumption. Alcohol withdrawal is a physiological response to the absence of alcohol, which the body may have become dependent on due to prolonged and excessive consumption.

Symptoms of Alcohol Withdrawal:

Alcohol withdrawal symptoms can vary in severity, ranging from mild to potentially life-threatening. They typically begin within hours of the last drink and can last for days or weeks. Common symptoms include:

1. **Mild Symptoms:**
   - Anxiety or nervousness.
   - Insomnia.
   - Shaking or tremors, especially in the hands.
   - Sweating.
   - Headache.
   - Nausea or vomiting.
   - Irritability or mood swings.
   - Increased heart rate.
   - Loss of appetite.
2. **Moderate Symptoms:**
   - Mild hallucinations (seeing or hearing things that aren't there).
   - Seizures.
   - Sweating.
   - Rapid heart rate.
3. **Severe Symptoms (Delirium Tremens – DTs):**
   - Delirium tremens (DTs) is the most severe form of alcohol withdrawal and can be life-threatening. Symptoms include severe agitation, confusion, vivid hallucinations, and delusions.
   - High fever.
   - Seizures.
   - Severe confusion or disorientation.
   - Profound changes in mental functions.

Causes:

Alcohol has a depressive effect on the brain. In chronic alcohol use, the brain adjusts to the depressant effects of alcohol by increasing its activity. When alcohol use is suddenly stopped or reduced, the brain's increased activity can manifest as withdrawal.

Risk Factors:

- Prolonged heavy drinking.
- Previous history of alcohol withdrawal.
- Presence of other health problems.
- History of seizures or DTs.
- Previous detoxifications from alcohol.

Treatment:

1. **Medical Supervision:** Severe cases of alcohol withdrawal, especially those involving DTs or seizures, require immediate medical attention and are often treated in a hospital.
2. **Medications:** Benzodiazepines are commonly used to reduce withdrawal symptoms. Other medications may be used to treat specific symptoms like nausea or insomnia.
3. **Fluids and Nutrition:** Replenishment of fluids and nutrients, as heavy alcohol use can lead to dehydration and vitamin deficiencies.
4. **Long-term Treatment:** After stabilization, long-term treatment typically involves alcohol abstinence, counseling, and support groups like Alcoholics Anonymous (AA).
5. **Prevention of Future Withdrawal:** Strategies include long-term treatment for alcohol dependence, lifestyle changes, and ongoing support to maintain sobriety.

It is essential for anyone experiencing alcohol withdrawal to seek medical help due to the potential severity of the symptoms and the risk of complications like seizures and DTs.

How long will the effects of AW last?

The duration of alcohol withdrawal (AW) symptoms can vary significantly from person to person, depending on several factors including the severity of alcohol dependence, the duration of alcohol use, individual health conditions, and the presence of any co-occurring mental health disorders. Generally, the timeline for alcohol withdrawal symptoms is as follows:

1. **Initial Phase (6-12 hours post-last drink):**
   - Mild symptoms typically begin within hours after the last drink.
   - These can include anxiety, shaking, nausea, insomnia, and gastrointestinal disturbances.
2. **Peak Intensity (24-48 hours post-last drink):**
   - Symptoms may worsen and peak during this time.
   - Individuals may experience increased heart rate, sweating, tremors, and heightened blood pressure.
   - Some people may experience hallucinations or seizures during this stage.
3. **Severe Symptoms (48-72 hours post-last drink):**
   - This is the period when the most severe symptoms, such as delirium tremens (DTs), may occur. DTs can include severe agitation, fever, seizures, and hallucinations.
   - DTs, while less common, are potentially life-threatening and require immediate medical attention.
4. **Resolution Phase (after 72 hours):**
   - For most people, the acute symptoms of alcohol withdrawal begin to subside after about 72 hours.
   - Some symptoms, like changes in sleep patterns and mood disturbances, can persist for weeks or even longer in a condition known as protracted or prolonged withdrawal.
5. **Protracted Withdrawal:**
   - Also known as post-acute withdrawal syndrome (PAWS), this phase can last for months or even up to a year.
   - Symptoms include chronic insomnia, emotional changes like anxiety or depression, cognitive difficulties, and reduced energy and enthusiasm.
   - PAWS symptoms tend to come and go and can be triggered by stress.

Factors Affecting Duration:

- **Severity of Alcohol Dependence:** Individuals with a long history of heavy drinking may experience more prolonged and severe withdrawal symptoms.
- **Health Conditions:** Co-occurring physical or mental health disorders can influence the duration and severity of withdrawal symptoms.
- **Age and Metabolism:** Older adults or those with slower metabolism may process alcohol more

slowly, potentially prolonging the withdrawal process.

Importance of Medical Supervision:

Due to the potential severity of symptoms, particularly in the case of severe alcohol dependence, it is crucial to undergo alcohol withdrawal under medical supervision. This ensures safety, as complications like seizures and DTs can be life-threatening. Treatment may involve medications to ease symptoms, as well as support and monitoring to address any complications that arise.

What are psychoactive drugs?

Psychoactive drugs, also known as psychotropic, are substances that affect the brain, altering a person's mood, perception, consciousness, cognition, or behavior. These effects are achieved through the alteration of neurotransmitter systems in the central nervous system. Psychoactive drugs can be used for therapeutic purposes, as in the case of prescription medications for mental health disorders, or recreationally, which can sometimes lead to substance abuse or dependency.

Categories of Psychoactive Drugs:

1. **Stimulants:**
   - **Effect:** Increase alertness, attention, and energy, as well as elevate blood pressure, heart rate, and respiration.
   - **Examples:** Caffeine, nicotine, amphetamines (used in ADHD treatment), cocaine, and methamphetamine.
2. **Depressants:**
   - **Effect:** Slow down the function of the central nervous system and can cause relaxation and drowsiness.
   - **Examples:** Alcohol, benzodiazepines (like Valium and Xanax, used for anxiety or insomnia), barbiturates, and opiates (like heroin and prescription painkillers such as morphine and oxycodone).
3. **Opioids:**
   - **Effect:** Primarily used for pain relief but also produce feelings of euphoria.
   - **Examples:** Morphine, heroin, oxycodone, hydrocodone, and methadone.
4. **Hallucinogens:**
   - **Effect:** Alter perception, thoughts, and feelings. They can cause hallucinations, or sensations and images that seem real though they are not.
   - **Examples:** LSD, psilocybin (magic mushrooms), peyote, and MDMA (Ecstasy or Molly).
5. **Dissociatives:**
   - **Effect:** Produce a sense of detachment from one's self and environment.
   - **Examples:** Ketamine, PCP (phencyclidine), and DXM (dextromethorphan, found in some cough syrups).
6. **Cannabinoids:**
   - **Effect:** Affect the user's perception, mood, consciousness, cognition, and behavior.
   - **Examples:** Marijuana (cannabis) and synthetic cannabinoids like Spice and K2.

Therapeutic Use:

Many psychoactive drugs have legitimate medical uses. For example:

- Stimulants are prescribed for attention-deficit hyperactivity disorder (ADHD).
- Depressants, such as benzodiazepines, are used for anxiety disorders.
- Opioids are effective for pain management.

Risks and Concerns:

- **Abuse and Addiction:** Psychoactive substances, particularly certain stimulants, opioids, and depressants, can be highly addictive.
- **Withdrawal:** Cessation can lead to withdrawal symptoms, which vary depending on the substance.
- **Mental Health Effects:** Some psychoactive drugs can exacerbate or trigger mental health disorders.
- **Physical Health Risks:** Long-term use or abuse of these substances can lead to various health issues, including heart disease, liver damage, respiratory distress, and neurological impairment.

Due to their powerful effects and potential risks, the use of psychoactive drugs, particularly for non-medical reasons, is a major public health concern. Their use and distribution are often regulated by law.

What are psychobiotics?

Psychobiotics are a relatively new and evolving area of study within the field of psychopharmacology and gut-brain axis research. They are a type of probiotic—live bacteria and yeasts that are good for health, especially the digestive system—believed to have a beneficial impact on mental health. The term "psychobiotic" was originally coined to describe probiotics that produce a health benefit in patients suffering from psychiatric illness.

Key Concepts of Psychobiotics:

1. **Gut-Brain Axis:** Psychobiotics operate on the principle of the gut-brain axis, the complex communication network linking the gut and the brain. This axis involves various biological systems including the gut microbiota, the immune system, and the central nervous system.

2. **Neurotransmitters and Hormones:** Certain gut bacteria can produce or stimulate the production of neurotransmitters and hormones like serotonin, GABA (gamma-aminobutyric acid), and dopamine, which are crucial for regulating mood and emotions.

3. **Impact on Mental Health:** Psychobiotics may influence brain function and, consequently, mental health and behavior. Research has suggested potential benefits in reducing symptoms of depression, anxiety, and stress-related disorders.

4. **Types of Psychobiotics:** These can include specific strains of bacteria commonly found in fermented foods like yogurt, kefir, sauerkraut, and kimchi, or in dietary supplements. Common strains studied include various species of Lactobacillus and Bifidobacterium.

5. **Mechanisms of Action:** The proposed mechanisms through which psychobiotics exert their effects include modulation of the gut microbiota, reduction of gut inflammation, direct effects on the central nervous system, and impact on the stress response system.

Research and Evidence:

The field of psychobiotics is still in its infancy, and much of the research is preliminary. While some

studies have shown promising results, more rigorous clinical trials are needed to better understand the efficacy, safety, and mechanisms of action of psychobiotics.

Potential Applications:

- **Mood Disorders:** Such as depression and anxiety.
- **Stress-Related Disorders:** Like irritable bowel syndrome (IBS), which has a strong brain-gut component.
- **Neurodevelopmental Disorders:** Some research is exploring the impact of gut health on conditions like autism spectrum disorder (ASD).

Considerations:

- **Supplementation:** While incorporating probiotic-rich foods into the diet is generally considered safe, the use of probiotic supplements should be discussed with a healthcare provider, especially for people with underlying health conditions or those who are immunocompromised.
- **Holistic Approach:** Psychobiotics are likely to be most effective when used as part of a holistic approach to mental health that includes a balanced diet, regular exercise, and other lifestyle factors.

As research in this field grows, psychobiotics may become a more prominent part of recommendations for managing mental health, potentially offering a novel and natural approach to treatment alongside traditional therapies.

What are the investigations in a case of seizures?

When a patient presents with seizures, a thorough and systematic approach is required to diagnose the underlying cause and determine the best course of treatment. The investigations for seizures typically include a combination of medical history evaluation, physical and neurological examinations, and various diagnostic tests. Here is an overview of the common investigations used:

1. **Detailed Medical and Seizure History:**
   - Understanding the circumstances surrounding the seizures, including potential triggers, frequency, duration, and any specific symptoms experienced before, during, and after the seizure (aura, types of movements, postictal state).
   - Family history of seizures or epilepsy.
   - History of head trauma, infections, or other neurological conditions.

2. **Physical and Neurological Examination:**
   - Assessment of mental status, motor abilities, and sensory function to check for any neurological deficits.

3. **Blood Tests:**
   - To check for metabolic or biochemical abnormalities that could cause seizures, such as electrolyte imbalances, low blood sugar

(hypoglycemia), liver or kidney dysfunction, and infections.

- Toxicology screening to rule out poisoning or substance abuse.

4. **Electroencephalogram (EEG):**
   - A key diagnostic tool in epilepsy that records the electrical activity of the brain. An EEG can identify characteristic patterns that suggest a seizure disorder.
5. **Neuroimaging:**
   - **Magnetic Resonance Imaging (MRI):** Used to detect structural abnormalities in the brain, such as tumors, stroke, or developmental anomalies that might be causing seizures.
   - **Computed Tomography (CT) Scan:** Often used in emergency situations to quickly rule out acute conditions like hemorrhage or stroke.
6. **Lumbar Puncture (Spinal Tap):**
   - In cases where an infection of the central nervous system (such as meningitis or encephalitis) is suspected.
7. **Video-EEG Monitoring:**
   - Continuous EEG monitoring while recording video to capture seizure activity. This helps in classifying the type of seizure and can be crucial for planning surgical treatment in drug-resistant epilepsy.
8. **Genetic Testing:**
   - Particularly in cases of familial epilepsy syndromes or when a genetic cause is suspected.
9. **Cardiac Evaluation:**
   - ECG (electrocardiogram) and other cardiac tests may be conducted to rule out cardiac syncope that can sometimes be confused with seizures.
10. **Developmental, Psychological, and Psychiatric Evaluation:**
    - Assessments to identify conditions like autism, ADHD, or learning disabilities in children, or to rule out psychogenic non-epileptic seizures (PNES), which are psychological in origin.

The choice of investigations is guided by the patient's specific symptoms, seizure type, and clinical history. The goal is to pinpoint the cause of the seizures as accurately as possible to guide effective treatment.

What is the Treatment is a case of seizure?

The treatment of seizures depends on the underlying cause, the type of seizures, their frequency, and the overall health of the patient. Here is an overview of the typical treatment approaches:

1. **Antiepileptic Drugs (AEDs):**
   - The primary treatment for epilepsy (a condition characterized by recurrent seizures) is medication with AEDs.
   - These drugs are chosen based on the type of seizures (focal or generalized), patient's age, side effect profile, and potential interactions with other medications.
   - Common AEDs include levetiracetam, valproate, lamotrigine, carbamazepine, and phenytoin, among others.
   - The goal is to control seizures with the least amount of medication and the fewest side effects.
2. **Dietary Therapy:**
   - The ketogenic diet (high-fat, low-carbohydrate) and modified Atkins diet have been effective in some patients, particularly children, in controlling seizures.
3. **Surgery:**
   - Considered in cases where seizures are drug-resistant and originate from a specific area of the brain that can be safely removed.
   - Types of surgery include resective surgery (removing the seizure focus), lesionectomy (removing a lesion causing seizures), and corpus callosotomy (severing the connection between the two hemispheres of the brain).
4. **Neurostimulation:**
   - Vagus nerve stimulation (VNS) and deep brain stimulation (DBS) are options for patients who do not respond to medication and are not candidates for surgery.
   - These involve implanting a device that sends electrical impulses to the brain or vagus nerve to help control seizures.

5. **Emergency Treatment for Acute Seizures:**
    - In the case of prolonged seizures (status epilepticus), immediate medical intervention is required.
    - Treatment usually involves intravenous (IV) administration of benzodiazepines (like lorazepam) and other AEDs.
6. **Treatment of Underlying Cause:**
    - If seizures are due to an underlying condition (like an infection, tumor, or electrolyte imbalance), treating that condition is paramount.
7. **Lifestyle Modifications:**
    - Regular sleep, stress management, and avoiding known seizure triggers (such as alcohol or flashing lights in some individuals) are important.
8. **Observation:**
    - In some cases, particularly for a single seizure with no clear cause, the approach might be to wait and observe without immediate treatment.
9. **Psychological Support:**
    - For seizures with a psychological component, such as psychogenic non-epileptic seizures (PNES), therapy and psychological support are crucial.

The choice of treatment is highly individualized, and managing epilepsy often requires coordination between a team of healthcare providers, including neurologists, dietitians, and sometimes surgeons. Regular monitoring and follow-up are essential to adjust treatment as needed and to manage any side effects.

What is the status of Pregnancy and seizures?

Pregnancy in women with epilepsy or who experience seizures presents unique challenges and requires careful management. It is crucial for the health of both the mother and the fetus. The key concerns involve the effects of seizures and antiepileptic drugs (AEDs) on pregnancy and the impact of pregnancy on seizure control.

Seizure Control During Pregnancy:

1. **Effect on Seizure Frequency:** Pregnancy can affect seizure frequency. Some women experience an increase in seizures during pregnancy, while others see no change or a decrease in frequency.
2. **Risks of Seizures:** Seizures during pregnancy, particularly generalized tonic-clonic seizures, can pose risks to both the mother and the fetus. Risks include trauma from falls, hypoxia (reduced oxygen), and increased risk of miscarriage or premature labor.
3. **Monitoring and Medication:** It is important to closely monitor and manage epilepsy during pregnancy. This may involve adjusting AED dosages due to changes in drug metabolism during pregnancy.

Antiepileptic Drugs and Pregnancy:

1. **Teratogenic Risks:** Some AEDs have teratogenic risks (risks of causing fetal malformations) and may also affect fetal growth and development. However, the risk varies between different medications.
2. **Balancing Risks:** The risks of uncontrolled seizures usually outweigh the risks from AEDs. The goal is to maintain seizure control with the safest and minimal effective dosage of AEDs.
3. **Folic Acid Supplementation:** Women on AEDs are generally advised to take higher doses of folic acid before conception and during pregnancy to reduce the risk of neural tube defects in the fetus.

Pregnancy Management:

1. **Preconception Counseling:** Ideally, women with epilepsy should have preconception counseling to discuss the safest treatment plans during pregnancy.
2. **Regular Monitoring:** Frequent prenatal check-ups are necessary to monitor the health of the mother and fetus, including assessment of AED levels.
3. **Vitamin K Supplementation:** Women on certain AEDs may be advised to take vitamin K supplements in the last month of pregnancy to prevent hemorrhagic disease in the newborn.
4. **Labor and Delivery:** Most women with epilepsy can have a normal vaginal delivery unless there are other obstetric indications for cesarean section. Seizure control during labor is crucial.
5. **Breastfeeding:** While most AEDs are found in breast milk, the benefits of breastfeeding often outweigh the risks. However, this should be discussed with a healthcare provider.
6. **Postpartum:** After delivery, there is a need for careful monitoring as the metabolism of AEDs

changes, requiring dose adjustments. There is also a focus on managing the risks of seizures and the effects of AEDs while breastfeeding.

Each case is unique, and management should be tailored to the individual's seizure type, epilepsy syndrome, medication regimen, and overall health. Collaborative care involving neurologists, obstetricians, and pediatricians is essential for optimizing outcomes for both the mother and the baby.

What about interactions of Contraception and anti-seizure medications?

Interactions between contraception and anti-seizure medications (ASMs), also known as antiepileptic drugs (AEDs), are an important consideration for women with epilepsy or on seizure medications for other reasons. These interactions can affect the efficacy of both the contraceptive method and the ASM, which is crucial for preventing unintended pregnancies and ensuring effective seizure control.

Key Points on Interactions:

1. **Enzyme-Inducing ASMs and Hormonal Contraceptives:**
   - Certain ASMs, like carbamazepine, phenytoin, phenobarbital, primidone, and topiramate at higher doses, are enzyme inducers. They can increase the metabolism of estrogen and progestin in hormonal contraceptives (like birth control pills, patches, and vaginal rings), potentially reducing their effectiveness and leading to contraceptive failure.
   - Women on these ASMs may require higher-dose hormonal contraceptives, or they might be advised to use non-hormonal methods of contraception like copper IUDs (intrauterine devices).
2. **Valproate and Lamotrigine:**
   - Valproate does not decrease the effectiveness of hormonal contraceptives.
   - Lamotrigine levels can be reduced by hormonal contraceptives, potentially decreasing seizure control. Conversely, stopping hormonal contraceptives can increase lamotrigine levels, risking toxicity.
3. **Effectiveness of Contraceptives:**
   - Women on enzyme-inducing ASMs may be advised to use contraceptives with a higher dose of estrogen, or to use alternative methods like the progestin-only pill, an IUD, or an implant.
   - Barrier methods (like condoms), IUDs, and sterilization are not affected by ASMs and can be reliable choices.
4. **Pregnancy Planning:**
   - For women planning pregnancy, it is important to balance effective contraception with seizure control while minimizing fetal exposure to potentially harmful ASMs.
   - Preconception counseling is essential for discussing these issues and adjusting medication regimens as needed.
5. **Emergency Contraception:**
   - The effectiveness of levonorgestrel (Plan B) as emergency contraception may be reduced in women taking enzyme-inducing ASMs. A copper IUD or a higher dose of levonorgestrel may be recommended instead.
6. **Monitoring and Adjustments:**
   - Regular monitoring and dose adjustments of ASMs may be required when starting, changing, or stopping hormonal contraceptives.

Recommendations:

1. **Consult Health Care Providers:** Women on ASMs should consult with their healthcare providers, including neurologists and gynecologists, to choose the most suitable contraceptive method.
2. **Regular Review:** Medication and contraceptive methods should be regularly reviewed to ensure they remain effective and appropriate, especially if there are changes in seizure control or ASM type.
3. **Individualized Approach:** The choice of contraception should be individualized based on the type of ASM, seizure control, the woman's overall health, and her plans regarding pregnancy.

Understanding and managing the interactions between contraception and anti-seizure medications are vital for women's health, particularly in managing epilepsy effectively while ensuring reproductive health and rights.

What should be advice to the patients of epilepsy about Personal safety?

Providing advice on personal safety is an essential aspect of managing patients with epilepsy. Ensuring safety can help reduce the risk of injury during a seizure and improve overall quality of life. Here are key safety recommendations for individuals with epilepsy:

1. **Medication Adherence:** Encourage strict adherence to prescribed anti-seizure medications to reduce the frequency and severity of seizures.
2. **Avoiding Triggers:** Identify and avoid known seizure triggers, which can include lack of sleep, alcohol consumption, stress, flashing lights (in photosensitive epilepsy), and certain medications or drugs.
3. **Bathing Safety:**
   - Use showers instead of baths to reduce the risk of drowning.
   - Avoid locking bathroom doors or have a safety mechanism in place to allow access in case of a seizure.
4. **Cooking Precautions:**
   - Use a microwave instead of a stove to reduce the risk of burns.
   - If using a stove, cook on back burners and turn pot handles away from the front.
5. **Driving:**
   - Follow legal guidelines and doctor's advice regarding driving. Most places have regulations about a seizure-free period before driving is allowed.
6. **Swimming and Water Activities:**
   - Always swim with a companion who knows about your epilepsy and what to do if a seizure occurs.
   - Avoid swimming in deep or unsupervised areas.
7. **Sleeping Arrangements:**
   - Consider using a seizure alarm or monitor, particularly for children or if nocturnal seizures are a concern.
   - Ensure a safe sleeping environment, free from hard objects or sharp edges.
8. **Working Safely:**
   - Inform employers about epilepsy for necessary workplace adjustments.
   - Avoid working at heights or with unguarded machinery.
9. **Wearing Medical ID:**
   - Wear a medical ID bracelet or carry an identification card that provides information about your epilepsy.
10. **Regular Exercise:**
    - Stay physically active, but choose safe exercises and environments. Supervised exercise is preferable.
11. **Alcohol and Recreational Drugs:**
    - Avoid excessive alcohol and recreational drugs, as they can provoke seizures.
12. **Regular Health Check-Ups:**
    - Regularly visit the healthcare provider for check-ups and management of epilepsy.
13. **First Aid Awareness:**
    - Educate family members, friends, and colleagues about seizure first aid.
14. **Pregnancy Considerations:**
    - Women with epilepsy should consult their doctors for preconception planning and management during pregnancy.
15. **Home Safety:**
    - Implement general safety measures at home, like cushioning sharp corners, securing rugs to prevent slips, and using stair gates if necessary.

It is also important for individuals with epilepsy to have a strong support network and access to resources and information about their condition. Empowerment through education can help individuals with epilepsy lead safer and more fulfilling lives.

What is Seizure first aid?

Seizure first aid is a set of simple steps that anyone can follow to assist someone experiencing a seizure. The primary goal is to keep the person safe until the seizure stops naturally. Here are the key steps to follow:

General Seizure First Aid:

1. **Stay Calm**: Keep yourself and others calm.
2. **Time the Seizure**: If possible, note how long the seizure lasts. This information can be important for medical professionals.
3. **Keep the Person Safe**: Move any hard or sharp objects away from the person to prevent injury.

4. **Position the Person Safely:**
    - If they are on the ground, try to lay them on their side to help keep their airway clear and prevent choking.
    - Place something soft under their head (like a folded jacket or a pillow) to protect it from hitting the ground.
5. **Do Not Restrain**: Do not try to hold the person down or restrain their movements.
6. **Do Not Put Anything in the Person's Mouth**: Contrary to a common misconception, you should never put anything into the person's mouth during a seizure. They cannot swallow their tongue, but placing objects in their mouth can cause injury or obstruct their airway.
7. **Check for Medical ID**: Look for any medical identification (like a bracelet) that might offer information about the person's medical condition.
8. **Stay with the Person**: Remain with the person until the seizure ends and they are fully awake.
9. **After the Seizure**: Once the seizure has stopped, help the person into a comfortable and safe position. Check if they are breathing properly. If they are not awake or have difficulty breathing, call for emergency medical help.
10. **Reassure the Person**: People can be confused or disoriented after a seizure. Offer comfort and reassurance as they regain full awareness.

When to Call for Emergency Help:

- The seizure lasts longer than 5 minutes.
- Another seizure starts soon after the first one.
- The person does not regain consciousness after the shaking has stopped.
- The person is injured during the seizure.
- The seizure occurs in water.
- The person has a health condition like diabetes or heart disease.
- It is the person's first seizure.

Special Considerations:

- For a person with known epilepsy who has a typical seizure, emergency services may not be necessary if the seizure stops within a few minutes and they recover as usual.
- For prolonged or repeated seizures, or if the person is pregnant, injured, or diabetic, seek medical help immediately.

First aid for seizures is mainly about ensuring safety and supporting the person until the seizure subsides. After a seizure, it is essential to encourage the person to seek medical advice, especially if they don't have an established diagnosis of epilepsy or if their seizures are not well-controlled.

Why seizures, epileptic or non-epileptic, are seen in psychiatry OPDs?

Seizures, both epileptic and non-epileptic, are observed in psychiatric outpatient departments (OPDs) for several reasons. Understanding the interplay between psychiatric conditions and seizures is crucial for providing comprehensive care to patients. Here are some key reasons why these conditions are seen in psychiatric settings:

1. **Psychiatric Comorbidities in Epilepsy**:
    - Many individuals with epilepsy also experience psychiatric conditions such as depression, anxiety, and psychosis. These comorbidities often require management by psychiatric professionals.
    - The stress of living with a chronic condition like epilepsy can also contribute to the development of psychiatric symptoms.
2. **Non-Epileptic Seizures (NES):**
    - Non-epileptic seizures, also known as psychogenic non-epileptic seizures (PNES), are episodes that resemble epileptic seizures but do not have the characteristic electrical discharges in the brain associated with epilepsy.
    - PNES are considered a psychological condition and are often a physical manifestation of psychological distress.
    - Patients with PNES typically require treatment from mental health professionals to address the underlying psychological issues.
3. **Side Effects of Anti-Epileptic Drugs (AEDs):**
    - Some AEDs can have side effects that include mood changes, depression, or even psychotic symptoms, necessitating psychiatric evaluation and management.
4. **Differential Diagnosis:**
    - In some cases, distinguishing between epileptic seizures and other conditions such

as panic attacks, dissociative episodes, or movement disorders can be challenging. Psychiatrists play a crucial role in this differential diagnosis.

5. **Psychogenic Precipitants of Epileptic Seizures:**
   - Emotional stress is known to be a precipitant for epileptic seizures in some individuals.

Thus, psychiatrists may be involved in helping patients develop strategies to manage stress.

6. **Treatment-Resistant Cases:**
   - Some individuals with epilepsy may not respond adequately to AEDs and could benefit from a holistic approach that includes psychiatric evaluation and treatment.
7. **Counseling and Psychotherapy:**
   - Counseling and psychotherapy can be beneficial for patients with epilepsy, helping them cope with the psychological impact of living with a chronic neurological condition.
8. **Psychiatric Disorders Mimicking Seizures**:
   - Certain psychiatric conditions like bipolar disorder, schizophrenia, and panic disorder can have symptoms that mimic seizures, leading to referral to psychiatric services for evaluation and treatment.

In psychiatric OPDs, a multidisciplinary approach involving neurologists, psychiatrists, psychologists, and other healthcare professionals is often necessary to provide comprehensive care for individuals with seizures, whether epileptic or non-epileptic. This collaborative care helps address the complex interplay between neurological and psychological factors in these patients.

Are dying patients optimistic?

The emotional and psychological state of dying patients can vary widely and is influenced by numerous factors, including the individual's personality, the nature and progression of their illness, their cultural and spiritual beliefs, and the support they receive from family, friends, and healthcare providers.

Some dying patients may indeed exhibit optimism. This optimism can manifest in various ways:

1. **Hope for Quality Time**: They might be optimistic about enjoying quality time with loved ones in their remaining days, focusing on making meaningful memories.
2. **Spiritual or Religious Beliefs**: Faith and spiritual beliefs can provide comfort and a sense of hope or peace, leading to optimism about what lies beyond death.
3. **Acceptance**: Some patients reach a stage of acceptance where they are at peace with their situation, which can be perceived as a form of optimism.
4. **Legacy and Impact**: Feelings of optimism can also arise from reflecting on the impact they have had on others' lives and the legacy they leave behind.
5. **Hope for Relief**: There may be optimism about the end of suffering, especially in cases of terminal illness accompanied by significant pain or disability.

However, it is important to recognize that not all dying patients feel optimistic. Many may experience a range of emotions, including sadness, anger, fear, and grief. The process of dying is deeply personal and can be emotionally complex.

It is crucial for caregivers and healthcare providers to offer empathetic and individualized support, respecting each patient's unique emotional experience. This support might include psychological counseling, spiritual care, ensuring comfort, and facilitating conversations about end-of-life wishes and concerns.

Ultimately, whether a dying patient feels optimistic, peaceful, troubled, or a mix of many emotions, their feelings are valid, and compassionate care is key to supporting them through this final phase of life.

What is transcranial magnetic stimulation (TMS)?

Transcranial Magnetic Stimulation (TMS), often abbreviated as TMS (not TCMS), is a non-invasive procedure that uses magnetic fields to stimulate nerve cells in the brain. It is primarily used as a treatment for depression, particularly in cases where traditional treatments like medication and psychotherapy haven't been effective. Here is an overview of how TMS works and its applications:

How TMS Works:

1. **Magnetic Pulses**: TMS involves delivering repetitive magnetic pulses to the brain. These pulses are generated by passing current through an electromagnetic coil placed near the scalp.
2. **Targeted Brain Areas**: The magnetic pulses induce an electrical current in the brain tissue beneath the coil, targeting areas of the brain thought to be involved in mood regulation, particularly the prefrontal cortex.

3. **Neuronal Activation**: This stimulation can activate regions of the brain that have decreased activity in depression.

Types of TMS:

1. **Repetitive TMS (rTMS)**: Involves a series of repetitive magnetic pulses. It is the most commonly used form of TMS for depression.
2. **Deep TMS (dTMS)**: Uses a different coil design that allows the magnetic pulses to penetrate deeper into the brain.

Clinical Uses:

1. **Treatment-Resistant Depression**: TMS is most often used for depression that has not responded to medications and psychotherapy. It is approved by regulatory agencies like the FDA for this purpose.
2. **Other Mental Health Disorders**: Research is ongoing for the use of TMS in treating other psychiatric conditions, including anxiety, bipolar disorder, schizophrenia, and obsessive-compulsive disorder.
3. **Neurological Disorders**: There is also interest in using TMS for conditions like stroke recovery, Parkinson's disease, and chronic pain.

Procedure:

1. **Outpatient Procedure**: TMS is typically done on an outpatient basis and does not require anesthesia.
2. **Session Duration**: Each session lasts about 30 to 60 minutes, and treatment usually consists of multiple sessions over several weeks.
3. **Side Effects**: TMS is generally well-tolerated. The most common side effects include scalp discomfort at the site of stimulation and headache. There is a small risk of seizure, but it is considered very low.

Effectiveness and Benefits:

1. **Non-Invasive and Drug-Free**: As a non-invasive procedure, TMS offers an alternative for those who cannot tolerate the side effects of antidepressant medications.
2. **Efficacy**: Clinical trials have demonstrated the efficacy of TMS in reducing the symptoms of depression, with many patients experiencing significant improvements.
3. **FDA Approval**: TMS is FDA-approved for the treatment of major depressive disorder and has been extensively researched in this context.

TMS represents a significant advancement in the treatment of psychiatric conditions, offering hope for individuals who have not found relief through traditional treatment methods. However, it is important to consult with a healthcare provider to determine whether TMS is an appropriate treatment option based on individual health needs and medical history.

What is artificial intelligence (AI)?

Artificial Intelligence (AI) refers to the simulation of human intelligence in machines that are programmed to think and learn like humans. The term is frequently applied to the project of developing systems endowed with the intellectual processes characteristic of humans, such as the ability to reason, discover meaning, generalize, or learn from past experiences.

Key Characteristics of AI:

1. **Learning**: The ability to acquire and apply knowledge or skills. This involves algorithms (set rules) to process data, detect patterns, and make adjustments to improve performance over time. Machine learning, a subset of AI, exemplifies this through systems that learn from data.
2. **Reasoning**: The ability to solve problems through logical deduction. AI systems can be designed to make decisions based on the data they gather.
3. **Problem-Solving**: AI can be used to solve complex problems in various fields by processing large amounts of data and recognizing patterns that are not immediately evident to humans.
4. **Perception**: AI systems can interpret the world around them by recognizing objects, text, and speech. Technologies like computer vision and natural language processing enable this.
5. **Language Understanding**: AI can understand, interpret, and respond to human language in a way that is both meaningful and natural, mainly through advancements in natural language processing and machine learning.

Types of AI:

1. **Narrow or Weak AI**: Systems designed and trained for a particular task. Virtual personal assistants, such as Apple's Siri, are a form of weak AI.
2. **General or Strong AI**: Systems or machines with the ability to perform any intellectual task that a human being can. This is a more theoretical type of AI and is not yet fully realized.

Applications of AI:

- **Healthcare**: From diagnostics to personalized medicine, and even robotic surgeries.
- **Business**: In automation, predictive analytics, and customer service (like chatbots).
- **Education**: For personalized learning and automated grading.
- **Finance**: Used for trading, risk management, and fraud detection.
- **Transportation**: In developing self-driving cars and optimizing traffic management.
- **Entertainment**: For recommendations in streaming services and creating realistic visual effects.

Challenges and Ethical Considerations:

- **Bias and Fairness**: AI systems can inadvertently perpetuate and amplify biases present in their training data.
- **Job Displacement**: Concerns about AI replacing jobs, necessitating new skills and training.
- **Privacy**: As AI systems process vast amounts of data, there are concerns about how this data is used and protected.
- **Accountability**: Determining who is responsible for decisions made by AI systems.

AI continues to advance rapidly, driving innovation across various sectors but also raising important ethical and practical considerations. The development of AI involves not only technical expertise but also an understanding of the broader impacts these technologies have on society.

How can AI be of use to the healthcare industry?

Artificial Intelligence (AI) has the potential to significantly transform the healthcare industry by improving outcomes, reducing costs, and enhancing patient and provider experiences. Here are some key areas where AI is being utilized or has the potential to be integrated into healthcare:

1. **Disease Diagnosis and Identification:**
   - AI algorithms can analyze medical imaging more quickly and often more accurately than human practitioners. This is especially true in areas like radiology, pathology, and ophthalmology.
   - AI can assist in identifying diseases from patterns in data, such as spotting early signs of conditions like cancer, diabetic retinopathy, or heart disease.
2. **Treatment Personalization (Precision Medicine)**:
   - AI can analyze data, including genetic information, to tailor treatment to individual patients, improving the effectiveness of therapies and reducing side effects.
3. **Drug Discovery and Development**:
   - AI accelerates the drug development process by predicting how different drugs will work in the body, identifying potential candidates, and analyzing clinical trial data.
4. **Predictive Analytics**:
   - Using AI to analyze large datasets, healthcare providers can identify patients at high risk of developing a condition and intervene earlier.
   - This is particularly useful in managing chronic diseases and preventing hospital readmissions.
5. **Robotic Surgery and Assistance**:
   - AI-powered robotic systems can assist surgeons in performing precise and minimally invasive procedures, reducing recovery times and improving surgical outcomes.
6. **Virtual Health Assistants and Telemedicine**:
   - AI-driven chatbots and virtual health assistants can provide basic healthcare support and information to patients, improving access to care, especially in underserved areas.
   - Telemedicine platforms, augmented with AI, can aid in remote diagnosis and monitoring.
7. **Administrative Workflow Automation**:
   - Automating routine tasks like patient scheduling, billing, and claims processing can reduce administrative burdens and costs.
8. **Clinical Trial Research**:
   - AI can help identify suitable candidates for clinical trials more efficiently, ensuring that trials are populated more quickly and with appropriate patients.
9. **Enhancing Patient Engagement and Adherence**:
   - Personalized AI-driven applications can remind patients to take medications, attend appointments, and follow their treatment plans.

10. **Healthcare System Analysis and Policy Planning**:
    - AI tools can analyze healthcare systems to identify inefficiencies and suggest improvements, aiding in policy development and resource allocation.
11. **Mental Health Support**:
    - AI applications can support mental health by providing early detection of mental health issues and supporting cognitive behavioral therapy.
12. **Remote Monitoring and Wearables**:
    - AI integrated with wearable technologies can continuously monitor patient health data, providing insights and early warnings about health issues.

While AI brings numerous benefits to healthcare, challenges like data privacy concerns, the need for high-quality data, potential biases in AI algorithms, and the requirement for integration with existing healthcare systems must be addressed. The future of AI in healthcare is promising, with ongoing advancements leading to more innovative applications and improved patient care.

Is data a prerequisite to building good AI models?

Yes, data is a fundamental prerequisite for building effective and reliable AI models. The quality, quantity, and relevance of the data directly influence the performance and accuracy of AI systems. Here is why data is so crucial:

1. **Training and Learning**: AI models, particularly those based on machine learning, require data to learn and make predictions or decisions. This process is known as training, where the model is exposed to large sets of data, allowing it to learn patterns, relationships, and features.
2. **Quality of Data**: The quality of the data is as important as the quantity. High-quality data is representative, unbiased, accurate, and relevant to the problem being addressed. Poor quality data can lead to inaccurate models and unreliable outcomes (garbage in, garbage out).
3. **Diversity and Volume**: A large and diverse dataset helps ensure that the model can generalize well to new, unseen data. This is particularly important for models deployed in dynamic and varied real-world scenarios.
4. **Feature Representation**: The way data is presented to the model (feature engineering) significantly impacts the model's performance. Good data includes meaningful features that effectively capture the essence of the problem.
5. **Validation and Testing**: Apart from training data, separate datasets are needed for validation (tuning model parameters) and testing (evaluating model performance). This helps in assessing the model's effectiveness and ensuring it works well in real-world conditions.
6. **Ethical Considerations**: Data must be collected and used ethically, respecting privacy and avoiding biases that could lead to unfair or discriminatory outcomes when the AI model is applied.
7. **Domain-Specific Data**: For specialized fields like healthcare, finance, or autonomous vehicles, domain-specific data is essential for building models that are accurately attuned to the nuances of these areas.
8. **Data Augmentation and Synthetic Data**: In cases where data is scarce, techniques like data augmentation or synthetic data generation can be used to expand datasets, though care must be taken to maintain the integrity of the data.
9. **Continuous Improvement**: AI models can continue to improve over time with the availability of new data, enabling them to adapt to changing conditions and learn from new examples.

In summary, data is the foundation upon which AI models are built. The success of AI applications in any field hinges on the availability of robust, high-quality data, making data collection, processing, and management key aspects of AI development.

Do you think doctors will trust AI-based technology in clinical settings?

Whether or not doctors will trust AI-based technology in clinical settings is a complex issue that depends on several factors. The adoption of AI in healthcare has been growing, but the level of trust varies among healthcare professionals. Here are some key considerations:

Factors Influencing Trust in AI:

1. **Accuracy and Reliability**: If AI systems demonstrate high accuracy and reliability, especially in diagnosing and predicting outcomes, they are more likely to gain the trust of doctors. Clinical validation and evidence of effectiveness are crucial.
2. **Transparency and Explainability**: AI systems that provide clear, understandable reasons for their recommendations are more likely to be trusted.

Doctors often want to know how the AI arrived at its conclusions.

3. **Clinical Integration**: AI tools that seamlessly integrate into existing workflows and complement the clinician's expertise are more likely to be trusted and used.
4. **Training and Familiarity**: Exposure and training in AI can increase trust among doctors. As medical professionals become more familiar with these technologies, their confidence in using them is likely to grow.
5. **Regulatory Approval**: AI applications that have undergone rigorous testing and received approval from regulatory bodies like the FDA (U.S. Food and Drug Administration) are more likely to be trusted.
6. **Ethical and Legal Considerations**: Concerns about patient privacy, data security, and legal responsibility in case of errors affect trust in AI systems.
7. **Clinical Evidence and Peer Reviews**: Published studies, clinical trials, and reviews by medical peers can significantly influence doctors' trust in AI technologies.
8. **Customization and Adaptability**: AI systems that can be tailored to the specific needs and practices of different medical specialties are more likely to be trusted and accepted.
9. **Patient Outcomes**: Ultimately, the impact of AI on patient outcomes is a major determinant of trust. If AI technologies demonstrably improve patient care, reduce errors, and enhance efficiency, they are more likely to be embraced by healthcare providers.

The Future of AI in Healthcare:

- **Complementary Role**: AI is generally seen as a tool to augment the abilities of doctors, not replace them. It can handle data-intensive tasks, allowing doctors to focus more on patient care.
- **Continual Learning and Improvement**: AI systems that continually learn and improve over time, adapting to new medical knowledge and individual patient data, could increase trust among medical professionals.
  - **Collaboration**: The development of AI tools in close collaboration with healthcare professionals can ensure that these systems meet the real needs of clinical practice.

In conclusion, while there is potential for AI to become a trusted tool in clinical settings, building this trust will depend on demonstrating clinical efficacy, ensuring safety and reliability, maintaining transparency, and providing proper training and support to healthcare professionals. As the field evolves and more evidence accumulates, it is likely that doctors' trust in AI will continue to grow, especially if these systems prove to enhance patient care and outcomes.

Do you believe AI can work with specialists to help them arrive at a diagnosis?

Yes, AI has the potential to work alongside specialists to assist in arriving at diagnoses. In many cases, AI is already making significant contributions in this area. Here are a few key points highlighting how AI can complement the expertise of medical specialists:

1. **Data Analysis and Pattern Recognition**: AI excels in analyzing large datasets, including medical images, lab results, and patient histories, more quickly and sometimes more accurately than humans. It can recognize patterns and anomalies that might be overlooked by human eyes, aiding specialists in diagnosis.
2. **Diagnostic Accuracy**: In fields like radiology, dermatology, pathology, and ophthalmology, AI algorithms have been developed to identify diseases such as cancers, skin lesions, and diabetic retinopathy with high accuracy.
3. **Time Efficiency**: AI can process and analyze data much faster than humans, which can significantly reduce the time taken to reach a diagnosis. This efficiency can be particularly valuable in acute and critical care settings.
4. **Decision Support Systems**: AI can serve as a decision support tool, providing specialists with diagnostic suggestions based on the integration of patient data. However, the final decision and clinical judgment are still made by the human specialist.
5. **Learning and Adapting**: Advanced AI systems can learn from each new case and continuously improve their diagnostic algorithms. This feature can be especially useful in rare or complex cases where human experience is limited.
6. **Personalized Medicine**: AI can help in tailoring diagnoses and treatment plans to individual patients by considering their unique genetic makeup, lifestyle, and other factors.
7. **Reducing Diagnostic Errors**: AI systems can help reduce human errors due to factors like fatigue, cognitive biases, or information overload.

8. **Enhancing Access to Care**: In areas with a shortage of specialists, AI can provide preliminary diagnostic assessments, improving access to healthcare for underserved populations.

Challenges and Considerations:

- **Integration with Clinical Workflow**: For AI to be effectively used by specialists, it must be well-integrated into existing clinical workflows and systems.
- **Training and Trust**: Specialists need to be trained in the use of AI tools and must trust the system's recommendations. This trust is built through transparency, reliability, and validation of the AI system.
- **Ethical and Legal Aspects**: The use of AI in diagnosis raises ethical considerations, including patient privacy, data security, and liability in case of diagnostic errors.
- **Complement, Not Replace**: AI is generally seen as a tool to complement, not replace, the expertise of medical specialists. The human element, including clinical judgment, empathy, and communication, remains irreplaceable in healthcare.

In conclusion, AI has the potential to be a valuable partner for specialists in the diagnostic process. Its ability to handle vast amounts of data and recognize complex patterns can greatly assist in making more accurate and efficient diagnoses. However, successful integration of AI in healthcare requires careful consideration of technical, ethical, and practical aspects.

What was your research programme using machine to detect diabetic retinopathy?

As an AI language model developed by OpenAI, I haven't conducted any research programs myself, nor do I create or use machines or AI systems. However, I can provide information on how AI and machine learning have been used in the research and development of tools for detecting diabetic retinopathy.

AI and Diabetic Retinopathy Detection:

1. **Automated Screening**: Researchers have developed AI algorithms that can automatically analyze images of the retina (taken with a retinal camera) for signs of diabetic retinopathy. These algorithms use pattern recognition to identify abnormalities such as microaneurysms, hemorrhages, and exudates that are indicative of diabetic retinopathy.
2. **Deep Learning Models**: Most of these systems use deep learning, a type of machine learning that involves neural networks with many layers (deep networks). These models are trained on large datasets of retinal images that are annotated with information about the presence or absence of diabetic retinopathy.
3. **Data Training**: The effectiveness of these AI systems depends on the quality and size of the dataset used for training. Ideally, these datasets include images from diverse patient populations and represent various stages of diabetic retinopathy.
4. **Validation and Testing**: Once trained, these models are validated and tested using separate sets of images to assess their accuracy and reliability. This process includes comparing the AI's performance to that of human experts.
5. **FDA Approval**: Some AI systems for diabetic retinopathy screening have received FDA approval. For example, IDx-DR became the first FDA-approved autonomous AI diagnostic system in any field of medicine. It can make a screening decision without the need for a clinician to also interpret the image or results.
6. **Benefits**:
   - **Increased Accessibility**: AI-based screening can be used in primary care settings, reducing the need for specialists and making screening more accessible to patients in remote or underserved areas.
   - **Efficiency**: Automated screening can process large volumes of images quickly, enabling more widespread and frequent screening.
   - **Early Detection**: By facilitating regular and accessible screenings, AI can help in the early detection of diabetic retinopathy, improving the chances of preventing vision loss.
7. **Challenges**:
   - **Data Bias**: If the training data is not diverse, the model might not perform well across different patient populations.
   - **Integration into Healthcare Systems**: Practical integration into existing clinical workflows is necessary for these tools to be widely adopted.

In summary, AI and machine learning are making significant strides in the field of ophthalmology, particularly in screening for diabetic retinopathy. These technologies have the potential to improve patient outcomes through early detection and more accessible care.